D1710626

FOUNDATIONS OF PSYCHIATRY

FOUNDATIONS OF PSYCHIATRY

KENNETH DAVIS, M.D.

Chairman, Department of Psychiatry
Mt. Sinai School of Medicine
New York, New York

HOWARD KLAR, M.D.

Director, Medical Education
Roosevelt-St. Luke's Hospital Center
New York, New York

JOSEPH T. COYLE, M.D.

Distinguished Service Professor of Child Psychiatry
Professor of Psychiatry,
Neuroscience, Pharmacology and Pediatrics
Division of Child Psychiatry
The Johns Hopkins University School of Medicine
Baltimore, Maryland

1991

W.B. SAUNDERS
Harcourt Brace Jovanovich, Inc.

Philadelphia   London   Toronto   Montreal   Sydney   Tokyo

W. B. SAUNDERS
Harcourt Brace Jovanovich, Inc.

The Curtis Center
Independence Square West
Philadelphia, PA 19106

Editor: Martin Wonsiewicz

Library of Congress Cataloging-in-Publication Data

Foundations of psychiatry/[edited by] Kenneth Davis, Howard Klar,
   Joseph T. Coyle.
       p.   cm.
   ISBN 0-7216-1341-1
   1.   Neuropsychiatry.   I.   Davis, Kenneth L.,   II.   Klar,
Howard,   III.   Coyle, Joseph T.
   [DNLM: 1.   Brain--physiology.   2.   Mental Disorders.   WM   100 F771]
RC341.F68   1991
616.89--dc20
DNLM/DLC
for Library of Congress   90-8866
                                                                         CIP

FOUNDATIONS OF PSYCHIATRY   ISBN   0-7216-1341-1

Printed in the United States of America

Last digit is the print number: 9   8   7   6   5   4   3   2   1

To our students
with the hope that
this book will enable them
to better serve their patients

Contributors

EMIL F. COCCARO, M.D.

Associate Professor of Psychiatry and Director, Outpatient Division, Department of Psychiatry, Eastern Pennsylvania Psychiatric Institute, Medical College of Pennyslvania, Philadelphia, Pennsylvania

Psychodynamic Aspects of Mood Disorders

JOSEPH T. COYLE, M.D.

Distinguished Service Professor of Child Psychiatry and Professor of Psychiatry, Neuroscience, Pharmacology and Pediatrics, Johns Hopkins University School of Medicine; Director of the Division of Child Psychiatry, Johns Hopkins Hospital, Baltimore, Maryland

Childhood Psychopathology: Diagnosis and Treatment

MICHAEL DAVIDSON, M.D.

Associate Professor of Psychiatry and Chief, Clinical Research Division, Department of Psychiatry, Mount Sinai School of Medicine, New York, New York

Neuropeptides

KENNETH L. DAVIS, M.D.

Professor and Chairman, Department of Psychiatry, and Attending Chief of Service, Mount Sinai School of Medicine, New York, New York

Delirium and Dementia; Pathogenesis of Mood Disorders; Biology of Schizophrenia

STEPHEN I. DEUTSCH, M.D., Ph.D.

Associate Chairman for Clinical Neurosciences, Department of Psychiatry, and Associate Professor of Psychiatry, Georgetown University School of Medicine; Associate Professor of Psychiatry, Howard University School of Medicine; Chief, Psychiatry Service, Department of Veterans Affairs Medical Center, Washington, D.C.

Neurophysiological and Neurochemical Basis of Behavior

GAIL A. EDELSOHN, M.D., M.S.P.H.

Assistant Professor and Director of Residency Training, Child and Adolescent Psychiatry, Johns Hopkins University School of Medicine, Baltimore, Maryland

Elementary-School-Age Child

LAUREN KANTOR GORMAN, M.D.

Instructor of Clinical Psychiatry, Columbia University College of Physicians and Surgeons; Assistant in Psychiatric Service, Presbyterian Hospital, New York, New York

Pathogenesis of Mood Disorders

BLAINE S. GREENWALD, M.D.

Assistant Professor of Psychiatry, Albert Einstein College of Medicine, Bronx, New York; Director, Geriatric Psychiatry, and Assistant Attending Psychiatrist, Hillside Hospital, Long Island Jewish Medical Center, Glen Oaks, New York

Biology of Schizophrenia

CHARLES S. GROB, M.D.

Assistant Professor of Psychiatry and Human Behavior and Director, Adolescent Psychiatry, University of California Irvine Medical Center, Irvine, California

Adolescence

RONNIE HALPERIN, Ph.D.

Associate Professor of Psychology, State University of New York at Purchase, Purchase, New York

Hypothalamic Control

LEONARD HANDELSMAN, M.D.

Assistant Professor of Psychiatry, Mount Sinai School of Medicine, New York, New York; Medical Director, Drug Dependency Treatment Program, Veterans Affairs Medical Center, Bronx, New York

Drug and Alcohol Dependency; Anxiety

VAHRAM HAROUTUNIAN, Ph.D.

Associate Professor of Psychiatry, Mount Sinai School of Medicine, New York, New York

Gross Anatomy of the Brain

JAMES C. HARRIS, M.D.

Director, Developmental Neuropsychiatry, and Associate Professor of Psychiatry, Pediatrics, and Mental Hygiene, Johns Hopkins University School of Medicine, Baltimore, Maryland

Developmental Perspective; The First Years of Life

THOMAS B. HORVATH, M.D.

Professor of Psychiatry, State University of New York Health Science Center at Brooklyn; Chief of Staff, Veterans Affairs Medical Center, Brooklyn, New York

Consciousness and Attention; Integrative Brain Mechanisms; Delirium and Dementia

EDWARD JOSEPH, M.D.

Professor of Psychiatry, Mount Sinai School of Medicine; Training and Supervising Analyst, New York Psychoanalytic Institute; Attending Psychiatrist, Mount Sinai Hospital, New York, New York

Psychodynamic Personality Theory

PHILIP KANOF, M.D., Ph.D.

Assistant Professor of Psychiatry, Mount Sinai School of Medicine, New York, New York; Attending Psychiatrist, Veterans Affairs Medical Center, Bronx, New York

Neurotransmitter Receptor Function; Pathophysiology of Pain

STEVEN E. KELLER, Ph.D.

Associate Professor of Psychiatry and Neurosciences, University of Medicine and Dentistry of New Jersey, Newark, New Jersey

Stress and the Immune System

KENNETH S. KENDLER, M.D.

Professor of Psychiatry and Human Genetics, Medical College of Virginia/Virginia Commonwealth University, Richmond, Virginia

Behavior Genetics

HOWARD KLAR, M.D.

Associate Professor of Clinical Psychiatry, Columbia University College of Physicians and Surgeons; Director of Education, Department of Psychiatry, St. Luke's–Roosevelt Hospital Center, New York, New York

DSM-III-R Classification of Mental Disorders; Personality Disorders

ARTHUR T. MEYERSON, M.D.

Professor and Chairperson, Department of Psychiatry, Hahnemann University; Chief of Psychiatry, Hahnemann University Hospital, Philadelphia, Pennsylvania

Psychodynamic Theories of Schizophrenia

RICHARD C. MOHS, Ph.D.

Professor, Department of Psychiatry, Mount Sinai School of Medicine, New York, New York; Psychologist, Psychiatry Service, Veterans Affairs Medical Center, Bronx, New York

Learning and Memory

MICHAEL MURPHY, M.D., Ph.D.

Director, Clinical Neuroscience, Hoechst-Roussel Pharmaceuticals, Inc., Somerville, New Jersey; Clinical Assistant Professor of Psychiatry, Mount Sinai School of Medicine, New York, New York; Clinical Assistant Professor of Psychiatry, University of Medicine and Dentistry of New Jersey, Piscataway, New Jersey

Neurophysiological and Neurochemical Basis of Behavior; Anxiety

ALLAN L. REISS, M.D.

Assistant Professor, Psychiatry and Pediatrics, Johns Hopkins University School of Medicine; Associate Director, Department of Developmental Neuropsychiatry, The Kennedy Institute, Baltimore, Maryland

Mental Retardation

ARTHUR RIFKIN, M.D.

Professor of Psychiatry, Albert Einstein College of Medicine, New York, New York; Assistant Director for Academic Affairs, Department of Psychiatry, Queens Hospital Center Affiliate, Long Island Jewish Medical Center, Jamaica, New York

Phenomenology of Mental Disorders

WILMA G. ROSEN, Ph.D.

Associate Clinical Professor of Medical Psychology, Columbia University College of Physicians and Surgeons; Associate Professional Psychologist, Columbia-Presbyterian Medical Center, New York, New York

Higher Cortical Processes

STEVEN J. SCHLEIFER, M.D.

Associate Professor of Psychiatry, University of Medicine and Dentistry of New Jersey; Director, Consultation-Liaison Service, University Hospital, Newark, New Jersey

Stress and the Immune System

LARRY J. SIEVER, M.D.

Associate Professor of Psychiatry and Director, Outpatient Psychiatry Division, Mount Sinai School of Medicine, New York, New York

Biological Rhythms and the Neuroendocrine System; Pathogenesis of Mood Disorders; Personality Disorders

JEREMY M. SILVERMAN, Ph.D.

Assistant Professor of Psychiatry, Mount Sinai School of Medicine, New York, New York; Director of Family Studies, Psychiatry Service, Veterans Affairs Medical Center, Bronx, New York

Behavior Genetics

BARBARA H. SOHMER, M.D.

Assistant Professor, Psychiatry and Pediatrics, and Director, Child and Adolescent Psychiatry Consultation/Liaison Service, Johns Hopkins University School of Medicine; Active Staff, Psychiatry and Pediatrics, Johns Hopkins Hospital, Baltimore, Maryland

Childhood Psychopathology: Diagnosis and Treatment

MARVIN STEIN, M.D.

Esther and Joseph Klingenstein Professor of Psychiatry, Mount Sinai School of Medicine; Attending in Psychiatry, Mount Sinai Hospital, New York, New York

Stress and the Immune System

Preface

Psychiatry has changed. Not long ago it was a specialty in which diagnoses were as unreliable as a gambler's luck, etiologies were a matter of personal opinion, and treatments were mere nostrums and wishful thinking.

So, what has changed?

Not long ago the brain was a black box, a tangled, incomprehensible jumble of nerves and tracts that aroused wonder and defied understanding; the brain is now the focus of intense medical research. Although we are still far from fully understanding the workings of the brain, we can at least ask more reasonable questions about its structure, its function, its ways of communicating with itself, and the neurochemicals that serve as the basis of this transmission of information. In addition, a growing technology and data base have begun to answer current questions and ask new ones.

Not long ago, human behavior—mesmerizing in its variability and complexity—seemed beyond classification and without plausible explanation. Today, we can reliably agree on characterizing behaviors, quantify many, and explain the basis of some. Certain behaviors are clearly linked to brain events; others are understandable in terms of individual life history; and most, not surprisingly, appear to be related to the complex interplay between a person's genetically endowed behavioral predilections and his or her developmental experiences.

Psychiatry, the medical specialty devoted to understanding these behaviors and treating people when behavior goes awry, has embraced these changes with a passion. Increasing understanding of mental function and human development, and how the relationship between them affects behavior, will do much to promote mental health and alleviate the suffering of troubled people.

In reality, the change that has taken place is that psychiatry has become a science. And, as we would hope, science has transformed mystery into mere confusion. This enables us to ask more precise questions about people's behavior and its biologic and developmental basis and to generate new theories of health and pathology. This book, while offering a foundation upon which to build a current understanding of human behavior, also hopes to prompt new and better questions.

We hope that in these chapters our readers will find, as well as information, new possibilities for thinking about behavior. Where controversies exist, we have tried to present the most forceful arguments for various points of view. No doubt, some people will feel that we have treated some subjects as noncontroversial while controversies remain. When data about neuroscience or behavior are unclear or unavailable, we have said so. We have left discussion of the treatment of psychiatric disorders to other sources.

We see this book as a first effort to integrate the explosion of neuroscientific and behavioral research into an introductory preclinical text of psychiatry and human behavior. As such, we hope our readers will treat it as we have intended, as the first word, not the last, and the start of a dialogue that will continue for a long time.

KENNETH L. DAVIS, M.D.

HOWARD KLAR, M.D.

JOSEPH T. COYLE, M.D.

Acknowledgments

The editors gratefully acknowledge the contributions of Marvin Stein, M.D., former chairman of the department of psychiatry at Mount Sinai Medical School, who created a clinical and educational environment in which the ideas presented in this book could take root and be applied; of George Ryan, whose editorial and literary skill enabled the authors to present their ideas with greater clarity; and of JoAnn Lawler-Fink, whose commitment and attention to detail enabled all of us to persevere through the many drafts and communications a book like this entails.

Contents

Part I
Introductory Concepts

Chapter 1
Psychodynamic Personality Theory

Edward Joseph, M.D.

Understanding human behavior requires an acceptance of the fact that not all phenomena are explicable in terms of neurobiological changes. Many aspects of human behavior require consideration at a purely psychological level. Over the years, many psychological theories have been advanced, and much research at a psychological level has been done in applying such theories to human behavior. This research has expanded psychological understanding and provided useful guidelines to comprehending human behavior. A complete approach to understanding human behavior requires, therefore, a combination of neurobiological and psychological aspects, since not all phenomena can be encompassed within any one frame of reference. At the same time, it is not possible to completely translate from a neurobiological frame of reference to a psychological one, nor conversely. An analogous situation occurs in physics, in which explanations of phenomena associated with light require the utilization of both a wave theory and a particle theory of the nature of light. Physicists have not been

able to combine the two theories into a unified theory; instead, they move from one frame of reference to the other with ease. The same applies to human behavior.

Of a number of current psychological theories, the psychodynamic frame of reference seems to have the widest explanatory power. It has been utilized for a number of years, has expanded in scope from its early form, and is probably as widely applied today as any theory. The psychodynamic theory is essentially derived from the work of Sigmund Freud and his followers. Many of its basic tenets have been so widely accepted that they are almost taken for granted, without either their origins or basic assumptions being considered. Many of its terms are familiar to individuals who have not studied any part of the theory and who use its terminology freely, without fully understanding the definitions and derivations. In this category come such terms as Freudian slip, unconscious, conflict, defense mechanisms, ego, id, superego, oedipus complex, primary process, and secondary process.

Before discussing the status of many of the

psychodynamic concepts used in the study of human behavior today, a brief historical background will be given to set the stage for the discussion of present concepts.

FREUD

Freud began his studies around the turn of the century. As a physician, he had an extensive background in embryology, histology, pharmacology, and neurology. Many of his publications in those fields remained classics for years, and he was among the first to explore the use of cocaine as a local anesthetic. Turning to the study of neurophysiological disorders, his clinical exposure was more to individuals with neuroses than psychoses. His contemporary Emil Kraepelin studied the psychoses extensively and laid the groundwork for their modern classification and understanding. Freud's work took him in a different direction, since the sources of his clinical observations were of a different order.

Freud was a keen clinical observer who utilized the clinical situation as an experimental laboratory. After trying various clinical approaches, he undertook a series of observations using the method called *free association*. This method required the patient to speak freely of whatever might come to mind and has formed the basis not only of the therapeutic application of psychoanalysis but of continued study and research into the nature of mental processes. Much of the so-called psychodynamic theory is derived from this experimental situation of free association.

Early in his work, Freud attempted to correlate his psychological findings with the neurophysiology of the nervous system, advancing a "scientific project" which attempted to explain one set of findings in terms of the other. He offered a number of hypotheses that attempted to bridge the neurophysiological knowledge of his time with his psychological findings. In so doing, he attempted to eliminate the dichotomy between mind and brain. That he failed to do so is related more to the lack of knowledge of brain neurophysiology at that time than to the fact that such a bridging cannot be achieved.

FREUD'S POSTULATES

Derived from his clinical observations and from the study of a number of other behavioral phenomena, such as dreams, slips of speech,

errors of behavior, wit and humor, and, of course, the neuroses, Freud made several basic hypotheses which have proven to have great explanatory power and opened the way for much research and development of concepts. These basic postulates are: unconscious mental activity, psychic continuity, and psychic energy.

Unconscious Mental Activity

This postulate holds that a great deal of mental activity goes on outside of consciousness and, in fact, that the most basic motives of human behavior are often unconscious. A characteristic of the inferred unconscious portion of mental activity is that unconscious mental processes and content cannot readily acquire consciousness. Moreover, the nature of unconscious mental activity is different from that of conscious mental acitivity. Evidence for this postulate was derived from dreams, hypnotic processes, and so on. The concept of unconscious mental activity has dynamic implications, since certain principles of unconscious mental functioning can be elucidated. These include (1) timelessness, (2) two elements of unconscious mental content can be contradictory to one another without either element being obliterated, (3) lack of negation, (4) a part can stand for a totality, and (5) symbolization may be used as a mode of expression of unconscious content.

Psychic Continuity

The concept of psychic continuity applies to thoughts, feelings, fantasies, and memories as they are registered in the mind. This postulate states that any of these mental phenomena can continue to exist throughout the lifetime of an individual. They may exist at an unconscious level but are always potentially available. Research on the developmental stages in the life cycle of individuals is based on this postulate. The earlier stages of development can, and often do, exert an influence on later levels of development and of mental functioning. In the clinical situation, thoughts, feelings, or actions that follow each other in temporal sequence have a relationship to each other (psychic determinism).

Psychic Energy

The postulate of psychic energy provides a quantitative factor as well as a connection between mental activity and its biological roots. Two sources of mental energy are assumed, a libidinal one and an aggressive one. These are regarded as deriving from somatic sources, the origins of which are unknown, and provide the necessary energy that activates many mental activities.

MODELS OF THE MIND

In his effort to understand the nature of mental life and its role in the production of various psychiatric illnesses, Freud developed several models of the mind. Two of his models continue to be used by students of the psychodynamic process. The first of these models utilizes the relationship to consciousness as the basis for differentiating regions of the mind. The model includes a conscious portion of the mind (that of which a person is aware at any given moment) and an unconscious portion of the mind (the inferred area described earlier). It was also recognized, from clinical observation, that an area lies between the conscious and unconscious portions of the the mind, the contents of which can easily acquire consciousness but which exist outside consciousness at any given moment. This intermediate region is called the preconscious, so that the three regions of the mind in this model are

- Conscious
- Preconscious
- Unconscious

The differentiating point between the unconscious and the other two regions is that the content of the unconscious region cannot readily acquire consciousness under most circumstances, and requires either special processes or special altered states of the mind, such as exist in the sleeping state or under hypnosis.

This model served for many years and is still often used descriptively; however, a number of clinical phenomena were observed that could not be explained within the confines of such a model. To account for these observations and to provide a broader scope for relating the mental activities that go on within an individual and between an individual and his or her environment, another model evolved which has a wider explanatory power and is in common use today. In this later model, the interactions between a range of mental activities and the outside world—reality—are interconnected. The model still has three portions, called *arbitrarily* the id, the ego, and the superego.

Id

The id is defined as that region of the mind which contains the mental representation of bodily needs. It is considered to be wholly unconscious, known to consciousness only by its effects and by inferences from behavior.

Ego

The region of the mind called the ego is believed to contain both conscious and unconscious parts, which serve a mediating role between bodily needs (id) and the external world. As the human organism develops, certain moral and ethical demands are acquired, which then have to be taken into account in this mediating function. Thus, the role of the ego ultimately is between needs and the outside world, on one side, and internal moral and ethical demands, on the other.

Superego

The superego is regarded as having both conscious and unconscious portions and is considered the internal representation of society's moral and ethical demands.

Role of Conflict

These models of the mind provide a motivational basis to explain human behavior, whether it occurs in normal circumstances, in neurosis, or in psychosis. They are based upon the assumption of a conflict theory of behavior. At first, the conflict was thought to be between a person's mode of thinking, feeling, or behaving and the environment in which he or she existed; however, clinical experience demonstrated that much human conflict exists not only in terms of the relationship to the environment, but within the mind.

The first model allows for the demonstration of conflict between the unconscious portions of the mind and the conscious portions. Thus, an unconscious thought might seek expression at a conscious level. There would be an opposition to the emergence or acceptance of this thought, and conflict would ensue between the unconscious and conscious levels. However, this conflict model was insufficient to account for a number of clinical phenomena, which led to the second model described above.

In terms of the second model, the concept of inner conflict continued, but the conflict was believed to exist between ego and id, ego and superego, id and superego, or ego and reality. With this change in model of the mind, a conflict theory of human behavior became applicable to normal, neurotic, or psychotic individuals, with a conflict being either internal—within the mind—or external. With the new model, it was possible to see that many aspects of human behavior arise and function without conflict; such nonconflictual behavior is termed autonomy. Conflict will be further discussed under the heading Psychic Conflict.

EGO FUNCTIONS

Careful examination of an individual's behavior indicates the operation of a number of mental activities coordinated in a variety of ways. Each of these mental activities can be separated out, and a series of individual functions can be determined. It can be shown that each of these mental functions has a developmental history from birth onward, arising out of an undifferentiated matrix. It is possible to differentiate an early primitive form that gradually evolves into a more mature adult form. A close interrelationship exists between the primitive and more developed forms of the ego functions, and it is possible, at various stages of development, to see the changing nature of the particular function.

The development of each ego function comes about through an interaction and interplay among three factors that arise, almost inevitably, in the course of growth and development: (1) innate maturational forces, (2) experiential events, and (3) internal conflicts. Although basic instinctual drives are approximately similar in all persons, the interplay among these three factors allows for an infinite variety of functioning in individuals.

Among the ego functions to be considered are those basic ones derived from neurophysiological processes: perception, memory, and motility. These ego functions are basic because the development of more complex mental activities depends upon their operation.

Perception

Perception is more than the neurological sensation which reaches the appropriate area in the brain from the periphery of the organism. In psychological terms, it is the mental registration of the sensation.

Memory

Memory includes the storage and encoding of the perception as a memory trace and the recall process. See Chapter 2: Learning and Memory.

Motility

Motility refers to the psychological or mental control of movement, which is initially an involuntary, unconscious act that later comes under a combination of conscious and unconscious control at a psychological level. Motility or action can be regarded as the end stage of a process that starts from perception and memory and leads to action based on the nature of the perception and the memories associated with it.

Affect

An important and very human mental function, affect is a combination of emotion, usually perceived in terms of pleasure or displeasure, and an accompanying physiological response. Affects can be thought of as existing along a pleasure-unpleasure continuum, ranging from complete satisfaction and gratification at one end of the scale to complete dissatisfaction, pain, and extreme discomfort at the other end. Affects start out in an all-or-none way and probably are experienced at an early age in terms of satiation or lack of satiation. With later development come varying degrees and modulations of affect, with more intermediate stages evolving.

Affect also operates on a love-hate continuum, which, again, early in life is probably experienced with an all-or-none quality and later modulates into varying degrees of liking or disliking. Another affective series that follows the pleasure-unpleasure continuum is the one of happiness vs. unhappiness, leading to extremes of loneliness and depression. These are prominent in affective disorders, particularly those of a depressive nature. See Chapter 27: Psychodynamic Aspects of Mood Disorders.

Thinking

The ego function of thinking is one of the most important mental activities. Thinking includes fantasy, daydreaming, reverie, and dreams during sleep, as well as the organized logical thinking characteristic of the mature person. Most thinking processes occur outside the consciousness. The thought of which an individual is aware is a relatively small portion of the thinking process and products. Thinking is obviously based on neurophysiological brain functioning.

The thinking process can be classified in another way as being primary or secondary process.

Primary process thinking is characterized by lack of logical connection between associated thoughts, the replacement of one thought by another, a part standing for a whole thought sequence, a marked use of symbolization, and contradictions occuring within the same context. Primary process thinking, which is characteristic of early forms of thinking, can occur in normal people under stress, in sleep, during illness, and so on.

Secondary process thinking is based on reality; it is logical, with connection between associated thoughts; abstract; and a total expression of an idea rather than only a part. Most adults use secondary process thinking, and the appearance of primary process thinking as a frequent occurrence is a sign of pathological regression of the thinking process.

Object Relations

Object relations is one of the most important ego functions. For simplicity, people, things, animals, and so forth are all collected together under the term *objects*. Objects, particularly people, are an absolute necessity for the survival of the newborn infant. The biological helplessness following birth makes the infant completely dependent on his environment. The environment is essentially made up of the people within it, particularly the caregiving people. The earliest relationship with people is called an *anaclitic* one, in which one's existence is dependent upon someone else. As an infant learns to distinguish the existence of an outside person, that outside person is regarded in terms of its ability to fulfill the needs of the infant. This is the stage of the *need-satisfying object*, in which the object is highly regarded only insofar as it satisfies the needs of the infant. With further development and further experiences, there is awareness of the totality of the object with its own needs as well as its ability to satisfy the needs of the infant itself. The object then becomes the recipient of feelings: love or hate.

Sense of Self

Another ego function evolving simultaneously is the development of a sense of self. Starting from an early matrix in which there appears to be no differentiation between one's self and the outside world, a gradual differentiation takes place between the boundaries of one's own body and one's surroundings; a *body image* is developed and also a sense of one's physical entity as separate and distinct from other entities in the environment. Gradually, one gains a sense of one's own sexual nature and the concept of one as a separate psychological individual as well as a physical individual.

In the course of developing a sense of one's self or an image of one's self, the process of *identification* plays an important role, in addition to the other maturational and developmental factors mentioned above. Identification is a mental process whereby the individual takes on as an integral part of his or her psychological self some or all of the attributes of an admired, or sometimes of a hated, person. This is a more global process early in life, becoming refined later. This mental process goes on throughout much of one's life, so that, at any stage in the life cycle, an individual can, and often does, identify with someone whom he or she admires a great deal. Identification also occurs when a loved object has been lost, either in fact or in fantasy. A common reaction to the death of a loved one is for the bereaved to unconsciously identify with some attributes of the dead person and become somewhat like him or her.

Reality Testing

Reality testing normally develops in the course of growth. Through perception, memories, and experiences, the individual learns the nature of the world around him or her. The individual learns to differentiate between his or her own inner thoughts and what exists outside him or her. This is a gradual process that takes many years and aids in adapation to the world. Having acquired or learned a *sense of reality*, the individual then begins to test perceptions against this sense of reality. The differentiation between objective reality and psychic reality is important. *Objective reality* is what most people would agree upon as existing in the world or in the environment around them. *Psychic reality* is what an individual believes exists, regardless of the objective reality. No one's sense of reality is 100 percent accurate; rather, it is always influenced by one's memories, experiences, affects, and fantasies, so that at best there is an approximation of psychic and objective reality.

Integrative or Synthetic Functions

All of the ego functions thus far described are manifest in the form of clinical phenomena observable in patients and normal individuals upon study of their mental activity. The clinical phenomena so derived often show such a close coordination and interaction among the ego functions that some infer that silent functions must be held responsible for the order and harmony. These are called integrative or synthetic functions.

PSYCHOSEXUAL DEVELOPMENT

In addition to the ego functions, there is a separate developmental sequence of sexual responses. The word "sexual" is used here in its broadest sense, ranging from any experiences associated with pleasure to adult sexual experiences. The psychosexual stages interact with the various ego functions in a circular or feedback mechanism; in the feedback mechanism, psychosexual development affects the development of ego functions and vice versa. The psychosexual stages unfold in a biologically, probably genetically, predetermined manner. However, the actual process is also affected by the nature of experiences at various stages of development.

There are two ways of regarding psychosexual development. The first of these is to regard the development from an autoerotic stage (narcissism) in which the individual is the source of his or her own satisfaction, often associated with masturbation as the principal form of gratification, to a later object-related stage, in which satisfaction is found in terms of a relationship or activity with an outside object.

In the second approach, psychosexual development is classified in terms of the principal zones of the body which serve at various times as chief areas from which gratification is obtained. Not that gratification obtained at one zone is ever wholly given up, but each zone gives way to the primacy of other zones in the course of development.

Oral

The first stage centers around the mouth as the orifice for obtaining physiological needs and, as these are met, the achieving of a degree of gratification. The mouth, like all other orifices of the body, is richly endowed with nerves. Stimulation of the mouth gives rise to many sensations which, through their perception and association with gratifying experiences, acquire the quality of pleasure. Mouthing and putting things in the mouth are characteristic of early infants as a way of exploring the environment. In later relationships with objects, mouth or oral activity often is part of the foreplay leading, ultimately, to genital contact. Too much gratification associated with oral activity, or too little, may affect later personality or character types.

Anal

Subsequent to the stage of oral primacy, there is a shift to the anal region as the zone of gratification. Often this shift is associated with the beginnings of toilet and bowel training. There is pleasure associated with expelling or retaining bowel contents. A certain amount of anal play predominates during this stage. Depending again upon gratifications and frustrations, permanent characteristics of the personality may derive from this level of development.

Phallic

The next shift is to the phallic region as the chief zone associated with gratification. This does not mean that the oral and anal gratifications are completely gone but that they are diminished in importance. The phallic level involves the penis in the male and the clitoris in the female; this level is associated with masturbatory activity as the principal source of gratification. Fantasies of varying nature (for instance, oedipal fantasies) often accompany such masturbatory acts.

Lesser Sources of Gratification

Accompanying the primacy of the body zones are other areas of the body which serve as lesser sources of gratification. These include tactile, visual, olfactory, and aural areas. Pleasure is also associated with looking at others and their activities, as well as being looked at or exhibiting oneself.

Genital

The pleasurable qualities of all body areas come together in the primacy of the genital area and in a desire for union with an outside object, more usually of the opposite sex but also of the same sex. This stage of genital primacy is one in which the genital activity is the chief aim of the sexual activity, with contributions from all other body areas.

PSYCHIC CONFLICT

As previously discussed, psychic conflict can occur among the id, ego, superego, and environment. The ego's mediating role and its reality function serve to keep such conflict within the mind. At times, various ego functions may conflict with each other; for example, a fantasy may conflict with the sense of reality.

Inner conflict may arise from many sources, but there are particular times in life when conflict is more prone to occur. In early stages of development, before the various control systems represented by ego functions are well established, the strength of wishes may produce conflict between wishes and external reality. At times of life marked by biological change, for example, at adolescence or menopause, a biologically strengthened series of wishes might threaten to overwhelm the control systems represented by the ego functions. Conflict may also be brought about by extreme degrees of stimulation, whether from the external world or not, giving rise to an unusual flood of perceptions, memories, affects, or combinations of all these, requiring great effort on the part of the control systems to contain the conflict.

If psychic conflict occurs at an unconscious level, and if it is successfully mastered and dealt with, the end result may be an *adaptation* to a combination of wish and reality. One adaptive measure utilizing the function of anticipation is the *postponement of gratification* until reality may be altered, after which the wish may be gratified. This can be an extremely adaptive process and makes possible concentrated periods of work for which the gratification is not immediately forthcoming. However, if attempts to solve the conflict are unsuccessful, the end result is a stimulation of the affect of *anxiety*, at which point other psychological mechanisms come into play. These mechanisms perform the function of defense and are an important component of mental activity.

DEFENSE MECHANISMS

"Defense" is a general term used to describe the struggles of the ego to protect itself against danger. The danger arises because of the threat of eruption into consciousness of a repressed wish which has become associated with some real or imagined punishment. This is signaled by painful feelings of anxiety or guilt, and these feelings impel the ego to ward off the wish or drive. Defenses always operate unconsciously, so that the person is unaware of what is taking place. The specific methods of warding off such dangerous drives or wishes are known as defense mechanisms. The operation of these mechanisms may result in a deletion or distortion of some aspects of reality.

Defense mechanisms also lend form to personality. For example, repression (keeping content out of consciousness) is associated with hysteria; isolation (separation of idea and affect) is associated with obsessive-compulsive personality; and projection (attributing one's thought to another) is connected with paranoid personality.

DREAMS AND DREAM PROCESSES

Early in his studies, Freud found that patients frequently reported dreams when free-associating. Rather than ignoring them, as previous students of human behavior had done, Freud studied the dreams and dream processing. His findings were of two kinds. The first kind relates to the content of dreams, in which he demonstrated that dreams are a kind of night thinking governed more by primary process. He felt that it was possible to show that dreams have meaning and significance, often in a disguised form. He distinguished between the manifest content—the dream as reported by the dreamer—and a latent content, which represents the unconscious thoughts or wishes that went into the dream formation. He believed that it is possible to understand the meaning of a dream through the free associations of the dreamer and that this meaning represents the gratification of an unconscious wish that arose in the course of the night. He felt that the function of the dream was to preserve sleep, if possible, through the gratification of this unconscious wish.

Freud's second finding was an explanation of the process of dream formation utilizing a combination of the neurophysiology of his time and the mental mechanisms he had been uncovering. He believed it was possible to show that dream formation occurred through the interaction of some portion of the day's experience (day residue) with unconscious mental content from the past, thereby gaining conscious representation, in a disguised form, as the manifest dream. His complicated postulations were, of course, based upon the knowledge of his time.

Later students of dreaming and dream processing have tended to accept that dreams have meaning and significance for the individual but that the processes of dream formation take into account more conscious processes, aspirations, problem-solving devices, and so on. No single theory of either dream processes or dream formation is fully accepted.

At a clinical level, particularly in relation to various forms of psychotherapy, dreams are often utilized for their significance in understanding the processes of the patient. The psychodynamic concept of the significance of dreams is a useful tool in those situations.

BIBLIOGRAPHY

Abend, S.: Psychological conflict and the concept of defense. Psychoanal. Quart. 50:67-76, 1981.

Blanck, G. and R.: Ego Psychology: Theory and Practice. New York, Columbia University Press, 1974, pp. 19-40.

Brenner, C.: Elementary Textbook of Psychoanalysis, ed. 3, New York, International Universities Press, 1984. Paperback.

Ellenberger, H.: The Discovery of the Unconscious. New York, Basic Books, 1970. Historical background.

Freud, A.: The Ego and Mechanisms of Defense. New York, International Universities Press, 1973.

Freud, S.: Introductory Lectures on Psychoanalysis, vols. 15 and 16, and New Introductory Lectures on Psychoanalysis, vol. 22, Complete Psychological Works, Standard Edition. London, Hogarth Press, 1963. Also available in other editions and paperbacks.

Horowitz, M.: Introduction to Psychodynamics. New York, Basic Books, 1988.

Joseph, E.: Memory and conflict. Psychoanal. Quart. 35:1-16, 1966.

Joseph, E.: Perception and reality, in Perspectives in Psychoanalysis, I. Marcus (ed.). New York, International Universities Press, 1972.

Marmer, S.S.: Theories of the mind, in Textbook of Psychiatry, J. Talbott et al. (eds.). Washington, D.C., American Psychiatric Press, 1988.

Chapter 2
Learning and Memory

Richard C. Mohs, Ph.D.

How people learn and remember is currently the focus of many investigations, both from psychological and biological perspectives. Learning is usually defined as a relatively permanent change in behavior that occurs as a result of experience. Learned behaviors are distinguished from those which occur entirely as a result of maturation (and thus require no experience) and from behavioral changes which are not long-lasting, such as those due to fatigue. Memory is the physical system used to store information during the learning process and to retrieve it when it is needed. Although some attempts have been made to describe the learning process without reference to memory, most current work is based on the premise that learning can best be understood by developing and testing theories of memory.

Many aspects of memory, particularly human memory, remain only poorly understood. Nevertheless, enough evidence exists to indicate certain features that must be included in any viable model of the human memory system. This chapter reviews some of the major lines of evi-

dence which have influenced contemporary theories of memory and outlines the principal features shared by most theories. Results on both psychological and biological aspects of memory are presented, but the emphasis is on fundamental principles of memory functioning rather than on applied research dealing with memory problems or memory improvement.

ATTENTION AND PATTERN RECOGNITION

In order for any environmental event to influence behavior, the organism must pay attention to the event and must, in some sense, recognize the event. Attention can be divided into two components: (1) maintenance of a general state of arousal or alertness, which sensitizes the organism to stimuli in general; (2) selective attention, which selects certain stimuli for additional processing. Factors that affect the selection of stimuli have been investigated in some detail; they include the physical characteristics of the stimulus, the observer's expectations, and the observer's familiarity with the stimulus. For present purposes, it is sufficient to note that, in order for learning to occur, the learner must be attentive in the general sense and must selectively attend to those stimulus events that are to be learned. For a fuller discussion of attention, see Chapter 6: Consciousness and Attention.

The first step in learning about stimuli or events to which the learner's attention has been drawn is to identify patterns that are already familiar. Numerous studies have demonstrated that a given learning task can differ according to the learner's familiarity with the material to be learned. One example of such a study investigated the rate at which subjects could learn sequences of binary digits (zeroes and ones). Some learners tried to learn the sequences by rote, while others knew how to recode groups of 2, 3, 4, or 5 binary digits into decimal equivalents. The rote learners performed most poorly, and the rate of learning increased with the size of the unit that could be recoded into a decimal number; that is, the learners who could recognize the largest units were able to learn more quickly, presumably because the number of units they had to store in memory was smaller. At least two important principles of memory functioning are illustrated by these results: (1) The learning task is, to a large extent, determined by the kinds of patterns the learner can identify in the environment. (2) A learning task that is difficult for one person may be quite simple for another who can identify many familiar patterns in the material to be learned.

SENSORY MEMORY

Experiments investigating memory for visually presented displays have shown that the visual system has the capacity to store images in relatively unprocessed form for very brief periods of time. The number of items a person can remember from a single glance at a visual display is quite small, usually five to seven items. This amount, called the span of apprehension, is limited because people can only remember as many items as they can identify and store in memory while the visual display is available.

Originally, it was thought that items were available to be identified only while the visual stimulus was present. However, a series of experiments in which subjects were asked to name letters presented visually for brief periods (less than 0.1 second) demonstrated that the visual image persists after the stimulus is removed. Displays of up to three rows of four letters each were presented. On some trials, subjects were simply asked to name as many letters as they could; on other trials, a spot of light appeared at varying intervals following the display to instruct the subjects to report only letters in the top, middle, or bottom row. On these partial-report trials, the number of letters available to the subject for identification is

$$N = np \times L$$

where N = number of letters available
n = number of letters per line
p = probability of a correct report
L = number of lines

When the spot of light was presented immediately following the letter display, N was 12, the size of the display. N decreased gradually as the light spot was delayed up to approximately 1 second, at which time N was 4.5 letters, the number reported when no light cue was given. The fact that N was greater than the number of items actually reported for 1 second indicated that a visual image was maintained for up to 1 second after the stimulus display was turned off. The memory system used to hold this image has been called iconic memory; an analogous system has been demonstrated in the auditory system and is called echoic memory.

The function of these two sensory memory systems is probably to provide more time for the organism to examine incoming sensory data to determine which stimuli should be processed further. For stimuli to enter these sensory memory systems, the organism must be attentive in the general sense but not in the selective sense. On the other hand, the cued recall data demonstrate that items are only read out from sensory memory to longer-term memory if the organism selectively attends to them. Unattended items rapidly decay from sensory memory and are lost.

SHORT-TERM AND LONG-TERM MEMORY STORE

One of the most obvious characteristics of human memory is its selectivity. The human memory system does not work like a tape recorder or videotape machine. Even if one tried, it would be impossible to remember a verbatim record of all that happened around one. Rather, the human memory system is organized so that it selectively remembers those things which have been studied or, for some reason, are highly salient. The sensory memory systems described above play an important role in enabling the memory system to be selective. The primary memory system, or, as it is often called, the short-term memory store (STS), also plays an important role in making memory selective. The existence of something like the STS was originally suggested by studies of limits on the span of memory. Although people do not remember most things the way a tape recorder does, they can recall a few items verbatim for a short period of time after they are presented. The number of items that can be recalled in order after a single presentation is called the memory span. It is determined by presenting a small number of items for immediate recall, say two digits, and then increasing the number of items to be recalled until the person can no longer recall them without error. For most people, the memory span is about seven items. Certainly, people can learn things that exceed the memory span, but to do so requires a series of repetitions or other kinds of study. The STS is that part of the memory system used in tests of memory span; it is a system of limited capacity used to hold small amounts of information for brief periods. To learn information that exceeds the capacity of the STS, it must be stored in the long-term memory store (LTS), a system of essentially unlimited capacity where information can be stored permanently.

Both psychological and biological data support the distinction between STS and LTS. Much of the psychological evidence comes from studies of free recall, a paradigm used to examine the way people learn and remember ongoing events. In a free-recall task, the subject is read a list of words (say 20) that exceeds the capacity of the STS; then the subject tries to recall all of the words in any order. Recall is usually best for the last words presented, next best for the first words presented, and poorest for the words from the middle of the list (Fig. 2-1). This pattern can be accounted for by assuming that the final words are recalled well because they are still in the STS, that the first words are recalled fairly well because they were most likely studied long enough to be stored in the LTS, and that the middle items are poorly recalled because they are no longer in the STS and are poorly represented in the LTS. If a delay of several seconds involving mental arithmetic is introduced between list presentation and recall, the last items are no longer well recalled; presumably this is

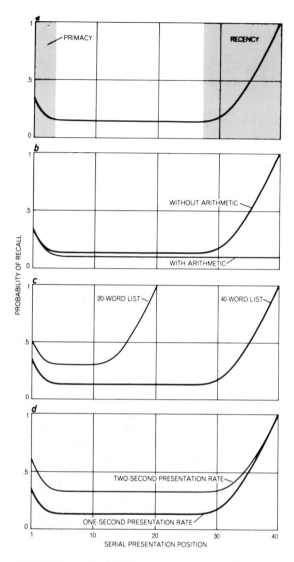

FIGURE 2–1. Probability of recall in free-recall experiments varies in a characteristic way with an item's serial position in a list: a "primacy effect" and a "recency effect" are apparent (a). If an arithmetic task is interpolated between presentation and recall, the recency effect disappears (b). Words in long lists are recalled less well than words in short lists (c). Slower presentation also results in better recall (d). The curves are idealized ones based on experiments by James W. Deese, Bennett Murdock, Lee Postman and Murray Glanser. (From Atkinson, R.C., Shiffrin, R.M.: The control of short-term memory. Sci. Am. 225:82–90, 1971. Copyright © 1971 by Scientific American, Inc. All rights reserved)

because mental arithmetic displaces these items from the STS. If the presentation rate is slowed, recall of early and middle items improves, while recall of the last items is unchanged; presumably this reflects the fact that a slower presentation rate enables more items to be stored in the LTS. These and a variety of other effects due to such things as word familiarity and list length can be accounted for by the STS-LTS distinction.

Studies of amnesic patients indicate that one or the other of these stores can be affected without dramatically impairing the other. Many patients with damage to the medial temporal regions have relatively normal memory spans but are greatly impaired on tasks requiring storage of information beyond the capacity of the STS. The most dramatic example of this phenomenon occurred in a patient with bilateral removal of the hippocampus, suggesting that this structure is critical for storing information in the LTS. A few patients with relatively normal learning ability but with markedly reduced memory spans have also been reported. These patients generally have cortical lesions of the parietal and occipital areas.

FACTORS AFFECTING LEARNING

Information or behaviors can be learned either well or poorly, and the learning can take place either quickly or slowly. Factors that can affect learning include characteristics of the learner, properties of the material to be learned, and the learning conditions themselves. Many of these factors have been investigated in some detail. One of the most important and most obvious is practice. In a verbal learning task such as free recall, repeated presentation of the list improves recall, and items within the list that receive more rehearsals are recalled better than items receiving fewer rehearsals. In manual tasks such as typing, most measures of learning such as speed and number of errors improve with practice. The distribution of practice is also important since the same amount of practice is usually more effective if it is spread out over several sessions rather than in one session.

Information that is familiar to the learner is considerably easier to learn than is unfamiliar information. This may appear to be almost a trivial statement, but work designed to investigate why this is true has shed considerable light on normal learning and on the performance of individuals who are highly skilled at certain tasks. For example, master chess players who were shown pictures from real chess games for only 5 seconds were usually able to recall the positions of about 90 percent of the pieces, while weak players could recall only about 40 percent of the positions. This difference was not due simply to the masters' greater familiarity with master play; when asked to guess the correct positions of pieces without seeing the picture of the game, masters were no more accurate than weak players. Furthermore, when shown the same number of pieces spread randomly around the board, both masters and weak players could recall only about 40 percent of the positions. Closer inspection of the masters' recall strategy for real games revealed that they tended to recall pieces in several chunks, each containing a few pieces in a familiar configuration. Weak players and masters confronted with randomly distributed pieces tended to recall pieces by rote. What enabled the masters to remember board positions from real games so easily was their knowledge of the game. More specifically, they were able to recognize a large number, estimated at approximately 40,000, different combinations of pieces that commonly occur during games. These kinds of results suggest that one component of skill in many activities such as computer programming or playing a musical instrument is the knowledge of familiar patterns stored in memory. They also indicate that the rate of learning will be determined to a large extent by the size of the familiar "chunks" which the learner can identify.

In nonhumans, the rate of learning is often governed primarily by reinforcement; that is, animals learn those behaviors which lead either to a positive reward such as food or water or to the cessation of pain. In humans, the effects of reinforcement are more complex, since few behaviors lead directly to biologically significant reinforcers and much human behavior is apparently motivated by success, self-esteem, and other kinds of satisfaction. Even though the actual reinforcers for much human learning are difficult to identify, many of the rules describing the effectiveness of reinforcing events apply to human as well as animal learning. Take a situation in which a person must repeatedly decide between two alternatives (for example, which of two routes to take to work or whether to trust a coworker). After each choice, the person receives feedback about whether the choice was correct. Formally, the situation is analogous to animal learning experiments in which the animal has two response alternatives and is rewarded a certain proportion of the time for each choice. The effect of feedback in these two choice situations can be described quite accurately by a simple linear "operator" model:

$$p_{n+1} = \lambda[p_n + \theta(1 - p_n)] + (1 - \lambda)(p_n - \theta p_n)$$

where p_{n+1} = probability of choosing the first
alternative on trial $n + 1$

p_n = probability of choosing the first
alternative on trial n

λ = probability of positive feedback
about the first alternative

θ = a constant between 0 and 1

Then, by simple algebra:

$$p_{n+1} = p_n + \theta(\lambda - p_n)$$

These models clearly have some limitations. Chief among them is the assumption that no information other than the positive feedback is available to the learner. Also, since they are probabilistic, they do not make exact predictions about the response on any trial. Nevertheless, they do make predictions which are generally true in both human and animal experiments. One is that, over the long run, the probability of selecting the first alternative will equal the probability that the first alternative leads to positive feedback. A second prediction is that, in the short run, the probability of selecting the first alternative will be heavily influenced by the outcome of the most recent trials. The biological mechanisms by which feedback or reinforcement changes memory traces and thus alters subsequent behavior are unknown.

Forgetting

Ordinary experience convinces almost everyone that memory traces, which are the biological structures where memories are stored, change over time. Forgetting is a common occurrence, as is the experience of suddenly remembering something which was previously forgotten. The way in which memory traces change over time and the factors affecting one's ability to retrieve them have been the subject of many investigations. The biological substrates of memory undergo changes over many years. In humans, this can be demonstrated most readily in patients receiving electroconvulsive therapy. Following electroconvulsive therapy, these patients have both an anterograde amnesia, which lasts for a few weeks, and a retrograde amnesia, which can last for several months. The retrograde amnesia is most severe for information that was learned immediately prior to the electroconvulsive therapy, and decreases in severity until 5 to 7 years

prior to the electroconvulsive therapy. Information that old can be recalled just as well by patients who have received electroconvulsive therapy as by controls, whereas information stored more recently is disrupted by electroconvulsive therapy. The process by which memory traces become more stable over time in the LTS is referred to as consolidation.

Normally, of course, the process of consolidation is not disrupted by events such as electroconvulsive therapy, but nevertheless forgetting occurs. Psychological research on forgetting has been concerned primarily with two factors, inhibition and loss of retrieval clues. These two factors produce most of the memory loss that occurs over time.

Inhibition

Inhibition refers to the fact that similar kinds of learning, either before or after the event to be remembered, interfere with later recall of that event. Experiments investigating inhibition typically have two groups of subjects, both of whom are asked to learn a set of items called paired associates. These items may be random pairs, such as *farmer-paper*, or more meaningful pairs, such as names with occupations: *John-painter*. After the initial learning, the experimental group learns a second set of items in which some of the original words are in new pairs, such as *John-farmer*. A control group either has no second learning task or has one that is completely unrelated to the paired-associate task. Following the second task, both groups are tested for recall of the original pairs. On this test, the performance of the experimental group is inevitably poorer than that of the control group. Since the second learning task interferes with recall of the first, this phenomenon is referred to as retroactive inhibition. An analogous phenomenon occurs when the experimental group participates in an interfering learning task prior to the learning task common to both groups. In this case, the poorer recall by the experimental group reflects proactive interference.

Interference of both types has been demonstrated with many different kinds of learning tasks. The changes that take place in memory to cause interference are not at all clear. Whether memory traces are actually lost as a result of inhibition or are simply inaccessible is a question that has concerned many investigators. The evidence on this point is inconclusive, but many memories lost through interference have been shown to be recovered over time.

Loss of Retrieval Cues

The question of whether memory traces are permanent or can be lost has also been of interest to investigators looking at the effect of different kinds of retrieval cues on memory performance. The common experience of suddenly being able to remember something, such as a name, which previously could not be recalled suggests that many instances of forgetting are due to retrieval failures rather than to loss of memory traces. One of the most important factors determining the amount that a person appears to remember is the manner in which the person is tested. Comparison of different testing methods indicates that the percentage retained is lowest when testing is by reproduction of the learned material as in free recall. The percentage retained is greater if testing is done by having the person relearn the original material, and the percentage retained is highest if the subject is tested for his or her ability to recognize the previously learned items.

Recall performance can be improved dramatically by providing appropriate cues to the subject. For example, if the learner in a free-recall test is given a list of 20 words taken from five semantic categories, recall will be improved if the subject is cued with the names of the categories. Most contemporary memory theories attribute the effectiveness of retrieval cues to the fact that they facilitate memory search processes. According to these theories, memory consists of a series of representations of familiar items connected by associations. Learning in a free-recall task involves establishing a new set of associations, and retrieval involves locating all of the associated words. Cues facilitate the process of locating learned words because they provide multiple entry points into the network of associations.

The fact that people can recognize as familiar more things than they can recall can easily be accounted for within this framework. In recognition testing, the subject must only decide whether or not each test item was studied before. Each test item provides a cue to its own representation in memory, and therefore no memory search through the network of associations is required. Recognition memory performance can usually be accounted for by assuming that the decision to say an item was studied is based on only two factors: a unidimensional measure of the item's familiarity in memory and a decision criterion. Familiarity depends primarily on how recently the test item was studied, while the decision criterion reflects the subject's estimate of the consequences involved in false positive or false negative decisions.

The biological mechanisms involved in memory search and decision processes are almost completely unknown, but studies of drug effects on retrieval indicate that the neurochemical state of the brain can serve to facilitate or impair retrieval much like other retrieval cues. Studies designed to investigate drug effects on retrieval typically employ four groups of subjects. Two groups learn following the administration of a drug, while the other two learn following the administration of a placebo. Later, when the drug is no longer active, retrieval from memory is tested. Two groups, one that learned in the drug state and one that learned following a placebo, are readministered the drug prior to retrieval testing. The other two groups receive a placebo before testing. For a variety of psychoactive drugs, the probability of correct retrieval has been found to be greater if the subject is in the same drug state during retrieval as during learning. Regardless of the drug's effect on learning, retrieval is impaired if the subject is not returned to the same drug state prior to the retrieval. Learning in which probability of correct retrieval depends on the similarity of the subject's drug state at learning and retrieval is said to be state-dependent.

PHYSIOLOGICAL THEORIES

To a large extent, the physiological basis of memory and learning remains a mystery. Much of the early work on the biology of memory was designed to identify the physiological or chemical units used to store individual items of experience. This research, often referred to as the search for the engram, was based on the premise that individual memories are stored in particular places in the brain. Learning new relationships between already familiar items was thought to involve the formation of associations between these isolated memories in the brain. The primary reason for the downfall of these "switchboard" theories of memory was that they could not account for the results of brain lesion studies conducted by K. S. Lashley and others. In these studies, animals were first trained on a task, and then cortical lesions were made in an attempt to determine the exact location of the memory trace for the learned habit. However, performance decrements were found to depend not so much on the exact location of the lesion but rather its size. The implication seemed to be that memory function depends upon the coordinated activity of a number of brain areas and that individual memories are not located in specific places.

Hippocampus

Identifiable brain structures and neurochemical systems may, however, play distinct roles in certain kinds of memory function. The hippocampus, in particular, has been identified as a structure that is necessary for the storage of new information beyond the capacity of the STS. Patients with bilateral lesions of the hippocampus are almost completely unable to learn either verbal or visual information beyond the five to seven items that can be held in the STS (Fig. 2-2). Certain kinds of learning, such as that involving motor skills, are preserved in these patients. This suggests a distinction between learning which does not involve specific propositions (that is, knowing how) and learning which involves a set of facts (that is, knowing that). Apparently these two kinds of learning are quite different, and the hippocampus is required only for the latter sort. See Chapter 12: Hypothalamic Control.

Acetylcholine

The neurochemical changes responsible for memory storage and retrieval are undoubtedly very complex, but evidence suggests that the neurotransmitter acetylcholine plays an important and somewhat specific role. Normal people who are given an anticholinergic drug develop a temporary anterograde amnesia for information that exceeds the capacity of the STS. The hippocampus has a high concentration of cholinergic neurons, and it seems reasonable that the amnesic effects of anticholinergics are due to blockade of acetylcholine receptors in this area. For further discussion of this neurotransmitter, see under the heading Acetylcholine in Chapter 8: Neurophysiological and Neurochemical Basis of Behavior.

The role of acetylcholine in memory is also

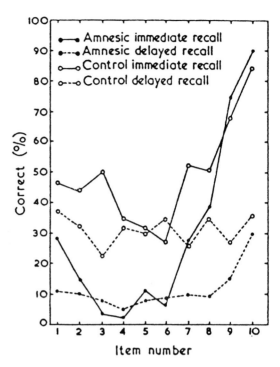

FIGURE 2-2. Immediate and delayed free recall in amnesic and control patients. Note that amnesics show a normal recency effect. (From Baddeley, A.D., Warrington, E.K.: Amnesia and the distinction between long- and short-term memory. J. Verbal Learning Verbal Behav. 9:176-189, 1970.)

supported by findings that patients with Alzheimer's disease have a dramatic loss of cholinergic neurons. This disease is characterized by a progressive loss of memory and other cognitive functions, including language and praxis. Neuropathologically, it is characterized by the development of neuritic plaques and neurofibrillary tangles, concentrated most heavily in the hippocampus and neocortex. The finding that patients with Alzheimer's disease have a loss of cholinergic neurons has raised the possibility that this and other conditions which cause memory loss might be treated with drugs that increase cholinergic activity. The short-acting cholinesterase inhibitor physostigmine has been shown to transiently enhance memory both in normal volunteers and in patients with Alzheimer's disease. Major efforts are being made to develop and test long-acting drugs that increase cholinergic activity. These efforts, along with studies of drugs affecting other neurotransmitters and neuromodulators, should lead to a better understanding of memory and to the development of treatments for memory disorders.

For a more detailed discussion, see under the heading Alzheimer's Disease in Chapter 22: Delirium and Dementia.

BIBLIOGRAPHY

Atkinson, R.C., Shiffrin, R.M.: The control of short-term memory. Sci. Am. 225:82-90, 1971.

Baddeley, A.D.: The Psychology of Memory. New York, Basic Books, 1976.

Bower, G.H., Morrow, D.G.: Mental models in narrative comprehension. Science 247:44-48, 1990.

Gazzaniga, M.S.: Organization of the human brain. Science 245:947-952, 1989.

Lashley, K.S.: Mass action in cerebral function. Science 73:245-254, 1931.

Squire, L.R.: Memory and Brain. New York, Oxford University Press, 1987.

Thompson, R.F.: The neurobiology of learning and memory. Science 233:941-947, 1986

Chapter 3
Behavior Genetics

Kenneth S. Kendler, M.D., and
Jeremy M. Silverman, Ph.D.

Behavior genetics is a relatively new science that combines aspects of psychology, psychiatry, physiology, and genetics. The goal of this science is to clarify the role that genetic factors play in the determination of behavior.

Before proceeding further, some definitions will be helpful. *Genotype* is the genetic constitution of an organism, which is coded in the base pairs of DNA. *Phenotype* is the overt manifestation of a particular trait of an organism. Eye color, height, visual acuity, and arm length are all examples of phenotypes. Behavior is also a phenotype. Genes do not directly code for behavior; rather, they code for enzymes, structural proteins, or "control genes" that alter the expression of enzymatic or structural proteins. Alterations in these proteins then can affect behavior.

Genotype is not the only variable that affects phenotype. All nongenetic factors that can influence a phenotype are termed *environmental variables*. These nongenetic factors are widely variable and include nutrition, infectious organisms, trauma, and various complex behavioral and social parameters, such as an overly de-

manding parent, a poor school system, or a stressful job.

In a simplistic fashion, phenotypes can be divided into three groups:

1. *Hereditary*. In this group, all the variation in a trait in the population is due to genetic factors. Examples of such phenotypes would be eye color and blood groups.

2. *Acquired*. These phenotypes are called acquired because genetic factors play no role in their expression. These traits are entirely controlled by environmental variables. Examples include language and hair style.

3. *Genetic-environmental*. The result of both genetic and environmental factors, these phenotypes include traits for which the relative importance of genetic and environmental factors vary considerably.

The concept of *heritability* quantitates the relative importance of genetic and environmental factors for a particular phenotype. "Broad heritability" is the proportion of total variability in a trait in the population that is due to genetic

19

factors. A fully "hereditary" trait would have a heritability of 1, while a fully "acquired" trait would have a heritability of 0.

Behavioral phenotypes of interest can be found in all three of the above categories. However, most of the psychiatric disorders of importance fall into the third group.

This brief overview of behavior genetics is divided into three major discussions. In the first discussion the genetic basis of several animal behaviors is reviewed. The second discussion examines the behavioral effects in humans of several reasonably well understood genetic abnormalities, including the XYY syndrome, phenylketonuria, and Huntington's disease. In the third discussion the genetic basis of several important psychiatric disorders is reviewed.

ANIMAL BEHAVIOR GENETICS

Animal models are useful in behavior genetics because the genetic manipulations possible are much greater in animals than in humans. Therefore an understanding of the role genetic factors play in animal behavior often exceeds that in human behavior. The two animal behaviors examined here are "emotionality" and ethanol intake.

Emotionality in Mice

Emotional behavior in mice is defined as the behavioral response to an open-field apparatus—a brightly lit open area into which the mouse is put for the first time. Its behavior in response to this novel environment is then measured. "Emotional" mice tend to freeze and defecate, whereas "nonemotional" mice spend much more time exploring.

Genetically Related Strains

In animal behavior genetics a number of different, and complementary, methods are available for exploring the genetic basis of a behavior of interest. One of the simplest methods, and one that has direct parallels in human behavior genetics, is the examination of the behavior in genetically related mice. Not surprisingly, the behavior of parents and offspring and siblings in the open-field apparatus correlates positively. This result is consistent with genetic effects on open-field behavior. However, since relatives share both genes and environment, such results do not equivocally demonstrate that genetic factors are operative.

Inbred Strains

Another way to examine the influence genetic factors have on behavior in animals is to use inbred strains. These strains are the product of intensive inbreeding over at least 20 generations, which produces individuals in the strain that are all genetically identical. Much work has been done in open-field behavior in two mouse strains: BALB and C57BL. Activity in the open-field apparatus indicative of low emotionality is over five times greater in the C57BL strain than in the BALB strain. This suggests that genetic factors are important in the control of emotionality in mice. However, it is possible that the difference in emotionality in the mice is not due to genetic effects but to differences in the intrauterine or postnatal experience of the two mouse strains.

Cross-Fostering

The best method for examining the possible importance of the postnatal environment is a cross-fostering study. This approach, which has direct parallels in human adoption studies, separates the influences of genetic and postnatal environment by taking the offspring of one biological set of parents and having them reared by another "adoptive" set of parents. If differences in rearing are important in producing emotionality in mice, a C57BL mouse taken at birth from its parents and reared by a BALB mother should be very emotional (have low ambulation in the open field). On the other hand, if rearing differences are not important in the production of emotionality in mice, a C57BL mouse reared by BALB parents should have the same low emotionality seen in a C57BL mouse reared by its own parents. When this study was done, it was found that the emotionality of the C57BL mouse reared by BALB parents was slightly greater than that found for a C57BL mouse reared by its natural parents, but much less than that of a BALB mouse reared by its natural parents. Rearing environment played some small role in the production of levels of emotionality, but genetic factors were much more important.

Paternal Half-Siblings

Cross-fostering does not rule out the unlikely possibility that intrauterine effects may be important in the production of emotionality in mice. One way to examine this is to look at paternal half-siblings, that is, mice sired by the same male mated to different females. Since the male does not contribute to the intrauterine environment, similarity between paternal half-sibling must be due to genetic factors. This approach can be used also in human behavior genetics.

Ovarian Transplants

Ovarian transplantation can be used only in animals. By various techniques, one can prevent tissue rejection and transplant ovaries from one female mouse to another. Therefore it is possible to have a fertilized egg from one mother grow in the uterus of another. In a complex experiment utilizing this approach, prenatal environment was shown to have no significant effect on emotionality in mice.

Selection Studies

The last method to be examined for exploring the role of genetic factors in behavior in animals is that of the selection study. In this approach the experimenter acts like natural selection in evolution by selecting animals to produce the next generation that possess the behavioral trait of interest. Thousands of years before the formal science of genetics began, animal and plant breeders were selecting species for characteristics of interest. Probably the best-known example of behavioral differences resulting from artificial selection is that of breeds of dogs. The friendliness of cocker spaniels, the "high-strung" disposition of fox terriers, and the aggressiveness of German shepherds are all the result of artificial selection, albeit not conducted by a trained behavior geneticist.

In the laboratory, bidirectional selection is usually the best methodological approach for determining the degree of genetic control over a trait of interest. Bidirectional selection in emotionality means that in the first generation one group is selected to breed because of low emotionality and the other group is selected because of high emotionality. From the offspring of these two groups, two lines are selected, usually for at least 10 generations. These "high" and "low" lines are then compared on the behavioral trait of interest.

Possessing such selected lines also has an additional advantage. These lines become excellent tools for exploring the neurobiological substrate of the behavioral trait in question. Unlike inbred lines, which, although they may differ in the behavior of interest, also differ in lots of other extraneous ways, lines produced from selection experiments essentially only differ for the trait in question. Therefore, neurobiological differences between them can help uncover the biological substrate of the behavior.

All these different methods show that genetic factors play an important role in the control of emotionality in mice. Although behaviorally the mouse is a much simpler species than humans, these results nonetheless suggest that genetic factors can be important in the control of complex behavioral traits such as emotionality.

Alcohol Tolerance and Intake in Mice

Although the relevance of emotionality in mice to human psychiatric disorders can be questioned, it is nonetheless a useful model for understanding some of the principles of behavior genetics. A behavior of more direct relevance to human psychopathology is ethanol (alcohol) tolerance and intake in mice. This behavior belongs to the discipline of psychopharmacogenetics, the study of the role of genetic variation in controlling the response to drugs that alter behavior.

Human individuals and ethnic groups differ considerably in their ethanol intake. Some individuals report that they drink little because ethanol produces an unpleasant subjective feeling. How much are differences in alcohol intake due to genetic variation? Although this is difficult to answer in humans, a great deal is known about the genetics of alcohol preference in mice. Differences in inbred strains have been found to be large. When mice are given two bottles, one with 10 percent ethanol (about the concentration found in wine) and the other with water, the percentage of total liquid consumed from the ethanol bottle ranges from 9 percent (DBA strain) to 76 percent (C57BL strain). Because of the interest in these mice strains as a model for human alcohol-related problems, much work has been done on examining the effect of different environments on the ethanol intake in different strains. For example, forcing the DBA strain to consume ethanol (by removing all other sources of liquid) for a period of time does not increase ethanol intake when the animals are given a choice. Thus, this strain does not "learn to like" ethanol. Most likely, genes not only partially control the initial response to ethanol but also the ability to learn to like it.

The effect of social environment on ethanol intake has also been examined in inbred mice strains. (In human terms, this might be seen as the effect of "hanging out with the wrong crowd.") When the low-ethanol-consuming DBA mice are housed after weaning with the high-consuming C57BL/6 mice, the ethanol intake of the DBA mice increases, although it still remains much lower than that of the C57BL/6 mice. Conversely, living with the "temperate" DBA mice constrains the ethanol intake of C57BL/6 mice, although they still drink much more ethanol than the DBA mice. The effect of social environment can interact with genetic factors to alter ethanol consumption.

Selection studies have also been used to further the understanding of the role genetic factors play in alcohol consumption in mice. These investigators measured ethanol preference in the following manner. They measured the water intake of mice and deprived them of water for 24 hours. The animals were then given only 10 percent ethanol to drink. The ratio of the amount of ethanol solution they drank to their average daily water intake was termed their ethanol acceptance index. At the start of the selection study the parent strain of mice had an acceptance index of about 0.8. After 14 generations of selection the line selected for low ethanol acceptance had a mean index of about 0.3. The line selected for high ethanol acceptance had a mean index of about 1.1. Even by the tenth generation the lowest ethanol acceptance index found in the "high" line was higher than the highest ethanol acceptance index in the "low" line. As with emotionality, this selection study provides powerful evidence for the importance of genetic factors in control of ethanol preference in mice.

Attempts have been made to determine the exact mode of the genetic transmission of ethanol preference. No large single-gene effect has been found, which suggests that preference for ethanol is controlled by multiple genetic loci, each of which has a small additive effect. Such a mode of transmission is called polygenic. Most behavioral traits of interest in animals, including learning ability, appear to be under polygenic control. The heritability of ethanol preference has in different strains and experimental paradigms been estimated to be between 0.40 and 0.70. A large proportion of the difference between strains of mice in ethanol preference is due to genetic factors.

Gene-Environment Interaction

It is commonly assumed that the interaction of genes and environment will be additive; that is, if strain A is better at a particular task than strain B in environment X, then A will also be better than B in environment Y. This is not always the case. The clearest demonstration of this is found in the mating behavior of different

strains of fruit flies. Some strains mate well at low temperatures, and others at high temperatures. Therefore, although mating in fruit flies is under strong genetic control, different environmental temperatures produce different performances in different strains.

A gene-environment interaction was demonstrated in mice by examining the effect of early rearing environment on learning speed in mice. Mice were housed either in the typical mouse cage or in a large cage with a more complex environment for them to explore and play in. Different strains responded in different ways to the enriched environment. For example, learning speeds in BALB and C57BL mice were similar when they were reared in the standard environment. When both strains were reared in the enriched environment, however, the C57BL mouse learned substantially faster than the BALB mouse did. In other words, the enriched environment improved the performance of the C57BL mouse much more than it did the BALB mouse. Thus, environments can affect different genotypes in different ways. The interaction of genes and environment, especially when one moves from the laboratory to the real world, can become quite complex. It is clear that for a number of behavioral traits of interest, important gene-environment interactions occur.

Neurochemical Genetics

Differences in behavior due to genes must reside in biological differences in the animal, usually in the brain. Increasing interest has focused on differences in brain function that are controlled by genes. As an example, genetic differences will be examined in one of the more important neurochemical systems, that of the neurotransmitter dopamine. Abnormalities of the brain dopamine system have been implicated in a number of human psychiatric disorders known to have a genetic basis, especially schizophrenia.

Levels of dopamine in the brain have been shown to differ in different mouse strains by as much as 30 percent. The rate of turnover of dopamine in the brain differs by as much as 100 percent between different strains. Histological studies have shown that strains differ in the actual number of dopamine neurons in the brain. Receptor proteins for a number of different neurotransmitters have now been identified and can be measured. As measured in the striatum, part of the basal ganglia, different mouse strains had substantial differences in the number of these receptors—the highest strain having over 50 percent more receptors than the lowest strain.

A number of drugs clinically used in humans have profound effects on the brain dopamine system. Not surprisingly, substantial differences in the behavioral and neurochemical response to these drugs have been found in different mice strains. Antipsychotic drugs, or neuroleptics, probably work in large part by blocking brain dopamine receptors. The acute behavioral responses to these drugs in different mouse strains differ considerably. Long-term administration of these antipsychotic drugs causes a "supersensitivity" of the dopamine receptors in the mouse brain that is probably related to tardive dyskinesia, a long-term side effect in humans that is frequently caused by these drugs. The ability of these antipsychotic drugs to produce this supersensitivity of brain dopamine receptors differs considerably in different mouse strains. Genetic differences have consistently been found in neurochemical systems. Although these genetically coded differences in brain function are far from being entirely understood, they probably underlie the genetic differences in behavior under discussion. For the human dopaminergic system, see Chapter 8: Neurophysiological and Neurochemical Basis of Behavior.

Research in human neurochemical genetics is just beginning. As outlined in the third discussion of this chapter, genetic factors are clearly important in the etiology of human psychiatric illness. However, until recently, little was known as to how the predisposition to psychiatric illness might be genetically transmitted. Animal studies have shown that neurotransmitter systems may be etiologically involved in psychiatric illness. Therefore it is logical to suspect that the genetic susceptibility to psychiatric illness in humans is expressed by abnormalities in neurotransmitter function. If these genetically transmitted neurotransmitter abnormalities in humans were possible to identify, important clinical implications would follow. For example, the glucose-tolerance test is used to detect someone who is genetically related to a diabetic and who may be at increased risk for developing diabetes. In a parallel fashion, it might be possible to detect individuals at high risk for psychiatric illness by testing certain parameters of neurotransmitter function. Then measures could be taken to help prevent illness in those identified to be at high risk. Furthermore, differences in the therapeutic response to psychopharmacological drugs in humans probably have as their genetic basis differences in neurotransmitter systems. Recent studies of drug response

in schizophrenic patients have suggested that this may indeed be so. As we learn more about these differences, it might be possible to tailor the specific form of pharmacological treatment to the genetic makeup of the individual's neurotransmitter systems.

EFFECTS OF WELL-UNDERSTOOD HUMAN GENETIC ABNORMALITIES

This section examines the behavioral effects of some well-characterized genetic abnormalities in humans (Table 3–1). One example is chosen from each of the three main kinds of genetic abnormalities: chromosomal anomalies, single-locus recessive traits, and single-locus dominant traits.

XYY Syndrome

The best characterized human chromosomal anomaly that affects behavior is Down's syndrome, which in most cases is due to nondisjunction during meiosis, resulting in three copies of chromosome number 21. Down's syndrome produces a variety of physical abnormalities and various degrees of mental retardation from relatively mild to quite severe.

Just as nondisjunction during meiosis can occur for autosomes, it can also occur for the sex chromosomes. However, strong selection must exist against sperm or zygotes with two Y chro-

TABLE 3–1. Chromosome Assignment of Human Neurological Disorders

1. Charcot–Marie–Tooth disease (one form)
   Gaucher's disease (β glucosidase)
3. Generalized gangliosidosis
4. Huntington's disease
5. Sandhoffs disease (hexosaminidase B)
6. Spinocerebellar ataxia (one form)
11. Acute intermittent porphyria
12. Phenylketonuria
13. Retinoblastoma
    Wilson's disease
15. Prader–Willi syndrome
    Tay–Sachs disease (hexosaminidase A)
17. Glycogenosis type II
19. Myotonic dystrophy
    Mannosidosis
21. Homocystinuria (cystathionine synthase)
22. Hurler syndrome (α L-iduronidase)
    Metachromatic leucodystrophy

From Harper, P.S.: The genetic approach to neurological disorders, in *Diseases of the Nervous System*, A.K. Asbury, G.M. McKhann, and W.I. McDonald (eds.). Philadelphia, Saunders, 1986.

mosomes, because among normal males only about 0.13 percent possess two Y chromosomes. Compared to other males, XYY individuals are taller, often have severe acne, and generally have low intelligence—although rarely in the retarded range.

In 1965, at a hospital for the criminally insane, 197 inmates were karyotyped; 7 (3.6 percent) were XYY. This incidence is 25 times greater than that expected in the normal population. Since this original study, numerous investigators have examined this finding. From a total of 18 studies, 103 of 5,342 (1.9 percent) institutionalized male prisoners had an extra Y chromosome. Thus, it has been fairly well demonstrated that XYY males are overrepresented in criminal or mental-penal institutions. What is the probable cause of this phenomenon?

First, it should be stated that less than 1 percent of XYY males are institutionalized, and most lead outwardly normal lives. The early popular theory was that XYY individuals were "supermales" and therefore had an extra dose of aggression. This view was supported by studies in animals that showed a close link between male sex hormones and aggressive behavior. However, levels of testosterone are not greater in XYY than in normal males. A second theory held that their greater height in some way led to their more frequent involvement in crime.

A third, quite different reason for the overrepresentation of XYY individuals in prison has been suggested. Investigators karyotyped the tallest 16 percent of all living males in Denmark born between 1944 and 1947. Intellectual function was measured by scores on the army selection test. Criminal records were examined for all karyotyped individuals. Of the 12 cases of XYY males found, five (42 percent) had been incarcerated, compared to 9 percent of the normal XY men. Thus they found that XYY males were at substantially increased risk for being imprisoned. However, the nature of the crimes they committed were, on the average, no more violent than crimes committed by normal XY males. In fact, only one XYY male was convicted of a violent crime against another person; the rest had committed rather minor offenses. Of interest, of the five incarcerated XYY males, four had scores on the army selection test of well below average intelligence, and the fifth was somewhat below average. In the normal XY males, those with criminal records also had substantially lower average intelligence as measured by the selection test. Increased height was not involved in the increased likelihood for the

XYY males to be imprisoned. Thus, neither increased aggression nor increased height, but perhaps decreased intelligence, led to the increased rate of imprisonment in the XYY males.

Phenylketonuria

Phenylketonuria (PKU) is due to a classically recessive single locus that codes for an abnormal form of the enzyme phenylalanine hydroxylase. This enzyme normally converts phenylalanine to tyrosine. When this enzyme is deficient, levels of phenylalanine and of some of its breakdown products, such as phenylpyruvic acid, accumulate to toxic levels in the body. This toxicity affects the developing nervous system and, when untreated, produces moderate-to-severe mental retardation. As expected from a recessive trait, affected individuals rarely have an affected parent; on the average, 25 percent of their siblings are affected.

Knowledge of the cause of PKU led to a possible treatment. If the intake of phenylalanine is kept low by a special diet, these toxic substances do not accumulate, and development can occur in a nearly normal fashion. When treated at an early age, individuals with PKU develop an intelligence that is, on the average, little different from that of the rest of the population. PKU is a good example of the fallacy of the commonly held belief that once a disorder is understood to be genetic, there is no available treatment.

PKU formerly was considered a completely recessive trait, meaning that individuals who are heterozygous for the gene are indistinguishable from the rest of the population. It has long been known that an extra high intake of phenylalanine caused these heterozygotes to have a higher phenylalanine level than normal. This phenomenon has been termed an endophenotype, that is, a phenotypic manifestation detectable only by special metabolic probes. However, recent investigations have shown that heterozygotes for the PKU gene, on the average, have lower IQs than individuals homozygous for the normal phenylalanine hydroxylase enzyme. So, a trait initially thought to be purely recessive is now, on closer examination, shown to have subtle but demonstrable abnormalities in the heterozygote. To conclude, PKU is a well-understood single-locus abnormality resulting in a deficient enzyme that, in the homozygous state, probably has a small but significant deleterious effect on intellectual functioning.

Huntington's Disease

Huntington's disease is an example of a well-characterized disorder often having profound behavioral effects in humans that is due to a single autosomal dominant gene. This disorder is named after the New York physician George Huntington, who described it in 1872. Huntington's disease is caused by a gene that is fully penetrant and age dependent. This means that the likelihood that the disease will become manifest in the individual who carries the gene is 100 percent, provided he or she does not die of some other cause first. Since Huntington's is usually a disease of the middle adult years, most individuals carrying the gene *will* live to get this disease. Furthermore, the disease typically does not emerge until after the individual has already reproduced and thus has passed on the disease gene to 50 percent of his or her offspring. Thus, except for those cases in which the gene-carrying parent has died early, before the emergence of disease, individuals with this disorder will have had an affected parent. Although apparent "sporadic" cases (new mutations) are possible, they are extremely rare and, in most cases, are due to incorrect assignment of paternity.

The most prominent manifestation of this disorder is abnormal involuntary movements. However, psychiatric symptoms are also often prominent. The average age of onset of the neurological symptoms is 45, with nearly all cases starting between the ages of 25 and 55. In most cases, "minor" psychiatric symptoms such as nervousness, irritability, or depression precede the onset of the movement disorder by several years. Not infrequently, the initial presentation of this disorder can be as a psychotic disorder, usually resembling paranoid schizophrenia. Cases can present without neurological symptoms, with typical paranoid delusions and hallucinations. Without a family history, it would be easy for a clinician to misdiagnose such cases as schizophrenia. However, other cases present with virtually no psychiatric symptoms.

The neuropathology of Huntington's disease has been well described. The brain is grossly atrophied, with marked neuronal cell loss in the cortex and basal ganglia. Recent evidence suggests that the GABA neurotransmitter system may be most affected in Huntington's disease. However, unlike PKU, the abnormal enzyme underlying the disorder has not yet been characterized.

The course of the illness is currently irreversible, leading to increasing neurological abnormality and dementia, usually ending in death 10 to 15 years after onset. Treatment with major neuroleptic drugs, such as haloperidol, produces some decrease in abnormal movements but does not alter the underlying course of the illness.

One of the most exciting recent advances in clinical genetics has been the identification of the region where the locus (that is, the specific location of a gene on a chromosome) for a Huntington's disease gene lies. Investigators conducting a "genetic linkage study" located this gene on the end of the short arm of chromosome 4. Essentially, this method assesses the statistical probability that a particular sequence of DNA, or a DNA product from a known location, is "segregating," or assorting, with family members who have a disease of interest, that is, the phenotype of the disease gene. Although the general methodology of linkage studies is not new, the range of possible applications of this method has been enormously expanded, so that now a large variety of the diseases, including psychiatric disorders, caused by a single or a small number of genes can be investigated for linkage to almost any locus in the human genome. This increased utility has largely come about because of the many technological gains made in the late 1970s and early 1980s in molecular and quantitative genetics. More recent progress is further strengthening the potential power of these investigative techniques.

It is important to remember that identifying linkage identifies a small region where the disease gene lies; it does not identify the gene itself. In the case of Huntington's disease, for example, although linkage was first determined in 1983 and the location of the gene has been even more finely resolved since that time, the gene itself has yet to be identified.

GENETICS OF HUMAN PSYCHIATRIC DISORDERS

This discussion reviews the contribution of genetic factors to four important human psychiatric disorders: alcoholism, schizophrenia, affective illness (mood disorder), and Alzheimer's disease. In these and other important psychiatric disorders, unlike PKU and Huntington's disease, the exact form of the genetic contribution has been difficult to ascertain, although there is strong evidence that genetic factors play some role in the etiology of these conditions.

Alcoholism

Alcoholism is defined as a pattern of heavy ethanol consumption accompanied by social, occupational, or physical dysfunction attributable to the ethanol intake. The frequency of alcoholism in the general population varies in different countries. Reasonable figures for the United States and most Western European countries are 3 to 5 percent in men and 0.4 to 0.8 percent in women.

Both conceptually and historically, the starting point in human behavior genetics has been family studies, that is, the examination of the distribution of the trait of interest in natural families. Family studies of alcoholism have consistently found that the close relatives of alcoholics have a higher incidence of alcoholism than does the general population. Most studies have found that over 25 percent of the fathers and brothers and 3 to 10 percent of the mothers and sisters of alcoholics are themselves alcoholics. However, as noted, close relatives share both genetic and environmental factors. Although the familial clustering of alcoholism in the relatives of alcoholics is consistent with the importance of genetic factors, it could also be due to nongenetic familial factors, so-called cultural transmission. Two major investigative methods in human behavior genetics can begin to untangle the relative importance of genetic and nongenetic familial factors in the transmission of disorders: twin studies and adoption studies.

Twin Studies

Twin studies are based on the fact that in humans there are two kinds of twins. Dizygotic twins (DZ) are the result of two separate eggs being fertilized by two separate sperm. Although DZ twins share the same uterus, they are no more genetically similar than are any two siblings. Monozygotic twins (MZ) result from a single egg fertilized by a single sperm that, early in development, split into two separate embryos. MZ twins are genetically identical. DZ twins can be of the same sex or different sexes; MZ twins are always of the same sex. Most studies have compared concordance of disorders of interest in MZ and same-sex (ss) DZ twins. A twin pair is called concordant when both members suffer from the same disorder in question.

In general, MZ and ss-DZ twins share about the same degree of their environment. It is true that, on average, MZ twins are more often treated in a similar fashion by parents, friends, and teachers than are DZ twins. This difference

has led many to suggest that a comparison of concordance in MZ and ss-DZ twins is not a valid technique for separating genetic from nongenetic familial factors, because MZ twins genetically are more similar *and* have more similar environments than ss-DZ twins. However, although it is possible that MZ twins are more similar because they are treated in a more similar fashion by their environment, it is also possible that they are treated in a more similar fashion because they *are* more similar. Several approaches have been used to attempt to answer this question, and all have suggested that the latter explanation is more likely correct. The greater behavioral similarity of MZ compared to DZ twins is the cause of, and not the result of, the greater environmental similarity in the MZ twins. Therefore, determination of differences in concordance between MZ twins and ss-DZ twins probably is a fairly accurate way of determining the importance of genetic factors in humans.

Several twin studies of alcoholism in humans have been conducted. In a Swedish study of 174 male twin pairs in which at least one member had been shown to have an alcohol problem, concordance for alcoholism was 58 percent in MZ and 28 percent in ss-DZ pairs. Preliminary data from the large U.S. National Academy of Sciences twin registry show a concordance for alcoholism of 26.3 percent in MZ and 11.9 percent in ss-DZ twins. Although the overall rate for concordance is different in the two studies, in both cases the concordance for alcoholism in MZ twins was about twice that found in ss-DZ twins. A number of other twin studies, most of them conducted in Scandinavia, have generally found that MZ twins are more likely than DZ twins to share similar patterns of alcohol use and related drinking behaviors. These results suggest that genetic factors are important in alcoholism in humans.

Adoption Studies

Another major method in human genetic studies to separate genetic from nongenetic familial factors is adoption studies, which are similar to the cross-fostering studies used in animal behavior genetics. Adoption in human societies is a "natural experiment" that the behavior geneticist can utilize. If an adopted child has been separated early in life from his or her biological parents, this child then has received his or her genetic endowment from one set of parents but his or her rearing from another set of parents. If genetic factors are important for a particular behavioral trait, an adoptive child should resemble his or her biological parents and not adoptive parents. However, if nongenetic familial factors, such as rearing habit or family environment, are important, an adoptive child should resemble his or her adoptive parents and not biological parents. Adoption studies also allow for an examination of the question of gene-environment interaction. As discussed above, gene-environment interaction occurs when the effect of an environment is different for different genetic constitutions.

One large adoption study of alcoholism was carried out in Sweden. Of 89 male adoptees whose biological fathers were alcoholic and 42 male adoptees whose biological mothers were alcoholic, 36 percent became alcoholic as adults, compared to about 14 percent of a large number of male adoptees whose biological parents had no history of alcohol abuse. When a subset of these control adoptees was carefully matched to the adoptees with alcoholic biological parents on a variety of parameters, such as age at adoption and socioeconomic level of adoptive parents, the difference in the frequency of alcoholism in the two groups was just as large.

Although family, twin, and adoption studies have all provided evidence to support the importance of genetic factors in the etiology of alcoholism in humans, little is known about the exact genetic mechanisms that may be at work. A variety of mechanisms have been proposed, including polygenic, sex-linked recessive, and autosomal single-locus with incomplete penetrance. One recent theory suggests there may be two distinct types of alcoholism, with differing patterns of inheritance. However, it is not possible, given the current state of knowledge in this area, to intelligently choose among these hypotheses. For further discussion of alcoholism, see Chapter 24: Drug and Alcohol Dependency.

Schizophrenia

No psychiatric illness has been the focus of so many genetic investigations as schizophrenia. This is understandable, because schizophrenia is both a common and severe psychiatric disorder. The lifetime risk for schizophrenia in the general population in most studies varies between 0.5 and 1.5 percent (Table 3–2). An average figure of 1 percent is usually accepted as fairly accurate. As with alcoholism, the earliest genetic studies of schizophrenia were family studies. A large number of such studies have

TABLE 3–2.   Risk to Relatives of Schizophrenics

Relation	Risk (%)
First-degree relatives	
Parents	4.4
Brothers and sisters	8.5
Neither parent schizophrenic	8.2
One parent schizophrenic	13.8
Fraternal Twin	
Opposite sex	5.6
Same sex	12.0
Identical twin	57.7
Children	12.3
Both parents schizophrenic	36.6
Second-degree relatives	
Uncles and aunts	2.0
Nephews and nieces	2.2
Grandchildren	2.8
Half siblings	3.2
General population	0.8

From Tsuang, M.T., Loyd, D.W.: Schizophrenia in the Medical Basis of Psychiatry, G. Winokur and P. Clayton (eds.). Philadelphia, Saunders, 1986. Adapted from Tsuang M.T., Vandermey R.: Genes and the Mind: Inheritance of Mental Illness. Oxford, Oxford University Press, 1980.

been done. On average, the frequency of schizophrenia in the siblings and children of a schizophrenic is 8 to 12 percent, or about 10 times that found in the normal population. However, in the parents of schizophrenics the rate of schizophrenia has been consistently found to be lower, usually around 5 percent. This initially seems puzzling, since parents, siblings, and children are all first-degree relatives, sharing 50 percent of genes on the average. This discrepancy is now fairly well understood and seems to stem from the fact that the parents of schizophrenics, unlike the siblings and children, have been selected for a certain degree of psychological health in that they have successfully had offspring. Up until the advent of modern psychopharmacological treatment, the overall fertility of schizophrenics was less than half that of the normal population. Therefore, only the healthier group of individuals with a genetic propensity to schizophrenia left offspring.

Although early investigators took this strong tendency for schizophrenia to run in families as evidence for genetic transmission, others favoring a psychoanalytic or family-dynamic viewpoint used the same data to support the hypothesis that schizophrenia was due to psychodynamic abnormalities resulting from certain forms of upbringing.

Twin Studies

Eleven major twin studies of schizophrenia have been conducted. All have consistently found that the concordance for schizophrenia in MZ twins was substantially higher than that found in ss-DZ twins. The concordance for schizophrenia in MZ twins in most studies ranged from 40 to 70 percent, whereas in ss-DZ twins it ranged from 8 to 20 percent. No study has found a concordance of 100 percent in MZ twins. This means that environmental factors must play some role in the etiology of schizophrenia.

Adoption Studies

In the last two decades three major and several minor adoption studies of schizophrenia have been carried out. These adoption studies have consistently found support for the hypothesis that genetic factors are important in the etiology of schizophrenia. Adoption studies have helped to shape current understanding of the genetic causes of schizophrenia in another way as well. In the now classic Danish adoption studies the genetic relationship observed extended beyond the full-blown manifestation of schizophrenia itself to include certain personality characteristics. These characteristics were less severe than those typically found in schizophrenia but nevertheless seemed to bear a close resemblance to the schizophrenic symptoms. Thus the biological relatives of adopted-away schizophrenic patients not only tended to have relatives with hallucinations, delusions, and bizarre behavior characteristics, indicative of schizophrenia, but many of their relatives experienced milder perceptual illusions, held odd beliefs, or displayed inappropriate interpersonal rapport. Thus these studies have led many investigators to hypothesize that the gene or genes related to schizophrenia may cause a larger spectrum of disorders, ranging from rather mild personality symptoms to severe, deteriorating, chronic psychosis.

Alternatively, adoption studies in schizophrenia have provided little evidence in support of family environmental factors as an important cause of this disorder. Hence, taken together, twin and adoption studies suggest that genetic factors explain better than environmental ones why schizophrenia runs in families.

Genetic Mechanism

Although the evidence that genetic factors are operative in schizophrenia is overwhelming, as with alcoholism it has been difficult to characterize the exact genetic mechanisms involved. It was clear from early family studies that schizophrenia does not fit into a simple recessive or dominant mendelian pattern. Two major hypotheses are currently the focus of most interest: (1) single autosomal locus with incomplete penetrance and (2) polygenic. Attempts have been made to distinguish between these two hypotheses by means of segregation analysis, a method that attempts to fit the distribution of cases in pedigrees to that expected on the basis of a particular mode of inheritance. In the absence of conclusive evidence for a particular mode of inheritance, there continues to be lively debate among investigators. Recently, leading research centers have begun to pursue genetic linkage studies for schizophrenia. Although such strategies hold great promise, there is no convincing evidence for such a marker to date. These studies may be hampered in part by the likely heterogeneity in schizophrenia; that is, schizophrenia may have multiple causes, perhaps even multiple genetic causes. See Chapter 28: Biology of Schizophrenia.

Genetic Aids to Psychiatric Diagnosis

In addition to finding the degree and mode of genetic determination of the disorder in question, genetic studies can also be of interest in psychiatry to help clarify the phenomenological boundaries of psychiatric disorders. Since definitive objective laboratory tests to aid in diagnosis in psychiatry do not as yet exist, as they do in most of the rest of medicine, it is not always possible, on the basis of symptoms alone, to clarify the relationship between one syndrome and another. Genetic studies can clarify which psychiatric syndromes are genetically related and which are not. Genetic studies are one of the best ways of constructing a rational system of psychiatric diagnosis.

Affective Illness (Mood Disorder)

Along with schizophrenia, affective illness (mood disorder) is the most important of the "severe" psychiatric disorders. There are two main forms of affective illness: unipolar, which consists of a single or several episodes of depression, and bipolar, which consists of episodes of both depression and mania (often called manic depression). The lifetime risk for unipolar illness in the general population is 6 to 10 percent, and for bipolar illness about 1 percent. Although unipolar illness is two to three times more common in women than in men, bipolar illness occurs about equally in the two sexes. Like most other psychiatric disorders, affective illness tends to cluster in families. The risk for affective illness in the children, siblings, and parents of an individual with affective illness is 15 to 25 percent (Table 3–3). Most studies indicate that the risk is somewhat higher in the relatives of someone with bipolar than with unipolar illness. Some but not all studies find that the subtype of affective illness tends to run in families; that is, that bipolar patients tend to have bipolar relatives, whereas unipolar patients have unipolar relatives. These results have been taken as evidence that unipolar and bipolar affective illness may represent, at least in part, different genetic disorders.

Twin Studies

Nine twin studies of affective illness have been conducted, all with fairly small sample sizes. The concordance for affective disorders was higher in the MZ twins than in the DZ twins in all nine studies. Averaged together, the concordance for bipolar illness in the twin studies was 72 percent in MZ twins and 14 percent in DZ twins; for unipolar illness, it was 40 percent in MZ twins and 11 percent in DZ twins. These results suggest that the familial clustering of affective illness is at least in part due to genetic factors.

Adoption Studies

Three adoption studies of affective illness have been carried out. In Iowa, 3 of 8 (37.5 percent) adopted away offspring of mothers with unipolar or bipolar illness themselves developed affective illness, compared to 4 of 43 (9.3 percent) of adopted offspring of psychiatrically normal mothers. A study in Belgium examined the frequency of affective illness in the biological and adoptive parents of adoptees who developed bipolar illness. They found that 18 of 57 (31.6 percent) of the biological parents of these adoptees had affective illness, compared to 7 of 57 (12.3 percent) of their adoptive parents. By comparison, the frequency of affective illness in the biological and adoptive parents of normal adoptees was respectively 2.3 and 7.1 percent. The most recent adoption study, employing the Danish adoption records, has also found evidence for genetic factors in bipolar disorder and major depression. The findings were strongest when adoptees with more minor depressions were not

TABLE 3–3. Unipolar Depression in First-degree Relatives

Index Cases	No. of Relatives	No. (%) Blindly Interviewed with Unipolar Depression
Unipolar (N = 203)	416	34 (8.2)
Control (N = 160)	541	25 (4.6)

	No. of Deceased Relatives	No. (%) with Unipolar Depression Confirmed by Charts
Unipolar (N = 203)	606	13 (2.1)
Control (N = 160)	322	1 (0.3)

From Winokur, G.: Unipolar depression, in *The Medical Basis of Psychiatry*, G. Winokur and P. Clayton (eds.). Philadelphia, Saunders, 1986.

included. These adoption studies support the conclusion from twin studies that genetic factors are important in the transmission of affective illness in humans.

Genetic Linkage

A number of studies examined possible genetic linkage between affective illness and other genetic markers. Their results tended to be disappointing. A 1987 study of a large Amish pedigree reported linkage for bipolar and related disorders to a locus on chromosome 11. Two years later, however, as additional branches of the same family became newly available for analysis, this finding was reversed; the chromosome 11 locus has now been rejected as a linkage marker for bipolar disorder. In another study, linkage between bipolar disorder and the X chromosome was reported in a series of Israeli families. Unlike the Amish study, independent investigators found quite similar results. Nevertheless, conflicting results have also been observed for this locus.

A number of efforts have been made to determine the mode of transmission of affective illness. The linkage studies noted above suggest a single-locus mode of inheritance. This interpretation has been supported by some studies but not by others. See Chapter 26: Pathogenesis of Mood Disorders; see also under the heading Depression and Altered Immunity in Chapter 5: Stress and Immune Function.

Alzheimer's Disease

Alzheimer's disease is the commonest cause of dementia in humans. Dementia is a syndrome characterized by difficulties in memory, language, and cognition that follows a progressive course. Compared to alcoholism, schizophrenia, and affective illness, little is known about the genetics of Alzheimer's disease. Almost all studies have found a familial aggregation of the disorder.

Alzheimer's disease, like Huntington's disease, is an age-dependent disorder. Unlike Huntington's disease, it occurs late in life rather than in midlife. Many individuals who carry a gene for Alzheimer's never get the disease because they die of other causes first. Using a statistical technique called survival analysis, investigators have assessed the risk that first-degree relatives of Alzheimer's patients face if they live through the full human lifespan. The risk for an Alzheimer's-like dementia was found mostly, though not always, to be about 50 percent by the ninth decade of life. Although these results have been surprisingly consistent across studies, questions nevertheless remain, since the methods employed rely on highly accurate diagnoses of the family members, as well as the initial patient, and on a sample of patients completely unbiased by the presence of a family history. Finally, because few relatives live through the ninth decade, the estimates of risk become more uncertain at these late ages.

Only one small twin study of Alzheimer's disease has taken place, and no adoption studies, so that it is difficult to determine conclusively whether the familial aggregation is in fact due to genetic factors. A recent linkage study of Alzheimer's disease in four families with rare early onset disease reported linkage to markers on chromosome 21. Although evidence in support of this finding has come from independent studies of other families, several other studies have rejected linkage to these loci in still other families. See under the heading Alzheimer's Disease in Chapter 22: Delirium and Dementia.

Because of space limitations, evidence for the importance of genetic factors in other psychiatric disorders has not been discussed. Such evidence exists in varying degrees for sociopathy, anxiety neurosis, hysteria, and phobic neurosis. Important advances remain to be made in understanding the role that genetic factors play in the etiology of human psychiatric disorders.

BIBLIOGRAPHY

Brietner, J.C.S., et al.: Familial aggregation in Alzheimer's disease: Comparison of risk among relatives of early- and late-onset cases, and among male and female relatives in successive generations. Neurology 38:207-212, 1988. A family history study employing elegant statistical methods to explore the heritability of this late-onset disorder.

Cadoret, R.J.: Adoption studies: Historical and methodological critique. Psychiatr. Dev. 4:45-64, 1986. A useful review of the adoption study method as it has been applied to investigations of psychiatric disorders.

Cloninger, C.R., et al.: Genetic heterogeneity and the classification of alcoholism. Advan. Alcohol Substance Abuse 7:3-16, 1988. Discusses the theory based on recent twin and adoption studies that there are two distinct subtypes of alcoholism with distinct clinical features and patterns of inheritance.

Ehrman, L., Parsons, P.A.: Behavior Genetics and Evolution. New York, McGraw-Hill, 1981. A more advanced text, covering a wide range of material, from fruit flies to humans, in the general context of evolutionary theory.

Fieve, R.R., Rosenthal, D., Brill, H. (eds.): Genetic Research in Psychiatry. Baltimore, Johns Hopkins University Press, 1975. A multiauthored work, providing a fairly good summary of the field of psychiatric genetics as of the date of publication.

Fuller, J.L., Thompson, W.R.: Foundations of Behavior Genetics. St. Louis, C.V. Mosby, 1978. Hard cover only. A more thorough treatment of the literature than found in the book by Plomin et al.

Gilliam, T.C., Gusella, J.F., Lehrach, H.: Molecular genetic strategies to investigate Huntington's disease, in Advances in Neurology, vol. 48: Molecular Genetics of Neurological and Neuromuscular Disease, S. DiDonato et al. (eds.). New York, Raven Press, 1988. A brief, somewhat technical, but excellent review of the latest molecular genetic strategies being employed to locate and characterize the gene for Huntington's disease.

Goodwin, D.W.: Genetic factors in the development of alcoholism. Psychiatr. Clin. North Am. 9:427-433, 1986. A good brief review of the major twin and adoption studies conducted in the United States.

Gottesman, I.I., Shields, J.: A critical review of recent adoption, twin, and family studies of schizophrenia: Behavioral genetics perspectives. Schizophrenia Bull. 2:360-398, 1976. Probably the best review of this area of research.

Kendler, K.S.: Overview: A current perspective of twins studies of schizophrenia. Am. J. Psychiatry 140:1413-1425, 1983. Consideration is given to the methodological power and limitations of this method as they apply to this disorder.

Kety, S.S.: Schizophrenic illness in the families of schizophrenic adoptees: Findings from the Danish national sample. Schizophrenia Bull. 14:217-222, 1988. The most recent summary of Kety's famous adoption study of schizophrenia.

Nurnberger, J.L., Gershon, E.S.: Genetics, in Handbook of Affective Disorders, E.S. Paykel (ed.). New York, Guilford Press, 1982. A useful review of the major twin, adoption, and family studies relating to mood disorders.

Pardes, H., et al.: Genetics and psychiatry: Past discoveries, present dilemmas, and future directions. Am. J. Psychiatry 146:435-443, 1989. Discusses the potential power that the new molecular and quantitative genetic techniques offer psychiatry.

Plomin, R.: Behavioral genetic methods. J. Pers. 54:226-261, 1986. A discussion of the utility of some new statistical genetic epidemiological methods, such as genetic model fitting and structural models.

Plomin, R., DeFries, J.C., McClearn, G.E.: Behavioral Genetics: A Primer. San Francisco, Freeman, 1980. Available in paperback. The best general introduction to both animal and human behavior genetics. Clearly written. The emphasis in the section on human behavior genetics is more on psychological traits than psychiatric disorders.

Chapter 4

Higher Cortical Processes

Wilma G. Rosen, Ph.D.

Higher cortical processes, or cognition, involve information processing: the initial selection and reception of the stimulus input, the successive and simultaneous active processing in the peripheral and central nervous systems, and finally the response of the organism. The processes of learning, memory, perception, language, thinking, attention, and so on are aspects of cognition. The examination of higher cortical processes within the framework of brain-behavior relationships attempts to relate psychological processes to the underlying physiological and structural substrates. This chapter discusses the relationship between cerebral asymmetries and functional asymmetries; the relationship between cortical dysfunction and the major forms of apraxia, agnosia, and aphasia; and language disturbances in schizophrenia and Alzheimer's disease.

CEREBRAL ASYMMETRIES, LANGUAGE, AND SPATIAL FUNCTIONS

Initially, information about the functions of specific brain regions and particular psychological processes was obtained from both clinical

observations and systematic studies of brain-damaged persons. As a consequence of increased interest, more sophisticated experimental methodologies, and technological advances during the past 20 years, additional evidence about the complexity of brain-behavior relationships has been obtained from neuroanatomy and psychological processes in normal and brain-damaged adults and children.

It is well established that the left cerebral hemisphere primarily subserves language functions in 95 to 99 percent of right-handers and in 60 to 70 percent of left-handers. Thus, in right-handers, the left hemisphere is said to be *dominant* for language functions; this nearly exclusive processing of language by the left hemisphere is thought to represent a *functional asymmetry*. The right hemisphere appears dominant for analysis of the characteristics of space (location, orientation), although this asymmetry is considerably less exclusive than the language-left hemisphere relationship.

Anatomical Evidence

Anatomical differences between the cerebral hemispheres before birth and in adulthood may

32

reflect functional asymmetry. One structure of potential significance is the planum temporale, because it is part of the classical speech area of Wernicke. The planum temporale extends on the superior surface of the temporal lobe from Heschl's gyrus (primary auditory cortex) to the Sylvian (lateral) fissure. When the length of the planum temporale was measured in 100 adult brains, it was found to be longer in the left hemisphere in 65 percent, longer in the right hemisphere in 11 percent, and equal in both hemispheres in 24 percent. A larger left planum temporale has been noted neonatally as early as 29 to 31 weeks of gestation in fetal brains. When the course of the Sylvian fissure was compared in left and right hemispheres in adult brains, the right lateral fissure angulated upwardly more anteriorly and more pronouncedly than the left lateral fissure in 86 percent of the cases. Thus, the right planum temporale was reduced in length, but the right inferior parietal area posterior to the lateral fissure was larger. These inherent anatomical asymmetries may reflect biological programming of left hemisphere specialization for language and right hemisphere dominance for spatial functions.

Perceptual Laterality in Normals

Perceptual laterality refers to the occurrence of more accurate perception of a particular type of material in one visual field or at one ear than in the other. The two experimental methods used most extensively in investigations of the relationship between perceptual laterality and cerebral dominance are dichotic listening and tachistoscopic viewing.

Dichotic Listening

The dichotic listening procedure involves simultaneous auditory presentation of different material to each ear. The language task used most frequently is dichotic presentation of digit pairs. For example, three pairs of digits, 1-5, 6-8, 9-2, are presented so that simultaneously the 1 is heard with the right ear and the 5 is heard with the left ear, and so on for the remaining pairs. The subject's task is to report as many digits as possible. In the auditory modality, although input at each ear is projected bilaterally in the brain, 65 percent of the pathways project to the hemisphere contralateral to the ear receiving the input. Thus, information received at the right ear is projected primarily to the auditory cortex of the left hemisphere, whereas input to the left ear is received primarily at the right hemisphere. In dichotic listening, the most consistent finding for right-handers is a right-ear advantage (more accurate reporting of material presented to the right ear) for verbal material and a left-ear advantage for nonverbal material, such as musical notes. The explanation of these perceptual asymmetries is that, in the case of language, input to the right ear is processed more efficiently because it travels directly to the left hemisphere for language processing, whereas input to the left ear must cross the corpus callosum for language processing. Conversely, for nonverbal material, information projected from the left ear to the right hemisphere is processed more efficiently than information presented to the right ear, which is transmitted from the left hemisphere via the corpus callosum to the right hemisphere for processing.

Tachistoscopic Viewing

In the tachistoscopic viewing procedure, stimuli are presented in the visual field either to the left or right of central fixation, thus creating a left visual field and a right visual field (Fig. 4–1). Stimuli located in the right visual field fall on the left temporal retina and right nasal retina, which project to the left hemisphere only. Stimuli in the left visual field fall on the right temporal retina and left nasal retina, which project to the right hemisphere only. The most reliable findings in normal right-handers are a more accurate report of verbal material appearing in the right visual field than in the left (right visual superiority) and more accurate recognition in the left visual field (left visual field superiority) for the spatial tasks of localization of dots in space and determination of the angle of orientation of lines.

APRAXIA

Apraxia is a disorder of learned skilled movements not attributable to weakness, sensory loss, abnormal movements, impaired comprehension, inattention, or uncooperativeness. The major types of apraxia include ideomotor apraxia, ideational apraxia, constructional apraxia, and dressing apraxia.

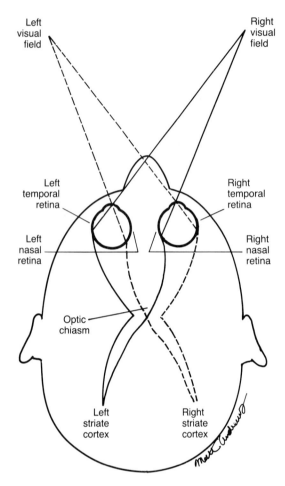

FIGURE 4–1. Projection of stimuli appearing in visual fields to nasal and temporal retinas and primary visual cortex (striate cortex).

Ideomotor Apraxia

The execution of simple, single gestures is disordered in this condition. Although these gestures may be performed automatically in appropriate situations, such as making the sign of the cross in church, the gesture is disturbed when the patient is required to perform it in an arbitrary situation, such as at an examination. Since the disorder is not usually apparent in everyday life, the presence of this type of apraxia only becomes obvious when the patient follows a verbal command or imitates the examiner. The examiner must be certain that a defective performance is not a consequence of impaired comprehension of the command.

Classification of the types of gestures used to demonstrate ideomotor apraxia, with examples of each, are shown in Table 4–1, in the generally accepted order of progressive difficulty for the apraxic patient. For types 1 to 3, the examiner either gives a command (such as "Show me how you wave goodbye" or "Pretend you are holding a hammer and show me how you would hammer a nail") or the patient imitates the examiner. On imitation of types 1 to 3, movements may be partially restored. Type 4 gestures can be done by imitation only.

Ideational Apraxia

In ideational apraxia, the mental representation or "idea" of a complex gesture or act is disturbed, although each of the individual movements is preserved. The patient has difficulty in the *planned* execution of the act and hence is unable to *sequence* the movements correctly. For example, if a patient with ideational apraxia has to light a candle with a match, errors might be attempting to light the wick with an unlit match or striking the wrong side of the matchbook. In the latter error, the individual movement of striking the match is executed correctly, but the planning of the act (where to strike the match) is impaired.

Another task used to demonstrate ideational apraxia is to fold a letter, put it in an envelope, seal the envelope, and stamp it. Patients usually show disorganization about the relationship of the letter to the envelope, sometimes placing an unfolded letter in the flap of the envelope. They may place the stamp on the letter, but the individual movements of licking and attaching the stamp are correct.

TABLE 4–1.   Types of Gestures Used to Demonstrate Ideomotor Apraxia

Gesture Type	Example
1. Expressive with symbolic content	Wave goodbye; blow a kiss
2. Expressive with conventional symbol value	Military salute; sign of the cross
3. Demonstration of object use with object absent	Hammer a nail; brush teeth with a toothbrush
4. Imitation of meaningless gestures	Fingers interlocked as rings; head postures relative to body; hand and limb movements relative to body

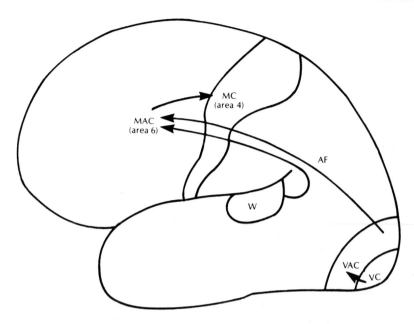

FIGURE 4–2.   Geschwind's schema. Lateral view of the left side of the brain. *AF* = arcuate fasciculus; *MAC* = motor association cortex; *MC* = motor cortex; *VAC* = visual association cortex; *VC* = visual cortex; *W* = Wernicke's area. The arrows indicate major connections of the areas shown. (From Heilman, K.M., Valenstein, E.: Clinical Neuropsychology, ed. 2. New York, Oxford University Press, 1985)

Mechanisms of Ideomotor and Ideational Apraxia

In ideational apraxia, the ability to organize a series of actions with an object (an often performed activity as in the preceding example) is impaired. This contrasts with ideomotor apraxia, where the overall plan is maintained but the individual movements are poorly executed. Ideational apraxia probably represents more severely compromised brain function than ideomotor apraxia. Ideomotor apraxia is frequently observed in the absence of ideational apraxia; however, ideational apraxia usually does not occur without ideomotor apraxia. Furthermore, ideational apraxia is always bilateral (left- and right-handed) and is most often present in conjunction with severe aphasia or dementia.

Ideomotor and ideational apraxias are associated with posterior left hemisphere bilateral lesions. One theory proposed as the mechanism of ideomotor apraxia is the "disconnection theory," which suggests that, in the case of apraxia to verbal command, the language areas are disconnected from the motor areas. Auditory input is projected to Heschl's gyrus and then to the posterior superior portion of the temporal lobe (Wernicke's area in the left hemisphere), an area

thought to subserve language comprehension (Fig. 4–2). The information is then relayed to the premotor cortex (motor association cortex) via the arcuate fasciculus and then finally to the primary motor cortex. Execution of a command with the right hand follows this pathway; with the left hand, the information must be transmitted from the left premotor area across the corpus callosum to the right premotor area. It is suggested that most ideomotor apractic disturbances are a consequence of disruption in the arcuate fasciculus pathway or in the corpus callosum. Although the patient comprehends the command, he or she cannot execute it properly because the language area can no longer relay information to the motor area or the two premotor areas are disconnected.

Constructional Apraxia

A constructional apraxia is an impairment in representation of space manifested as a deficiency in drawing geometric forms or simple objects (graphomotor tasks) or organizing blocks or sticks to create a design or form (manipulatory tasks). In graphomotor tasks, the patient draws by copying models or to verbal command. In manipulatory tasks, the patient constructs a copy of a pattern with blocks of different colors, sticks in particular configurations, or different-shaped blocks organized in three-dimensional configurations.

Constructional apraxia appears primarily in patients with posterior lesions (temporal, parietal, or occipital lobes). With a left parietal lobe lesion, constructional apraxia may be associated with aphasia, ideational, or ideomotor apraxia, and components of the Gerstmann syndrome. The four components of this syndrome are acalculia (impaired mathematical ability), agraphia (impaired writing), right-left disorientation, and finger agnosia (impaired finger identification). The most obvious error made following right parietal lobe lesions is failure to reproduce the left part of the model, which is consistent with the neglect of the side of space contralateral to the lesion. However, neglect does not always accompany right posterior lesions.

Typical errors indicative of a constructional apraxia are simplification of the model, lack of integration of the parts, substantial rotations (for example, the form is rotated 90 degrees from the vertical axis), and "closing in" (placing the construction close to, touching, or overlapping the model).

Dressing Apraxia

In dressing apraxia, the patient has difficulty in orienting and placing clothes properly on his or her own body. The clothes are manipulated incorrectly, so that they may be reversed or handled unsystematically. Even if the patient manages to put the clothes on properly, it requires considerably more effort and time than normal. Dressing apraxia appears with right-hemisphere lesions and is associated with a constructional apraxia when both sides of the body are involved (bilateral) or with neglect of the left half of the body (hemisomatagnosia) when the apraxia is unilateral.

A summary of the types of apraxias and related cortical structural damage is shown in Table 4–2.

AGNOSIA

Agnosia is defined as a failure to recognize perceptually the stimulus, which is not attributable to impaired sensory processing, intellectual functioning, or naming ability. Agnosia is most frequently specific to one modality and oc-

TABLE 4–2. Apraxias and Associated Cortical Structures

Apraxia Type	Cortical Structure
Ideomotor	Posterior left hemisphere or bilateral lesions
Ideational	Posterior left hemisphere or bilateral lesions; diffuse brain damage
Constructional	Posterior left or right lesions; diffuse brain damage
Dressing	Right posterior lesions; diffuse brain damage

TABLE 4–3. Agnosia and Associated Cortical Structures

Agnosia Type	Cortical Structure
Visual object	Left occipital lobe lesion, including subcortical white matter
Color	Left occipital lesion
Prosopagnosia (agnosia for faces)	Bilateral mesial occipitotemporal lesions
Spatial	Bilateral lesions
Auditory	
Word deafness	Superior temporal gyrus lesion
Amusia (music)	Bilateral temporal lobe lesions; unilateral right temporal lobe lesions
Tactile	Unilateral and bilateral lesions

curs most commonly in the visual, auditory, and tactile modalities. A summary of the major types of agnosias and related cortical structural damage is shown in Table 4–3.

Visual Agnosia

A patient with visual agnosia fails to respond appropriately to visually presented material. An appropriate response is elicited when the patient is permitted to handle the object or listen to the sound it makes. It is important to distinguish visual agnosia from a naming difficulty (anomia). If the patient cannot name the object but is able to give a description of it, demonstrate its use, or choose it from a group of objects when the examiner names it, the patient is considered to have an anomia rather than an agnosia.

Visual agnosias for objects and colors are thought to be indicative of an associated language disorder due to left hemisphere lesions. Visual agnosias for faces and spatial information are associated with somatosensory defects due to right hemisphere lesions.

Visual Object Agnosia

The patient sees the object but is unable to appreciate its meaning. In associative visual agnosia, the patient may describe its physical attributes and copy it. In apperceptive agnosia, the patient is totally unable to describe or copy the object. The necessary anatomopathological condition of visual object agnosia is a left occipital lobe lesion with extension into subcortical white matter. Also important are bilateral occipital lesions affecting the angular gyrus and perhaps the corpus callosum. Those areas of the right hemisphere necessary for perception of shape, space, and faces are spared.

Color Agnosia

In color agnosia, color perception is preserved, but there is an impairment in the ability to select all colors of the same hue, select colors on command, name colors, and give the color of specifically colored objects (for example, the sky or a tomato). Impaired color recognition is usually the result of left occipital lobe lesions.

Prosopagnosia (Agnosia for Faces)

The patient is unable to recognize the faces of people well known or newly introduced to him or her. Prosopagnosia is found in cases with bilateral lesions of the central visual system (the mesial occipitotemporal region).

Spatial Agnosia

Spatial agnosias include disorders of spatial perception and loss of topographical memory. Disorders of spatial perception include impaired localization of objects, impaired size perception, and impaired depth perception, and are usually associated with right posterior lesions. Deficient manipulation of spatial information is usually manifested as unilateral spatial neglect or loss of topographical concepts. The latter is apparent when the patient is unable to locate significant geographical locations on an unmarked map. Unilateral neglect and loss of topographical concepts are usually associated with right hemisphere lesions. Loss of topographical memory is a disorder of spatial orientation where the patient is unable to orient himself or herself in space due to an inability to use the cues around

him or her. The majority of cases with this impairment have bilateral lesions.

Auditory Agnosia

Auditory agnosia is an impairment in recognition of auditorially presented nonverbal acoustic stimuli in the presence of adequate hearing. An agnosia for sounds is manifested as an inability to recognize the meaning of nonverbal sounds, and it usually occurs in association with word deafness or amusia. Pure word deafness is characterized by an inability to comprehend and discriminate spoken language, although reading, writing, and speaking are relatively preserved. The lesion associated with this condition is located in the superior temporal gyrus, but does not impinge on Wernicke's area. Agnosia for music (receptive amusia) includes tone deafness, melody deafness, and disorders in the perception of rhythm. Some auditory agnosias may be associated with bilateral temporal lesions or unilateral right-sided lesions.

Tactile Agnosia

Tactile agnosia is apparent in the patient who is unable to recognize objects by tactile means, that is, by handling the objects without seeing them. In some cases, patients may match to sample objects as they palpate them but are unable to recognize what the object actually is. In other cases, the full meaning of the object is lost. Both unilateral and bilateral lesions have produced tactile agnosia.

APHASIA

Aphasia is a loss or impairment of language as a consequence of brain damage. Historically, the work of Paul Broca, Karl Wernicke, and others in the 1860s indicated that language impairments were associated almost exclusively with damage to portions of the left hemisphere. Later clinical investigations revealed that specific patterns of language dysfunction were associated with damage to particular regions within the left hemisphere.

Many classification schemes for types of aphasia have been developed in attempts to define specific syndromes of language disturbances. For the most part, particular clusters of symptoms define each syndrome and are associated with a particular brain region.

Speech output is characterized as either fluent or nonfluent. In nonfluent speech, the flow of speech is interrupted and marked by impairments in initiation, articulatory movements, and grammatical sequences. Nonfluent speech is associated with anterior cortical involvement. Fluent speech is characterized by long sequences of words with various grammatical constructions and intact articulation. Fluent speech usually appears with lesions posterior to the fissure of Rolando.

Paraphasia is the production of unintentional syllables, words, or phrases during speech. Phonemic (literal) paraphasia is the production of syllables in the wrong sequence or distortion of words with additional sounds, for example, "lubali" for "lullaby." Phonemic paraphasia is characteristic of conduction aphasia. Semantic (verbal) paraphasia is the unintentional substitution of one word for another, where that substituted word is related in meaning to the intended word, for example, "chair" for "table." In Wernicke's aphasia, semantic paraphasia predominates, although phonemic paraphasia may also be present. Transcortical sensory aphasia is marked by extended jargon, which is phrases or sentences containing neologisms (unintelligible words grossly changed by phonemic paraphasia).

Auditory comprehension refers to the ability to understand spoken language. In Wernicke's aphasia, the meaning of spoken words is impaired. In transcortical sensory aphasia, auditory comprehension is severely compromised, although the patient can correctly repeat long sentences and may echo the examiner's question instead of answering it.

Anomia, or word-finding difficulty, is impairment in the ability to produce words selectively. Almost all aphasias are characterized by anomia, although the specific nature of the deficit may vary depending upon the type of aphasia.

Repetition refers to the patient's ability to repeat what has been said. Broca's aphasics may be unable to initiate articulatory movements. Wernicke's aphasics may repeat without understanding and with paraphasia. Conduction aphasia is marked by the severity of a repetition difficulty which is disproportionately impaired compared with adequate auditory comprehension and fluent speech.

Clinical Testing

The purposes of the examination for aphasia are (1) to determine the pattern of deficits and spared functions so that changes over time can be detected, (2) to provide a thorough assessment for speech and language therapy, and (3) to identify the aphasic syndrome in order to increase knowledge about brain-behavior relationships. Clinical testing for aphasia includes the following:

- *Conversational speech:* The patient's output is assessed for fluency, paraphasia, grammatical form, word finding, articulation, and auditory comprehension.
- *Repetition:* The patient repeats orally presented single-syllable words, phrases, and complex sentences.
- *Comprehension of spoken language:* The patients is asked questions requiring minimal responses ("yes" or "no") in order to eliminate confounding by expressive speech disturbances.
- *Word finding:* The patient names common and uncommon objects, body parts, colors, and so forth.
- *Reading:* The patient reads simple words, phrases, and complex sentences; the patient's comprehension of the material is assessed.
- *Writing:* The patient writes to dictation simple words, phrases, and complex sentences; the patient is also asked to produce a spontaneous writing sample ("Write about your family or job or anything you want to").

LANGUAGE DISTURBANCES IN SCHIZOPHRENIA

One characteristic of many patients with schizophrenia (but not all) is the presence of a formal thought disorder. Although there is no generally accepted definition of thought disorder, various characteristic language disturbances in the speech of persons with schizophrenia are considered to be indicative of a thought disorder. These disturbances can include disordered communication skills, for example, steady slippage off the topic or a totally irrelevant answer to a question; disordered language in itself (syntactic and semantic rules are violated); and indications of disordered thought, for example, illogicality. Additionally, all persons with a formal thought disorder do not present with identical symptoms, and there is some overlap between language disturbances in schizophrenia and neurological disorders.

The language disturbances in schizophrenia sometimes mimic the symptoms of aphasia. Fluent paraphasic speech in schizophrenia is most frequently confused with aphasia due to severe posterior superior temporal lobe damage. Patients with damage to this region do not have a hemiplegia or focal signs of motor weakness and consequently may be misdiagnosed as having schizophrenia. Characteristics of this sort of speech in schizophrenia include incoherence (also known as "word salad," jargon aphasia, schizophasia, paragrammatism), neologisms, and semantic and phonemic paraphasias. This speech is incomprehensible (varying in frequency of occurrence) because there is a lack of coherence in a portion of the sentence or individual words, for example, "Beauty is in the eye of the beholder of the money of the producer." The neologisms may be completely made up words ("I'm in geet") or fusions of separate words. Examples of semantic paraphasias are "You just *subsided* to that," instead of "surrendered"; "I *demand* you by a look," instead of "command."

A few guidelines are helpful in the differential diagnosis. In an older adult with no history of a psychiatric disorder, the disturbance is probably aphasic, and a neurological examination should ensue. If there is a *sudden onset* of the speech disturbance in an older adult with a psychiatric history, the possibility of structural damage should be investigated. With fluent paraphasic speech, the presence of intact auditory comprehension is characteristic of schizophrenia. Good comprehension will be manifested in the ability to follow commands, attempts to answer the questions appropriately, echoing the examiner's speech, or incorporating the examiner's speech into his or her own speech. See Chapter 28: Biology of Schizophrenia.

LANGUAGE DISTURBANCES IN ALZHEIMER'S DISEASE

Alzheimer's disease is a progressive, degenerative dementia, which affects persons under 65 (presenile onset) and over age 65 (senile onset). Major symptoms of Alzheimer's disease include impaired intellectual functioning, deficits in memory for recent events, disordered visuospatial skills, and language impairments. In the early stages of Alzheimer's disease, the characteristic language disturbance is word-finding difficulty in spontaneous speech, which is manifested on formal neuropsychological testing as decreased verbal fluency. In order to compensate for the word-finding difficulty, the patient may circumlocute (talk around the point) or use a semantically related but off-target word. As the dementia progresses, the word-finding difficulty becomes more pronounced, testing for object naming is impaired, deficits in auditory comprehension become apparent, and phonemic and semantic paraphasias are evident. Some patients show decreased verbal output, echolalia (repetition of the examiner's speech), and eventually mutism. For other patients, speech evolves into jargon, so that there is fluent but often incomprehensible speech which is irrelevant to the current conversation. Impairments in reading aloud and repetition are apparent in the later stages of the dementia. Although the patient with Alzheimer's disease shows language disturbances that can be characterized as aphasic, the symptoms do not typify a singular aphasic syndrome. Instead, the progressive language impairments appear to reflect increasing compromise of left hemisphere functioning as the disease becomes more widespread in the cortex.

For a more detailed discussion of this condition, see under the heading "Alzheimer's Disease" in Chapter 22: Delirium and Dementia.

BIBLIOGRAPHY

Andreasen, N.C.: Thought, language, and communication disorders. Arch. Gen. Psychiatry 36:1315-1321, 1979.

Benson, D.F.: Disorders of verbal expression, in Psychiatric Aspects of Neurologic Disease, D.F. Benson and D. Blumer (eds.). New York, Grune & Stratton, 1975.

De Renzi, E.: Disorders of Space Exploration and Cognition, New York, Wiley, 1982.

Gazzaniga, M.S.: Organization of the human brain, Science 245:947-952, 1989.

Geschwind, N.: Disconnexion syndromes in animals and man. Brain 88:237-294, 585-644, 1965.

Geschwind, N., Levitsky, W.: Human brain: Left-right asymmetries in temporal speech region. Science 161:186-187, 1968.

Goodglass, H., Kaplan, E.: The Assessment of Aphasia and Related Disorders. Philadelphia, Lea and Febiger, 1972.

Hecaen, H., Albert, M.: Human Neuropsychology. New York, Wiley, 1978.

Heilman, K.M., Valenstein, E. (eds.): Clinical Neuropsychology, ed. 2. New York, Oxford University Press, 1985.

Perecman, E. (ed): Integrating Theory and Practice in Clinical Neuropsychology, Hillsdale, N.J., Lawrence Erlbaum Associates, 1989.

Rubens, A.B., Mahowald, N.W., Hutton, J.T.: Asymmetry of the lateral (Sylvian) fissures in man. Neurology 26:620-624, 1976.

Chapter 5

Stress and the Immune System

Marvin Stein, M.D., Steven J. Schleifer, M.D., and Steven E. Keller, Ph.D.

There has been increasing interest in the role that stress plays in the onset, course, and outcome of illness. Abundant evidence has accumulated indicating that stressful life events are related to adverse health effects; however, the mechanisms involved require clarification and elaboration. An extensive literature links stress and the central nervous and endocrine systems with health and illness.

The immune system is another major integrative network involved in biological adaptation; in the past several decades, striking advances have been made in immunology which are relevant to further understanding of stress and health and disease. Considerable evidence demonstrates that a variety of stressful experiences influence the central nervous system and, thereby, may result in suppression or enhancement of immune function. Accordingly, changes in immune function may increase or decrease the risk of onset as well as alter the subsequent course of a wide variety of clinical disorders. This chapter reviews the influence of stress effects on the immune system and some of the psycho-

biological mechanisms that may be involved. A brief review of the concepts of stress and of the immune system provides the background for considering specific aspects of stress effects on immune function.

CONCEPT OF STRESS

The term stress has been used to encompass several different components in a broad consideration of the effects of various stimuli on biological systems. *Stress* is frequently used interchangeably with *stressor* to refer to an event or stimulus to which an organism is exposed. At other times, it refers to the response to a stressor; frequently, stress is defined as encompassing the process of stressor, reaction, and consequence.

The early work of Walter Cannon on the effects of stress on the body demonstrated the importance of the sympathetic-adrenal medullary system in maintaining a steady state in the body, or homeostasis, in response to stressful physical or psychobiological events. Hans Selye reported that the pituitary-adrenal cortical axis also responds to stressful stimuli. Selye subsequently developed a theory based upon a series of studies which postulated that the pituitary-adrenal cortical response was nonspecific and any noxious stimulus or stressor would produce the response.

The emphasis on the nonspecific biological response to stressors has not been substantiated by further investigation. Others have shown that the nature of the stress conditions may determine the specific pattern of response. If physical stressors, for example, are not perceived as noxious or alarming, the physiological response induced may be smaller than the classical *stress response* or may be in the opposite direction. Both public speaking and physical exercise produce increased plasma concentrations of norepinephrine and epinephrine. Norepinephrine, however, is higher than epinephrine during exercise, while epinephrine is considerably higher than norepinephrine during public speaking. Such findings emphasize the necessity of considering the specificity of the stressor and the response and also call into question the exclusive utilization of specific biological responses as the basis for defining stress.

Recently, it has been proposed that three primary elements be delineated in a framework for considering stress, health, and illness: an activator in the environment, the reaction to the activator, and the consequence of the reaction. A subset of activators are sufficiently intense or frequent to be considered as stressors. This conceptualization permits the identification of potential stressors for specific settings or individuals, and the consideration of conditions which make a potential stressor stressful. The suggested framework also provides an approach to mediators which may be involved in the sequence of activator to reaction to consequence.

IMMUNE SYSTEM

Before specific aspects of the effect of stress on the immune system are considered, it is important to have a general understanding of the various components of the immune system and of the methods utilized to measure and evaluate immune function.

The immune system is responsible for the maintenance of the integrity of the organism in relation to foreign substances such as bacteria, viruses, and neoplasia. The immune system can be divided into two major aspects: cell-mediated immunity and humoral immunity. The basic cellular unit of both cell-mediated and humoral immunity is the lymphocyte; however, there are differences in the lymphocytes in each immune component. The T-lymphocyte is primarily involved in cell-mediated immunity, and the B-lymphocyte is primarily involved in humoral immunity. Both T- and B-lymphocytes derive from pluripotent stem cells in the bone marrow, with T-cells maturing in the thymus and B-cells in the bone marrow. Several subsets of T-lymphocytes have been described and include helper T-cells, suppressor T-cells, and cytotoxic T-lymphocytes. In addition to T- and B-lymphocytes, other cell types are involved in immune processes and include monocytes, macrophages, mast cells, and neutrophils.

In the development of an immunological response, antigens—substances recognized as foreign—attach to lymphocytes. Each lymphocyte is committed to recognize a specific target antigen which binds to its cell-surface receptor and, thereby, stimulates the cell. B- and T-lymphocytes initially contain the same genetic information as every other cell in the body. Each commits itself to develop a specific receptor by genetically programmed rearrangement of the DNA sequence which encodes the receptor structure. The end result is an immune system of extensive diversity such that in humans and other animals B- and T-lymphocytes can recognize 10 million different antigenic structures. When an antigen binds to the surface of a specific lymphocyte, a process of cell division and differentiation occurs which results in a permanent increase in the number of circulating lymphocytes with that particular antigen-binding specificity. This clonal expansion results in a more rapid and extensive secondary reaction upon reexposure to the antigen. A subset of the lymphocytes involved in the proliferative response is committed to terminal differentiation as effector cells. The immune system thus provides a wide range of diversity, accompanied by exquisite specificity.

In humoral immunity, sensitized B-lymphocytes, following activation by signals from macrophages and helper T-cells, proliferate and differentiate into plasma cells, which synthesize antigen-specific antibodies. Antibodies are immunoglobulins (Ig) and include five major classes: IgG, IgM, IgA, IgE, and IgD. The immunoglobulins IgM and IgG are produced in response to a wide variety of antigens, with the production of relatively small amounts of IgM soon after antigenic stimulation, followed by large amounts of IgG. IgA is involved in the protection of external surfaces of the body, and is found in mucous secretions of the gut and respiratory tract and in colostrum and milk. IgE is the reaginic antibody that binds to mast cells, when a specific antigen combines with IgE, the mast cells release the mediators of immediate hypersensitivity. These mediators include histamine, kinins, and the slow-reacting substance of anaphylaxis (leukotrienes).

The primary protective function of humoral immunity is against infections by encapsulated bacteria, for example, pneumococci and streptococci. At times, however, the response can be pathological, such as in anaphylaxis, in asthma, and, occasionally, in response to the organism's own tissues, in an autoimmune disorder such as systemic lupus erythematosus.

In contrast to the B-cell, whose role is primarily secretory, the T-cell itself participates in the cell-mediated immune response. T-lymphocytes passing through the tissues are sensitized to a specific antigen peripherally and then progress to a local lymph node, where they enter the free areas of the cortex follicles. The T-cells proliferate and are transformed into larger lymphoblasts. After several days, the T-lymphocytes become immunologically active. Effector T-lymphocytes mediate delayed-type hypersensitivity such as occurs in chemical contact sensitivity or in the tuberculin reaction. T-cells are also involved in cytotoxicity reactions; cytotoxic lymphocytes, also known as killer T-cells, are a subset of effector cells in cell-mediated immunity. They recognize, bind, and lyse target cells bearing the inducing foreign antigen. In addition, T-cells release lymphokines such as macrophage migration inhibitory factor (MIF), chemotactic factors, cytotoxic factors, and interferon that are involved in the destruction of antigen. Cell-mediated immune responses include protection against viral, fungal, and intracellular bacterial infection; transplantation reactions; and immune surveillance against neoplasia.

It is now recognized that the classic division of the immune system into cellular and humoral immunity is oversimplified. The immune system consists of highly fine-tuned and self-regulatory processes with T- to T- and T- to B-lymphocyte interdependence and interactions. Subsets of the T-cell population, helper T-cells and suppressor T-cells, have important regulatory functions that serve to control the initiation and termination of both T- and B-cell effector responses. A shift in the number or function of these cell types may result in either impaired or exaggerated immune responses with consequent pathological effects.

Furthermore, it has been demonstrated that exposure to antigen is not sufficient to stimulate T-cell division. Macrophages or other accessory cells are required for T-cell activation and produce a lymphocyte-activating factor, known as interleukin-1 (IL-1). IL-1 does not directly stimulate T-cell division but induces helper T-cells to produce a T-cell growth factor, interleukin-2 (IL-2), and to express cell-surface receptors for IL-2. The IL-2 lymphokine then stimulates T-cells to proliferate. It appears that regulation of B-cell proliferation and differentiation is similar to that of T-cells. A B-cell growth factor produced by T-cells and IL-1 appears to be required to evoke the division of activated B-cells. Specific differentiation factors are then required to elicit specific antibody production. The immune system thus operates by means of highly specific responses which incorporate an amplifying component involving a complex interplay of nonspecific chemical signals for growth and differentiation. These regulatory functions may have both protective and pathological effects on the organism.

In addition to T- and B-lymphocytes, a subpopulation of lymphocytes that spontaneously recognize and selectively kill some virally infected cells and cancer cells has recently been described. These cells are known as natural killer (NK) cells, since they mediate a cytotoxic reaction without the need for prior sensitization.

Various techniques and assays are available which permit detailed evaluation and investigation of the immune system in relation to brain and behavior. Cells of the immune system can be identified by surface markers with antigenic properties. The unique surface markers for the various cell types can be detected in vitro by specific monoclonal antibodies and the number of specific cells thereby enumerated. Monoclonal antibodies are available to assess the total number of T- and B-lymphocytes, as well as helper T-cells and suppressor T-cells. Cell markers are also available for natural killer cells. The quantitation of cell types provides information about the composition of lymphocyte subpopulations in the peripheral blood but not about lymphocyte function and other aspects of the immune response, including immunoregulatory processes.

A range of functional measures is available which can be employed in the study of stress effects on the immune system. The in vivo measurement of an antibody response to a specific antigen provides evidence of the ability to acquire specific immunity. This procedure involves exposure to a novel antigen and measurement of specific antibody production. As an experimental paradigm in humans, immunization is limited by its invasiveness, and it also cannot be utilized in longitudinal studies, since a second immunization will alter the pattern of antibody response compared with that of the primary immunization. In view of these limitations, many studies investigating the immune system in behavioral states have used in vitro assays of immune function.

Lymphocyte stimulation is an in vitro technique which is commonly used to assess the in vivo function and interaction of lymphocytes participating in the immune response. In the procedure, sensitized lymphocytes involved in the immune response are cultured and activated with specific antigens, or nonsensitized cells are activated with nonspecific stimulants, known as mitogens. A number of plant lectins and other substances have been utilized as mitogens. Phytohemagglutinin (PHA) and concanavalin A (ConA) are predominantly T-cell mitogens, and pokeweed mitogen (PWM) stimulates primarily T-dependent B-lymphocytes.

When lymphocytes are stimulated, there is an increase in DNA synthesis which eventually results in cell division and proliferation. The measurement of DNA synthesis is made by labeling stimulated cultures with a radioactive nucleoside precursor, such as tritiated thymidine, which is incorporated into newly synthesized DNA. The determination of the amount of precursor incorporated provides a measure of DNA synthesis and is employed as the standard measure of lymphocyte responsiveness.

B-cell function may be assessed by the determination in plasma of immunoglobulin secreted by differentiated B-lymphocytes or plasma cells. Each of the Ig classes may be readily assessed in plasma utilizing a simple precipitation reaction. Ig levels provide a global index of B-cell function, but do not provide information at a cellular level or about immunoregulatory mechanisms involved in B-cell function. PWM-induced differentiation of human B-cells in vitro can be employed to assay cellular immunoregulatory mechanisms and, in particular, the functional effects of helper and suppressor T-cells on PWM-activated B-cell differentiation.

In addition to evaluating cellular immunoregulatory mechanisms, it is possible to assess interleukins and their receptors by utilizing lymphocyte stimulation techniques and monoclonal antibodies. The availability of procedures to assess immunoregulatory processes at a cellular and chemical level provides a means to further understand brain and behavior in relation to immune function.

Natural killer cell activity is assayed in vitro by the insertion of ^{51}Cr into specific established tumor cell lines and evaluating the lysis of the tumor cells by the release of the radioisotope following the addition of natural killer cells.

Many of the measures described above are influenced by day-to-day variations, diurnal rhythms, sex, age, and a range of nonimmunological factors, such as medication effects. Special attention and controls for confounding influences must, therefore, be carefully considered in studies of the effects of stress on the immune system. These considerations are noted in the review of the various paradigms described in this chapter.

STRESS AND IMMUNE SYSTEM

A variety of stressors have been found to alter humoral and cell-mediated immunity. Early studies of stress and humoral immunity indicated that avoidance-learning stress decreases the susceptibility of mice to passive anaphylaxis and that the production of specific antibody can be suppressed in a variety of species by distressing environmental stimuli such as noise, light, movement, and housing conditions. Both primary and secondary antibody responses can be suppressed. In contrast, exposure to other stressors such as repeated low-voltage electric shock were found to enhance antibody responses.

More recent studies have tended to support the observation that although acute exposure to a stressor can suppress humoral immune responses, repeated exposure results in an apparent adaptation of the animals to the stressor and, in some cases, in an enhanced immunological response. For example, restraint or crowding, presented in a single session of varying lengths, induced suppression of antibody responses, but after 3 days of repeated presentation of the stimulus, the response returned to prestress levels. Exposure of mice to sound stress for up to 20 days suppressed the response of splenic lymphocytes to the B-cell mitogen lipopolysaccharide (LPS), but more extended exposure resulted in an enhanced response. The complexity of stress effects on humoral immunity are further highlighted by a study which found differential effects of different stressors on antibody responses in rats depending upon the sex of the animal. These studies suggest that the effect of stress on the humoral immune system are related to the nature and intensity of the stimulus, as well as to the biological and social characteristics of the organism.

A series of studies have investigated stress and cell-mediated immune function. Sound stress suppressed the response of murine splenic lymphocytes to ConA stimulation following short-term exposure to the stressor and an enhanced response with extended exposure which paralleled the findings with lipopolysaccharide. Separation experiences in primates have been studied, and decreased T-cell mitogen responses have been found following peer separation for 2 weeks in pigtailed monkeys raised together from early infancy. Mitogen responses returned to baseline within several weeks of reunion. A relationship has been demonstrated between the intensity of an acute stressor and the degree of suppression of T-lymphocyte function in rats. A graded series of stressors applied over 18 hours, including restraint in an apparatus, low-level electric tail shock, and high-level shock, produced a progressively greater suppression of both the number of circulating lymphocytes and of PHA-induced stimulation of peripheral blood lymphocytes.

Stress-induced suppression of lymphocyte stimulation may be related to the psychological state of the animal. PHA and ConA stimulation of lymphocytes was suppressed in rats exposed to inescapable, uncontrollable electric tail shock for 80 minutes, followed by several minutes of tail shock 24 hours later. However, animals receiving the same total amount of shock, by use of yoked paradigm, but able to terminate the stressor, did not have decreased lymphocyte activity compared with nonstressed controls. These findings are consistent with the hypothesis that the ability to cope with a stressor protects against its noxious effects. Although provocative, the studies of the effect of stress on the immune system are somewhat limited in their generalizability because of small sample size, lack of replication, and species-to-species variability. Further research is required to more fully evaluate the effect of stress on the immune system in animals.

Bereavement and Lymphocyte Function

Conjugal bereavement is among the most potentially stressful of commonly occurring life events and has been associated with increased mortality. Investigation has been made into the effect of bereavement on immune measures in a prospective longitudinal study of spouses of women with advanced breast carcinoma. Mitogen-induced lymphocyte stimulation was measured in 15 men before and after the death of their wives. Responses to PHA, ConA, and PWM were significantly lower during the first 2 months of postbereavement compared with prebereavement responses (Fig. 5–1). The number of peripheral blood lymphocytes and the percentage and absolute number of T- and B-cells during the prebereavement period were not significantly different from the postbereavement period. Follow-up during the remainder of the postbereavement year revealed that lymphocyte-stimulation responses had returned to prebereavement levels for most but not all of the subjects. Moreover, prebereavement mitogen responses did not differ from those of age- and sex-matched controls. These findings demonstrate that suppression of mitogen-induced lymphocyte stimulation is a direct consequence of the bereavement event.

It is important to emphasize, however, that these immune alterations associated with bereavement do not adequately explain the epidemiological findings of increased morbidity and mortality following bereavement. It remains to be determined whether stress-induced immune changes such as decreased mitogen responses are related to the onset or course of physical illness following life stress.

The processes linking the experience of bereavement with effects on lymphocyte activity are complex and require further investigation. Changes in nutrition, activity, exercise levels, sleep, and drug use, which are often found in the widowed, could influence lymphocyte function. The subjects, however, did not report major or persistent changes in diet or activity levels or in the use of medication, alcohol, tobacco, or other drugs, and no significant changes in weight were noted. Further study is required to determine if subtle changes on these variables are related to the effects of bereavement on lymphocyte function.

The effects on lymphocyte function of death of a spouse could result from centrally mediated stress effects. Stressful life experiences may be related to changes in central nervous system activity associated with psychological states such as depression. Bereaved subjects have been characteristically described as manifesting depressed mood, and a subgroup of bereaved individuals has been reported to have symptom patterns consistent with the presence of a major depressive disorder. There is some evidence that the severity of depressive symptoms accom-

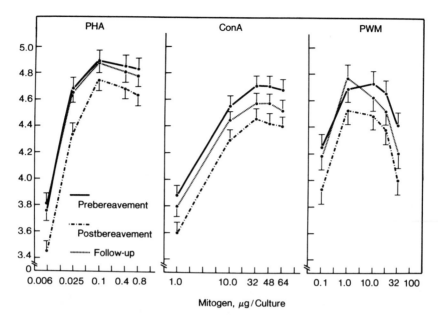

FIGURE 5–1. Mitogen-induced lymphocyte stimulation before and after (1 to 2 months) bereavement. Each point represents group mean ± SEM (n = 15) of each subject's mean log Δ counts per minute (CPM) for each period. (Adapted from Schleifer, S.J., et al. Suppression of lymphocyte stimulation following bereavement. J.A.M.A. 250:375, 1983. Copyright 1983, American Medical Association.)

panying bereavement may be related to decreased mitogen proliferative responses and to decreased NK-cell activity. It also appears that among subgroups of bereaved individuals with a depressive disorder there may be neurobiological alterations such as disturbances in the hypothalamic-pituitary-adrenal (HPA) axis that could influence immune responses, since it is well-known that corticosteroids are immunosuppressive. These findings taken together suggest that both depressive symptoms and major depressive disorders may be related to alterations in measures of the immune system.

Depression and Altered Immunity

In the past decade there has been considerable interest in the investigation of syndromal depressive disorders and the immune system. An association between depression and altered immunity has been suggested by a number of studies but has not been consistently demonstrated. Lymphocyte-stimulation responses to the mitogen PHA have been reported to be lower in hospitalized depressed patients during the acute phase of their illness than following clinical remission. Decreased lymphocyte responses to mitogens and decreased circulating lymphocytes have been found in patients with major depressive disorders. Some studies, however, report no immune changes in patients with major depression.

A series of studies has been conducted to determine if depressive disorders are associated with altered immunity. Significantly lower PHA, ConA, and PWM mitogen responses were found in drug-free hospitalized depressed patients compared with age- and sex-matched controls. These changes were not found in a sample of ambulatory patients with major depressive disorder who did not differ from controls in mitogen response. These observations suggest that some but not all patients with major depressive disorder may show immune changes. Since the depressed patients in whom decreased lymphocyte responses were found were hospitalized, more severely depressed, older, and predominantly male, these factors may be related to immune changes in depressed patients. Studies with nondepressed hospitalized patients suggested that hospitalization itself does not alter immune function.

In a recent study, immune function was measured in a not previously studied sample of 91 drug-free hospitalized and ambulatory patients with major depressive disorder representative of a range of ages, illness severity, and sex. No significant mean differences were found between the depressed patients and age- and sex-matched controls in the number of peripheral blood lymphocytes, T- and B-lymphocytes, or

T4- or T8-cells. Mitogen-induced lymphocyte-stimulation responses to PHA, ConA, or PWM for the depressed patients were similar to those of the matched controls, with no significant mean differences between the depressed and control groups. Natural killer cell activity also did not differ between the depressed and control subjects.

In order to investigate the contribution of age, sex, severity of depression, and hospitalization status to altered immunity in depressed patients and in controls, multiple regression analyses were undertaken. These analyses revealed significant age-related differences between the depressed patients and controls in mitogen responses and in the number of T4-lymphocytes. In contrast to age-related increases in mitogen response and in T4-cells in controls, depressed patients did not show increased lymphocyte responses or T4-cell numbers with advancing age. Severity of depression was associated with suppressed mitogen responses independent of age. Although altered immune system measures do not appear to be a specific biological correlate of a major depressive disorder, there may be subgroups of depressed patients with specific behavioral and biological characteristics who have immune alterations. Further investigation of the possible underlying biological mechanisms is required. An understanding of these mechanisms may allow a more focused evaluation of specific subgroups of depressed patients who may exhibit immune alterations based on the presence or absence of relevant biological abnormalities. Several biological alterations characterize certain patients with major depressive disorder that may be relevant to immune function, for example, disturbances in central nervous system (CNS) neurotransmitter function and abnormalities in the HPA axis. Both neurotransmitters and corticosteroids have potent immunoregulatory effects, and further investigation of these neuroimmune interactions is needed.

CNS AND IMMUNE SYSTEM INTERACTIONS

For many years the immune system was considered an autonomous self-regulatory network of cells and cell products that maintained immunological homeostasis. Recently, findings and techniques derived from the neurosciences and immunology have provided evidence of the following reciprocal interactions between the CNS and immune system:

- The effect of lesions of the hypothalamus and other areas of the brain on immune responses
- The presence on lymphocytes of receptors for hormones and neurotransmitters
- The influence of hormones, neurotransmitters, and peptides on immune function
- Neuroanatomic and neurochemical evidence of direct innervation of lymphoid tissues

A series of observations has suggested that the relationship of the CNS and neuroendocrine system with the immune system is not unidirectional and that immune processes can modulate CNS function and neuroendocrine activity.

Effects of Hypothalamus on Immune System

Some of the earliest reports linking the CNS and immune system investigated the effect of destructive lesions of specific areas of the brain on immune function. Systematic investigation of the relationship between the brain and immune function was initiated in a series of studies concerned with the effects of lesions on lethal anaphylaxis. Anaphylaxis is a humoral immune response related to severe allergic and asthmatic reactions in humans. In experimental models of anaphylaxis, animals are sensitized to an antigen that induces a specific antibody, usually IgE or IgG, which attaches to cells such as mast cells in the lung. On reexposure of the animal to the antigen, an immune reaction between the antigen and tissue-fixed antibody occurs. This reaction releases a variety of chemical mediators from the mast cell that, in guinea pigs and in humans, induce bronchiolar obstruction, resulting in dyspnea, wheezing, asphyxiation, and death.

Following a report that bilateral midbrain lesions in the guinea pig inhibited anaphylactic death, attention was directed primarily to the effect of lesions of the hypothalamus on anaphylaxis. Multiple pathways link limbic and higher cortical areas with the hypothalamus, which is involved in the regulation of endocrine and neurotransmitter systems. Both of these systems participate in the modulation of humoral and cell-mediated immunity.

Lethal anaphylactic shock in the guinea pig and rabbit can be prevented by bilateral focal lesions in the anterior hypothalamus. There is significant protection against lethal anaphylaxis in guinea pigs with electrolytic lesions in the anterior hypothalamus, with use of either picryl chloride or ovalbumin as the sensitizing antigen. Median and posterior hypothalamic lesions have no significant effect on lethal anaphylaxis. The effects of hypothalamic lesions on anaphylaxis could be explained both by antigen-specific and nonspecific changes in the immune system, as well as by changes in tissue factors and target-organ responsivity.

Brain lesions have also been shown to have an effect on cell-mediated immunity. Anterior hypothalamic lesions in the guinea pig suppress the delayed cutaneous hypersensitivity response to picryl chloride and to tuberculin. Median and posterior hypothalamic lesions do not alter the response. Hypothalamic lesions in guinea pigs also alter in vitro lymphocyte function. Anterior hypothalamic lesions suppress in vitro lymphocyte stimulation by the antigen purified derivative (PPD) in sensitized animals and by PHA, demonstrating that the hypothalamus can directly influence lymphocyte function. The effects of brain lesions on cell-mediated immune function in the rat have been shown to be short term. Animals with bilateral anterior hypothalamic lesions have fewer splenic lymphocytes than controls do 4 days after the placement of lesions but do not differ from controls 14 days after the procedure. The response of spleen cells to ConA is also suppressed 4 days after hypothalamic lesioning but not at 7 or 14 days after lesion placement. In contrast, lesions in the amygdaloid complex or hippocampus increase mitogen responses. To explain the immunologic mechanisms by which brain lesions alter immunity, the role of splenic macrophage suppressor function has been studied following the placement of anterior hypothalamic lesions. Although no increase in the number of splenic macrophages occurs following the placement of lesions, macrophages from animals with an anterior hypothalamic lesion have more suppressor activity than those from control rats. It thus appears that anterior hypothalamic lesions may produce quantitative changes in macrophages and, thereby, influence lymphocyte function.

Anterior hypothalamic lesions in rats also decrease splenic NK-cell activity, which returns to normal activity by 14 days following lesion placement. The effect of hypothalamic lesions on NK-cell activity is not related to cytotoxic macrophages, nor is the altered NK-cell function due to macrophage suppression. Different mechanisms therefore appear to be involved in the effect of CNS perturbations on various aspects of the immune system.

Neurotransmitters and Immune System

Considerable experimental evidence supports neurotransmitter involvement in the modulation of immune function. The demonstration of receptors for neurotransmitters on surface membranes of lymphocytes is in keeping with the possibility that neurotransmitters play a major role in the regulation of immunity. It has been shown that pharmacological manipulation of norepinephrine in postganglionic sympathetic nerve fibers innervating lymphoid tissue alter immune function. It has also been demonstrated that serotonin has both enhancing and inhibitory effects on immunity.

Most of the research concerned with neurotransmitter regulation of immune function has involved peripheral or systemic manipulation of lymphoid tissues and has not investigated the effect of central neurotransmitter processes on immune reactivity. Recently, it has been shown that humoral immune responsiveness is impaired by the injection of 6-hydroxydopamine (6-OHDA) into the cisterna magna. Administration of 6-OHDA significantly reduces norepinephrine in the hypothalamus, midbrain, and pons-medulla. The treatment with 6-OHDA decreases the primary antibody response to sheep red blood cells and also impairs the development of immunological memory. If 6-OHDA was administered prior to immunization, it did not have an effect on the antibody response. These findings suggest that norepinephrine may play a role in the modulation of the afferent limb of the immune response.

Direct Noradrenergic Innervation of Lymphoid Tissue

Considerable evidence has accumulated demonstrating direct autonomic innervation of parenchymal lymphoid tissue in the spleen, lymph nodes, thymus, appendix, and bone marrow. Noradrenergic fibers innervate both the vasculature and parenchyma in lymphoid organs. This structural link between the nervous and immune systems provides another possible route for the neuromodulation of the immune system. The effect may be related to catecholamine neurotransmitters' altering blood flow and regulating humoral factors entering lymphoid tissue. Direct interaction with lymphocytes is also possible in view of the availability of noradrenergic and peptide receptors on the cell-surface of lymphocytes and could thus have a direct effect on lymphocyte function. Further in vitro and in vivo investigations of the effects of neurotransmitters on lymphoid tissue are required; however, the demonstration of direct sympathetic innervation of lymphoid tissue further supports the concept of CNS modulation of immunity.

Neuroendocrine and Immune System Interactions

Recently, a series of observations has suggested that the relationship of the CNS and the neuroendocrine system with the immune system is not unidirectional and that immune processes can modulate CNS function and neuroendocrine activity. Rats with a concomitant primary immune response to sheep red blood cells had increased levels of corticosterone and decreased levels of thyroxine with the development of the antibody response. These findings suggest that the primary immune response can influence the neuroendocrine system, perhaps by its effects on the CNS. An increase in the firing rate of neurons in the ventromedial nucleus of the hypothalamus has been found during the course of an immune response in rats, as well as the altered hypothalamic noradrenergic activity concurrent with the immunization process. Alpha interferon (IFN) applied microiontophoretically into the rat brain increases the firing of neurons of the cortex and hippocampus in a dose-related manner, whereas in the ventromedial hypothalamus low doses of interferon tended to suppress firing, and high doses enhanced the firing rate. In contrast, IFN did not alter the activity of thalamic systems. These results suggest the presence of a feedback loop between specific components of the immune response and specific structures in the CNS.

A possible mechanism of immune-neuroendocrine feedback has been the focus of a number of recent studies. Mitogen-stimulated lymphocytes produce a factor that increases glucocorticoid levels by pituitary processes, and it has been suggested that IL-1 stimulates corticosterone in rats following the onset of an immune response. As previously noted, IL-1 is a monokine produced by monocytes and has a role in the regulation of immune, metabolic, and nervous system functions. IL-1 was first described in the 1940s and initially was designated endogenous pyrogen for its role in the production of fever. IL-1 is derived primarily from activated phagocytic cells but is produced by other cells, including other immunocytes and astrocytes and microglia of the CNS. It is the principal activator of lymphocytes and in general increases intracellular metabolism. CNS effects of IL-1 stem from its actions on the hypothalamus and pituitary and include fever production, increased slow-wave sleep, and increases in neuropeptides, for example, endorphins. It has been demonstrated that IL-1 also increases plasma levels of corticosterone and elevates plasma ACTH concentrations. It is not clear, however, whether the site of action of IL-1 is in the hypothalamus with the release of CRF or in the pituitary with the release of ACTH. IL-1 produced by cells of the immune system thus may be mediating between the immune, central nervous, and endocrine systems.

Another area of research has suggested that the immune system may also influence neuroendocrine activity by mechanisms not involving the classic hypothalamic-pituitary axis. It has been reported that lymphocytes can secrete an ACTH-like substance following viral infection. Hypophysectomized mice infected with Newcastle disease virus had increased corticosterone and IFN production. Furthermore, splenic cells from infected animals showed positive immunofluorescence with antibodies to ACTH, suggesting that the lymphocytes were secreting an ACTH-like substance along with the lymphokine IFN. The virus-induced increase in corticosterone, but not in IFN, was blocked by dexamethasone.

It has also been shown recently, with molecular cloning techniques, that mitogen activation of T-helper cells of mice induces the preproenkephalin gene in T cells. The production of a peptide neurotransmitter from activated T cells may provide a means by which T cells may be involved in the modulation of the CNS. Furthermore, the neurohypophyseal peptides, oxytocin and neurophysin, have been identified in human thymus, providing additional support for the notion of integrated neuroendocrine functions and immune processes. These findings, taken together, suggest a regulatory feedback system involving the CNS, the neuroendocrine system, and the immune system.

Conditioning of Immune Processes

An association between the central nervous system and immune processes is further suggested by a series of studies concerned with behavioral conditioning of immune responses. This research is of considerable importance in that it considers a behavioral effect involving higher cortical function. Studies from eastern Europe over the past 50 years based on pavlovian concepts have attempted to condition a variety of immune responses with variable results. More recently several groups of investigators have pursued the investigation of conditioning effects on the immune system and have demonstrated that antibody responses can be suppressed by conditioned stimuli (CS) that had been paired previously with a pharmacological immunosuppressant (US). The paradigm employed used taste-aversion learning, a passive-avoidance paradigm, in which saccharin, the CS, was paired with cyclophosphamide, the US. Three days after the conditioning procedure, which can be accomplished by a single pairing of CS and US, the animals were immunized with sheep red blood cells (SRBC) and then exposed to the CS, US, or placebo. Six days later, hemagglutinating antibodies to SRBC were measured and found to be significantly lower in the conditioned animals than in controls, although not as low as in animals injected with cyclophosphamide.

Since the humoral immune response to SRBC involves helper T-cell function, a study was undertaken to determine if B-cell function is subject to conditioning effects independent of effects on T-cells. Using the saccharin/cyclophosphamide conditioning paradigm, they found that the antibody response to the T-cell–independent antigen trinitrophenyl-lipopolysaccharide was attenuated by exposure to the CS, although the findings were less consistent than those obtained with SRBC in rats.

Two other models of immune responsivity have also been found to be subject to conditioning effects. The graft-vs.-host response, a function of cellular immunity, was found to be lower in conditioned rats than in controls. This response was assessed by measuring the size of draining lymph nodes after injection of splenic leukocytes from donor rats. Conditioning effects have also been reported in relation to cyclophosphamide-induced suppression of autoimmune glomerulonephritis in mice, an animal model of systemic lupus erythematosus. Both proteinuria and mortality were significantly reduced by conditioning.

Cell-mediated immune responses in humans may be subject to conditioning effects. In an interesting study, subjects were skin-tested monthly with tuberculin, with antigen placed on one arm and saline on the other. At the sixth trial, the placement of tuberculin and saline was reversed without the knowledge of the subject or of the nurse who applied the antigen. A markedly diminished or absent delayed cutaneous response was found for the tuberculin placed on the arm where saline was expected. When the subjects were then informed of the identity of the test substances and the tuberculin again applied to the "saline" arm, a brisk response, comparable to that of the first five trials, was obtained. These findings may represent conditioning effects in which the skin-testing protocol was the CS and the tuberculin response the US. Alternatively, the effects may have been related to the subjects' cognitive state of expectation and unrelated to conditioning effect per se. In keeping with such a possibility is the observation that the tuberculin reaction can be inhibited by hypnotic suggestion. According to either hypothesis, the data demonstrate an association between higher cortical function and an immune response.

MEDIATION OF STRESS EFFECTS ON IMMUNE FUNCTION

A variety of biological factors may be involved in mediating the associations among the brain, stress, depression, and the immune system. The endocrine system is highly responsive to both life experience and psychological state and has a significant although complicated effect on immune processes. The most widely studied hormones are those of the HPA axis. A wide range of stressful experiences is capable of inducing the release of corticosteroids and, as noted, cortisol secretion is increased in major depressive disorder. Corticosteroids have extensive and complex effects on the immune system. Of particular interest is the demonstration that glucocorticosteroids can suppress mitogen-induced lymphocyte stimulation and induce a redistribution of T-cells and of helper T-cells from the circulating pool to the bone marrow.

Secretion of corticosteroids has long been considered to be the mechanism of stress-induced modulation of immunity and related disease processes. The regulation of immune function in response to stress, however, may not be limited to corticosteroids. As previously noted, unpredictable, unavoidable tail shock in rats suppressed immune function as measured by the number of circulating lymphocytes and PHA stimulation.

In an effort to determine if the adrenal is required for stress-induced suppression of lymphocyte function in the rat, the effect of stressors in adrenalectomized animals was investigated. The four groups of rats studied were non-adrenalectomized, adrenalectomized, sham-ad-renalectomized, and adrenalectomized animals given a corticosterone pellet. The four be-havioral conditions (home-cage control, appa-ratus control, low shock, and high shock) were identical to those used in the previous study. There was a progressive increase in corticoste-rone, with increasing stress in both of the groups with adrenals; no corticosterone was detected in the adrenalectomized group; and the concen-tration of corticosterone in the adrenalec-tomized group that received the corticosterone pellets was constant. A progressive stress-induced decrease in the number of lymphocytes (that is, lymphopenia) was found in the nonad-renalectomized and sham-adrenalectomized groups, but no stress-related changes in lym-phocyte number were found in the adrenalec-tomized groups.

Lymphopenia following exposure to stress was described as early as 1937 and has been asso-ciated with adrenal hypertrophy and involution of the thymus and spleen. It has been shown that stress-induced leukopenia can be prevented by adrenalectomy in mice. The overall findings of these studies demonstrate that stress-induced lymphopenia in the rat occurs in association with stress-induced secretion of corticosteroids and can be prevented by adrenalectomy.

The stressful conditions suppressed the stimulation of lymphocytes by PHA in the adrenalectomized animals (Fig. 5–2). The stressors similarly suppressed PHA responses in non-adrenalectomized animals, in sham-adren-alectomized rats, and in adrenalectomized ani-mals with steroid replacement. These findings demonstrate that stress-related adrenal secre-tion of corticosteroids and catecholamines is not required for the stress-induced suppression of lymphocyte stimulation by the T-cell mitogen PHA in the rat. It may well be that there is an adrenal-independent, stress-induced depletion of functional subpopulations of T-cells or a se-lective redistribution of lymphoid tissues. A va-riety of other hormonal and neurosecretory systems may be involved in the adrenal-inde-pendent, stress-induced modulation of T-cell function.

These findings of adrenal-dependent, stress-induced lymphopenia and of adrenal-indepen-dent effects on lymphocyte stimulation indicate that stress-induced modulation of immunity is a complex phenomenon involving several, if not multiple, mechanisms. Changes in thyroid hor-

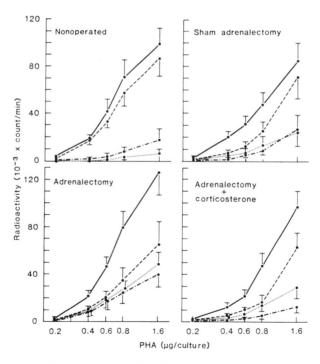

FIGURE 5–2. Stimulation of isolated peripheral blood lymphocytes by PHA for each of the four operative groups and four treatment procedures. Means ± SEM are presented as Δ CPM. (From Keller, S.E., et al.: Stress-induced suppression of immunity in adrenalectomized rats. Science 221:1302, 1983. Copyright 1983 by the AAAS.)

mones, growth hormones, and sex steroids have been associated with exposure to stressors, and all have been reported to modulate immune function. Further, as previously noted, the hypothalamus plays a central role in neuroendocrine function and modulates both humoral and cell-mediated immunity. These findings suggest that a range of neuroendocrine processes may be involved in stress-induced altered measures of the immune system.

Since a variety of hormones under pituitary control have been associated with immunoregulatory processes, the role of the pituitary in mediating stress-induced alterations of immunity has been investigated. The effect of a stressor on immune function has been studied in hypophysectomized rats. Three groups of rats were studied, including nonhypophysectomized, sham-hypophysectomized, and hypophysectomized. The two treatments, home-cage controls and tail-shocked animals, were similar to those in previously described studies. Plasma ACTH and corticosterone were increased in the stressed groups with pituitaries and were below detectable levels in the hypophysectomized animals.

In both the nonhypophysectomized and sham-hypophysectomized groups a stress-induced peripheral blood lymphopenia was found, as well as a stress-related decrease in the number of T-cells and helper T-cells but not in the number of suppressor T-cells. The number of B-cells was not altered by the stressful condition. No stress-related changes were found in the absolute number of lymphocytes or lymphocyte subpopulations in the hypophysectomized animals. These findings indicate that the stress-induced lymphopenia in the rat is selective for T-cells, specifically helper T-cells, and that stress-induced lymphopenia is pituitary dependent and associated with increased levels of plasma ACTH and corticosterone, consistent with the observation that the number of circulating immunocompetent cells in response to a stressor is regulated by the HPA axis. The stress-related decrease in lymphocytes from the peripheral blood may be related to vascular margination or migration into the interstitial compartment, the lymphatics, or lymph nodes.

The stressful condition suppressed PHA-induced stimulation of peripheral blood lymphocytes in the hypophysectomized animals as well as in both control groups. These findings demonstrate that factors of other than pituitary origin mediate the stress-induced suppression of peripheral blood lymphocyte proliferation. In addition to the hypothalamic-pituitary axis, the autonomic nervous system is another major stress-activated system, and stress-induced modulation of lymphocyte function may be related to neurotransmitter alterations. With the use of a stressor similar to that employed in the hypophysectomy study, a marked depletion of norepinephrine has been found in various regions of the rat brain, including the hypothalamus and locus coeruleus. It may well be that the findings of a pituitary-independent, stress-induced suppression of peripheral blood lymphocyte proliferation is related to the involvement of central and peripheral catecholamine systems, which as previously discussed have been shown to regulate immune processes.

It is of note that in the study of stress-induced alterations of the immune system in hypophysectomized rats the magnitude of the stress-induced suppression of lymphocyte function in the hypophysectomized animals was significantly greater than in animals with pituitaries. These findings demonstrate that pituitary processes are involved in countering stress-induced immunosuppressive mechanisms. Although the specific pituitary-dependent mitigating or compensating processes are not known, the findings suggest that there is a regulatory network of hormonal and nonhormonal systems involved in the maintenance of immunologic capacity following exposure to stressors. The pituitary's restraining influence on stress responses may be relevant to the understanding of homeostatic maintenance of critical body functions.

The findings of a stress-induced, pituitary-dependent lymphopenia, of pituitary-independent stress effects on peripheral blood lymphocyte stimulation, and of the pituitary's restraining influence on the stress-induced suppression of peripheral blood lymphocyte proliferation indicate that stress-induced modulation of immunity is complex and involves a range of mechanisms. Interactions between the nervous system and the immune system are extensive and include hormones, catecholamines, monoamines, neuropeptides, and opioids. Each of these systems requires consideration in the elucidation of the processes involved in stress-induced modulation of the immune system.

BIBLIOGRAPHY

Ader, R., Cohen, N.: Immune system interactions: Conditioning phenomena. Behav. Brain Sci. 8:379-426, 1985.

Elliott, G.R., Eisdorfer, C.: Stress and Human Health. New York, Springer, 1982.

Guillemin, R., Cohn, M., Melnechuk, T.: Neural Modulation of Immunity. New York, Raven Press, 1985.

Keller, S.E., et al.: Stress-induced alterations of immunity in hypophysectomized rats. Proc. Natl. Acad. Sci. U.S.A. 85:9297-9301, 1988.

Schleifer, S.J., et al.: Major depressive disorder and immunity: Role of age, sex, severity, and hospitalization. Arch. Gen. Psychiatry 46:81-87, 1989.

Schliefer, S.J., et al.: Suppression of lymphocyte stimulation following bereavement. J.A.M.A. 250:374-377, 1983.

Stein, M.: Stress, depression, and the immune system. J. Clin. Psychiatry 50(suppl.):35-40, 1989.

Stein, M., Keller, S., Schleifer, S.J.: The hypothalamus and the immune response, in Brain, Behavior and Bodily Disease, H. Weiner, M.A. Hofer, and A.J. Stunkard (eds.). New York, Raven Press, 1981.

Stein, M., Keller, S., Schliefer, S.J.: Stress and immunomodulation: The role of depression and neuroendocrine function. J. Immunol. 135:827s-833s, 1985.

Stein, M., Schiavi, R.C., Camerino, M.: Influence of brain and behavior on the immune system. Science 191:436, 1976.

Stein, M., Schleifer, S.J., Keller, S.E.: Psychoimmunology in clinical psychiatry, in Annual Review of Psychiatry, R.E. Hales and A.J. Francis (eds.). Washington, D.C., American Psychiatric Press, 1987.

Chapter 6
Consciousness and Attention

Thomas B. Horvath, M.D.

CONSCIOUSNESS AND ITS DISORDERS

Consciousness has been defined as a state of awareness of self and environment. The experience of consciousness consists of its *contents:* the sum of cognitive, affective, and conative mental functions; and of its *process:* arousal, activation, and attention. Arousal is used here in two senses: (1) as a *phasic* responsiveness to stimuli and (2) as activation, or *tonic* or *basal* arousal, the readiness to respond.

Disorders of the *contents* of consciousness form the major component of the work of the psychiatrist and psychoanalyst and constitute a large group of disorders influenced by genetic, developmental, cultural, and psychodynamic factors.

Disorders of the *process* of consciousness constitute a phenomenologically and neurophysiologically fairly homogeneous group. The phenomena consist of the *experience* of decreasing awareness and alertness, increasing drowsiness and confusion, with increasing misinterpretation

and finally oblivion of external reality; and in the disintegration of complex *behaviors*, release of primitive reflexes, and diminishing or inappropriate *responses* to external stimuli.

Four levels of consciousness have been described: alert, lethargic, semicomatose, and comatose. It is recommended that these terms be accompanied by specific descriptions of the stimuli applied (from weak to strong and from complex to simple) and the nature of the patient's response: (1) degree and quality of movement, (2) content and coherence of speech, and (3) eye opening and eye contact with the examiner.

Alert State

The ordinary, awake state of consciousness is generally taken for granted in a naive manner. William James, in his *Principles of Psychology*, correctly perceived, however, that

The mind is at every stage a theater of simultaneous possibilities. Consciousness consists in the compari-

53

son of these with each other, the selection of some, and the suppression of others, by the reinforcing and inhibiting agency of attention. The highest and most celebrated mental products are filtered from the data chosen by the faculty next beneath, out of the mass offered by the faculty below that, which mass was in turn sifted from a still larger amount of yet simpler material. . . . The world of each of us, however different our several views of it may be, all lay embedded in the primordial chaos of sensations. . . . My world is but one in a million, alike embedded and alike real.

In his *Varieties of Religious Experience,* James noted that "our normal waking consciousness is but one special type, whilst all about it, parted from it by the filmiest of screens, lie potential forms of consciousness entirely different."

From an experiential, experimental, and information system point of view, there appears to be a variety of ways of inducing these "altered states": hypnosis, concentrative meditation, "opening up" meditation, going to sleep (the hypnagogic state), physiological alterations (hypocapnia, hypoglycemia, sleep deprivation, sensory deprivation), and pharmacological induction (the psychedelic experience).

Abnormalities of awake, alert consciousness include the following categories from the American Psychiatric Association's revised third edition of the *Diagnostic and Statistical Manual* (DSM-III-R):

Depersonalization: an alteration in the perception or experience of the self so that the feeling of one's own reality is temporarily lost.
Derealization: a changed perception of the world, a "spaced-out" feeling; objects lose their normal characteristics.
Psychogenic amnesia: a sudden inability to recall important personal information.
Fugue: sudden travel from home, with assumption of a new identity and an inability to recall one's previous identity.
Multiple personality: two or more relatively distinct and coherent patterns of experience and behavior, with variable degrees of mutual awareness.

Hilgard proposed a useful psychological model to explain the above disorders as well as hypnosis and some forms of meditation. Following Pierre Janet, he proposed a "vertical" split or dissociation in consciousness instead of (and perhaps in addition to) the Freudian concepts of "horizontal" layers of the conscious, preconscious, and unconscious. It is not clear how these partitions of experience and behavior can come about, but physiological recordings and cerebral-event-related potential patterns appear to differentiate between some of these states.

The differences emerge in those areas normally influenced by attentional factors.

In medical practice, abnormalities of consciousness characterized by lethargy progressing to coma are more common than the above, somewhat esoteric alterations and dissociations of consciousness. Obtundation, reduction of awareness, clouding of consciousness, confusional state, stupor, and semicoma are some of the descriptive terms used, at times interchangeably, with presumed etiological terminology such as metabolic encephalopathy, acute brain syndrome, and toxic confusion. The DSM-III-R attempts to resurrect the old and honored term "delirium" and to imbue it with a specific meaning *not* limited to the florid state of excitement, hallucinations, and disorientation commonly described in medical textbooks.

Delirium

Delirium is characterized by the rapid evolution of impaired attention and a fluctuating state of awareness, with perception, thinking, and memory all disturbed to varying degrees. It often presents with a disturbance of the waking-sleeping cycle with frequent nightmares. These episodes may merge into illusions and hallucinations in the waking state. Delusions are usually secondary to illusions and hallucinations and represent an attempt to make sense of confusing and bizarre mental experiences. Delusions are often fragmentary and not logically coherent but may still lead to disturbed behavior. Some patients exhibit psychomotor overactivity with autonomic arousal, but many others show stupor, apathy, and somnolence, and progress toward a coma.

Delirium is primarily a disturbance of the polysynaptic reticular formation and related structures subserving arousal and attention. There is increasing evidence that cholinergic transmission in the reticular formation, cortex, and hippocampus is impaired first in the course of many metabolic encephalopathies. The dorsal tegmental pathway from the mesencephalic reticular formation to the tectum and thalamus seems to be the site of action. Acetylcholine synthesis at synaptosomes is easily disrupted by anoxia and related conditions. Physostigmine can improve the mental state in some deliria. Delirious states associated with alcohol and sedative withdrawal are complicated by a rebound hyperactivity of the locus coeruleus. Other delirious, confused states come about due to pontine and midbrain structural events or massive bilateral cortical disasters. See Chapter 22: Delirium and Dementia.

Comatose States and Comalike States

The differential diagnosis of *coma* from a behavioral point of view is discussed in *Neurology for Psychiatrists* by C. E. Wells and G. W. Duncan.

In *psychogenic coma*, there are no pathological neurological signs, no significant changes in respiratory pattern, and no pupillary or oculomotor changes; at times, there is evidence of some awareness of the surroundings. However, some patients with psychogenic unresponsiveness may not swallow their secretions or fluid placed in their mouths and may exhibit urinary and fecal incontinence and complete apparent insensitivity to pain.

In *catatonic stupor*, the distinction between "organic" and "functional" becomes blurred. Low-grade fever, tachycardia, tachypnea, sweating, and dilated pupils may occur. Choreiform movements, perseveration, rigidity, and *gegenhalten* and waxing flexibility have been described. Catatonic states occur in schizophrenia, in severely retarded depression, occasionally in response to overwhelming psychological stress, and very occasionally in response to a significant organic insult to the cerebrum.

In *akinetic mutism* a persistent severe lack of movement and mutism exist in the presence of alert-appearing eye movements. In the lethargic form, there are periods of sleep and reduced wakefulness; the lesion is generally in the midbrain. Septal lesions are associated with a "coma vigil," a persistent wakefulness with some behavioral outbursts.

In the *persistent vegetative state* the eyes open in response to stimuli, sleep-wake cycles exist, and blood pressure and respiratory control are maintained. But motor responses are absent, and there is no evidence of meaningful contact with the environment. Usually there is massive cortical damage.

The *locked-in syndrome* superficially resembles the above in that there is a paralysis in all four extremities and of the lower cranial nerves. However, the presence of voluntary blinking and vertical eye movements can be used by the patient to indicate awareness of self and environment. "Locked-in" patients have been taught to communicate by blinking Morse code messages. Most such patients had midbrain or pontine structural lesions.

This brief review of the clinical disorders of the process of consciousness points to a need to understand the concepts of arousal, activation, and attention, and their corresponding neurophysiological substrates.

ATTENTION AND ITS DISORDERS

Contemporary psychology approaches attention from three aspects: intensity, selectivity, and voluntary control.

1. The *intensity* component is the same as tonic or basal *arousal* or activation: a nonspecific background drive that prepares the organism to meet any challenge in the environment.

2. The *selectivity* of attention represents a mechanism that brings certain aspects of the environment into focus, treats them as stimuli, and reduces responsiveness to changes in the rest of the field, which are relegated to background. Attention is usually compelled to certain novel or pleasurable or painful stimuli.

3. Human beings evolved a *voluntary control* of their attentional system and learned to direct it according to certain plans of action.

Attention processes may be inferred from behavioral observations, including measurement of reaction times and errors of omission and commission in response to simple and complex stimuli. Physiological methods are also used; EEG, computer-derived averaged evoked potentials, heart rate, blood pressure, skin resistance and conductance, and electromyograms are some of the common methods. The data are interpreted through use of neurophysiological constructs, and hypotheses are supported by animal experiments and stimulation or lesions of certain tracts. Mathematical information theory and signal-detection techniques have been applied.

Disturbances of attention are seen in many psychiatric syndromes and, in some, contribute heavily to psychopathology (schizophrenia, delirium, anxiety states).

Intensity Dimension: Tonic or Basal Arousal or Activation

Stimulation of the reticular formation releases most of the peripheral physiological changes described for *visceral activation*. The activity of the reticular formation determines the cortical EEG pattern and the state of consciousness as well.

Implicit in the theories of activation is the concept of an arousal continuum, starting with sleep and ending in "overarousal," as in a state of terror, anxiety, or ecstasy.

Selectivity Dimensions

In both voluntary and involuntary attention there is a *central area* to be brought into focus, and there is a background that needs to be largely but not completely ignored. In voluntary vigilance tasks, extraneous signals are suppressed, whereas in involuntary attention the startle, phasic arousal, or *orienting responses* are followed by *habituation* if the novelty of the stimuli wears off.

Selectivity Dimension: Voluntary Selective Attention, Vigilance

The classic experiment in the selective attention field is the "cocktail party" paradigm. In this paradigm the task is to listen to and select one of many simultaneous conversations. The more two simultaneous messages resemble each other, the less they are separable. Messages presented separately to two ears are better perceived than two messages presented to the same ear. Messages from the two ears are rarely mixed up. Message continuity is important in keeping the two sets of signals separate. The physical characteristics of voice and the semantic content of the message are monitored and handled separately. Speech-shadowing experiments showed that if a person attended closely to one of two messages, only the physical characteristics of the rejected message were retained. Although words were not recalled from the rejected message, conditioned galvanic skin responses to some of them could be obtained, and the subject's name could often override the selective attention mechanism. Voluntary selective attention is disturbed in schizophrenia and delirium, in which patients may experience a "booming, buzzing confusion" of sense impressions.

Selectivity Dimension: Involuntary Attention, Phasic Arousal, Orienting and Its Habituation

In 1927 I.P. Pavlov introduced the term *orienting reflex* to describe the behavioral and physiological phasic arousal changes in animals confronted with new stimuli. At other times, he called this the "investigating" and the "what-is-it" reflex. He wrote

It is this reflex which brings about the immediate response in man and animals to the slightest changes in the world around them. The biological significance of this reflex is obvious. If the animal is not provided with such a reflex its life would hang at any moment by a thread.

The components of the orienting response include the following:

1. Increase in the sensitivity of sense organs
   a. Pupillary dilation
   b. Lowered threshold for light and sound
2. Muscle and skeletal changes
   a. General skeletal and musculature changes: arrest of ongoing reactions; increased electromyographic activity
   b. Changes in the muscles orienting the sense organs, for example, turning of the head, pricking up of the ears, sniffing
3. EEG changes toward faster and lower amplitude activity
4. Autonomic changes
   a. Changes in skin conductance and skin potential: the galvanic skin response
   b. Vasoconstriction in the limbs, vasodilation in the head
   c. Changes in the respiration rate and in the heart rate

The stimulus characteristics that evoke an orienting response include the following:

- Novelty, surprise, complexity, incongruity
  or
- Conflict, discrimination
  or
- Special significance, intensity, aversive effect

The size of the orienting responses depends on the magnitude of these sets of stimuli. The person's name always elicits an orienting response. If a neutral tone is associated with an aversive or appetitive stimulus, orienting reactions to the tone tend to persist. If a motor or mental response is required to a stimulus, the orienting response tends to continue. Variations in the stimulus result in alterations in the magnitude of the orienting reflex or in its persistence. In the absence of such variations in the stimulus the orienting response diminishes, or habituates, after 10 to 20 repetitions of the stimulus.

Habituation is the gradual diminution of responses to continued or repeated stimuli. Habituation is a fundamental biological mechanism, for if an organism is to survive, it must be able to suppress irrelevant stimuli and avoid irrelevant responses. If learning is understood as a process that manifests itself by adaptive changes in the individual's behavior as a result of experience, then habituation is simply learning not to respond to stimuli that tend to be without significance in the life of the animal. It is the simplest form of learning and can be demonstrated at a cellular and even synaptic level.

Habituation is a long-term, stimulus-specific waning of a response. It is not a permanent state, however, since the original stimulus should be able to evoke the response again if enough time has elapsed, and an interpolated stimulus should be able to renew the responses to the original stimulus. This process of dishabituation depends on the lapse of time or on the interpolation of a fresh stimulus. Thus, reversibility is one of the criteria for habituation.

Seven general propositions concerning habituation seem to be true for most organisms, including humans:

1. The decrease in response is a negative exponential function of the stimulus presentation.
2. The habituation rate is faster for regular stimuli.
3. Habituation is faster for weak stimuli.
4. The response recovers when the stimulus is omitted for a while.
5. Habituation of one response may generalize to another similar one.
6. A different stimulus may dishabituate the original response; habituation occurs to the dishabituating stimulus if it is frequently repeated.
7. If the stimulus requires a decision, a discrimination, or an action, habituation is delayed.

Thus, although orienting or phasic arousal alerts the organism to significant stimuli in the environment, the repetition of these stimuli in the absence of consequences leads to habituation and the return of the organism to a baseline level of tonic activation. Primates show habituation of the orienting and exploratory activity quite readily. Their habituation is a function of the intensity and interest value of the stimulus and of the individual's previous experience. Older animals and those individuals reared in perceptually enriched environments habituate faster; chimpanzees reared in captivity show more prolonged orienting behavior than wild members do.

Some withdrawn schizophrenics and some depressives fail to show any orienting reaction at all. Other schizophrenics and patients with delirium who have difficulty in controlling their attention react with large orienting responses to trivial stimuli and fail to habituate to them even after many repetitions. Other schizophrenics show heightened tonic activation—increased muscle tension, heart rate, skin sweating—yet

appear not to respond to novel stimuli, exhibiting a dissociation between phasic and tonic activation or arousal. Thus, problems in the control of passive selective attention or phasic arousal may be demonstrated in various forms of this illness.

Voluntary Dimension: Effort, Self-Directed Attention, Action

The concept of *effort* can now be added to that of phasic arousal and tonic activation. It takes effort to uncouple automatic motor responses from stimulus-generated phasic arousal; it takes effort and foresight to look beyond the immediate concrete stimulus to the context in which the stimulus is embedded. Pribram speculates that there is some voluntary, effortful control over the relationship between phasic arousal, tonic activation, and motor action and that this voluntary effort is related to activities of the frontal lobes. Inability to exert effort and failure to plan or to follow a plan are manifested in frontal lobe disorders. Patients with frontal lobe lesions often appear apathetic, "unmotivated," and "lazy."

There also appears to be an effortful component to remembering. Depression and schizophrenia are associated at times with memory failures due to an insufficient expenditure of effort on mnemonic strategies. Other failures of voluntary attention, similar to those seen in frontal lobe disorders, are also seen in these disorders.

HOW DO ORIENTING AND ITS HABITUATION AND THE REGULATION OF TONIC AROUSAL LEAD TO CONSCIOUSNESS AND THE VOLUNTARY DIRECTION OF ATTENTION?

The self-generated activity of the nervous system and the external and internal background stimuli impinging indirectly on the reticular formation summate in that structure to define the fluctuating level of tonic arousal or activation. This background arousal is expressed as basal autonomic and skeletal muscle activity and as a variable readiness for behavior and is experienced by the subject as awareness and attentiveness. Metabolic impairment of these polysynaptic neuronal networks in the reticular formation or their structural destruction leads to variable impairments of these physiological functions, from lethargy to coma.

When a change takes place in the external or internal environment, this may be perceived as a stimulus by the nervous system. Signals rapidly proceed via the thalamus to the primary sensory cortex, from there to the secondary association areas, and eventually to the tertiary association area, the posterior parietal cortex. But on their way, in the brainstem, the signals collaterally stimulate the reticular formation as well. Some of the output of the reticular formation goes via the mammillotegmental and mammillothalamic tracts and, with the collaboration of the prefrontal cortex, stimulates the retrieval of cortical memory traces for comparative purposes. Some of the other output goes via the medial forebrain bundle to the limbic striatum.

At the same time as the medial dorsal thalamic-frontal system is searching for a cortical match for the image evoked by the sensory-association system, the anterior-thalamic-cingulate-posterior parietal system is searching for emotional significance for it. If a previous cortical representation does not exist, or if there is affective significance attached to it, the frontotemporal system via the amygdala stimulates the limbic striatum (nucleus stria terminalis) and the reticular formation, reinforcing its phasic arousal and inducing it to emit the orienting reaction with its autonomic and cortical activating components.

As the stimulus is repeated, it loses its information or novelty value, unless it becomes coupled to visceral or affective experiences. The repeated stimulus without significance goes through a repeat of the processing described above. This time, however, an emerging cortical representation is found after the memory search, and the parietal control area, probably via the cingulate, stimulates the hippocampus, which has an inhibitory effect on the limbic striatum (nucleus accumbens) and on the reticular formation. Through several repetitions, the inhibition equals and exceeds the excitation, the stimulus-activated phasic arousal in the reticular formation is inhibited, and the orienting response gradually diminishes and finally habituates.

During the period of orienting, enhancement of collateral inhibition at the primary sensory cortex, mediated by the effect of secondary and tertiary association areas, improves and sharpens sensory receptiveness. In delirium, this is impaired. The frontal-amygdala complex provides a stop mechanism, increasing the likelihood of registration of the stimulus configuration. In delirium, memory formation is interfered with. When habituation commences, increasing self-inhibition at the sensory cortex diminishes the signal-to-noise ratio. The hippocampal system remains available via the inhibition of this self-inhibition to dishabituate the organism, if a subtle change should happen in the stimulus configuration. This effect is probably mediated through the limbic striatum and its outflow to the substantia innominata and, through that, to the tertiary association/posterior parietal cortex.

The voluntary directing of attention takes effort; it is mediated via the hippocampus but is ultimately controlled by the frontal lobes. Abnormalities are manifested as lack of motivation, lack of activity, and forgetting how to remember, without an impairment of consciousness. This is seen in schizophrenia, in some forms of depression, and in cases of frontal lobe damage by alcohol or head injury.

This neuroanatomical and physiological summary illustrates that the work of attentional mechanisms is the result of complex interactions of many different central nervous system modules. Impairment of several different systems may lead to defective attention and impaired arousal and orienting behavior, the same behavioral manifestations seen in disorders of consciousness.

BIBLIOGRAPHY

Brazier, M.A., Hobson, J.A.: The Reticular Formation Revisited. New York, Raven Press, 1980.
Hilgard, E.: Neodissociation theory of multiple cognitive control systems, in Consciousness and Self-regulation, G.E. Schwartz and D. Shapiro (eds.). New York, Plenum Press, 1976.
James, W.: The Principles of Psychology. New York, Henry Holt and Co., 1890 and 1918.
John, E.R.: A model of consciousness, in Consciousness and Self-regulation, vol. 1, G.E. Schwartz and D. Shapiro (eds.). New York, Plenum Press, 1976.
Lynn, R.: Attention, Arousal and Orientation Reaction. New York, Pergamon Press, 1966.
Norman, D.A., Shallice, T.: Attention to action: willed and automatic control of behavior, in Consciousness and Self-regulation, vol. 4, R.J. Davidson, G.E. Schwartz, and D. Shapiro (eds.). New York, Plenum Press, 1986.
Pavlov, I.P.: Conditioned Reflexes. Oxford, Clarendon Press, 1927.
Plum, F., Posner, J.B.: The Diagnosis of Stupor and Coma. Philadelphia, F.A. Davis, 1980.
Pribram, K.H.: Languages of the Brain. Englewood Cliffs, N.J., Prentice-Hall, 1971.
Pribram, K.H., McGuinness, B.: Arousal, activation and effort in the control of attention. Psychol. Rev. 82:116-149, 1975.
Strub, R.L., Black, F.W.: Neurobehavioral Disorders: A Clinical Approach. Philadelphia, F.A. Davis, 1988.
Tart, C.: States of Consciousness. New York, E.P. Dutton, 1975.
Wells, C.E., Duncan, G.W.: Neurology for Psychiatrists. Philadelphia, F.A. Davis, 1980.

Part II
Physical Functioning of the Brain

Chapter 7

Gross Anatomy of the Brain

Vahram Haroutunian, Ph.D.

The brain is the part of the nervous system contained in the cranial cavity. The brain is usually described as having the following six major parts:

1. Cerebrum $\left.\right\}$ Forebrain
2. Diencephalon
3. Mesencephalon Midbrain
4. Cerebellum $\left.\right\}$
5. Pons   Hindbrain
6. Medulla

CEREBRUM

The cerebrum is divided into right and left cerebral hemispheres, which constitute the main bulk of the human brain. Each hemisphere is divided into five lobes (Fig. 7–1):

1. Frontal lobe
2. Parietal lobe
3. Occipital lobe
4. Temporal lobe
5. Insula (insular lobe)

The cerebral hemispheres are connected at several points. The two main connections are the massive *corpus callosum* (Fig. 7–5) and the much smaller *anterior commissure*, both bands of nerve fibers.

Cerebral Cortex

The cerebral cortex is a thin layer of gray matter just beneath the surface of the cerebral hemisphere. This layer follows the convolutions of the hemisphere surface, which increases its surface area, much in the way a convoluted coastline has more shore. Beneath the layer of gray matter lies a core of white matter. Gray matter is so called because the nerve cell bodies of which it is composed look gray to the eye. White matter gets its color from the myelin sheaths of the nerve fibers of which it is chiefly composed. The gray-matter nerve cell bodies of the cerebral cortex are thought to be the actual thinking structures of the brain, whereas the white matter is more involved with the transmission of messages.

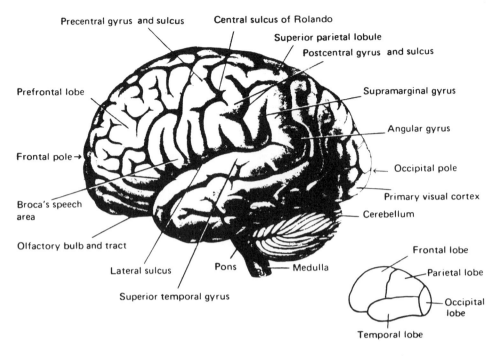

FIGURE 7–1. Lateral surface of the brain. (From Noback, C.R., Demarest, R.J.: The Nervous System: Introduction and Review. New York, McGraw-Hill Book Co., 1972, with permission.)

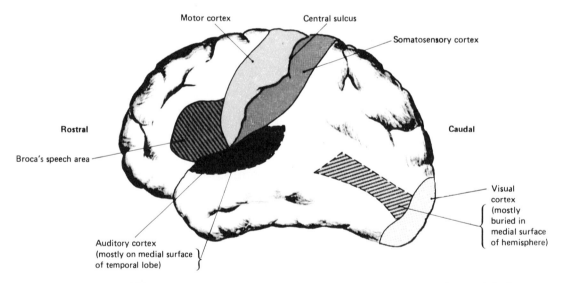

FIGURE 7–2. Schematic lateral view of brain, showing some of the important cortical areas. Only the more prominent sulci and gyri are shown. (From Neil R. Carlson, Physiology of Behavior. Copyright © 1977 by Allyn & Bacon. Reprinted with permission.)

Input Areas of Cortex

Particular areas of the cerebral cortex are known with reasonable certainty to be involved in certain mental processes. The following types of incoming messages from the peripheral nerves, carried to the brain by afferent nerves, are processed by different parts of the cerebral cortex (Fig. 7–2):

1. Visual: occipital lobe
2. Auditory: upper anterior temporal lobe

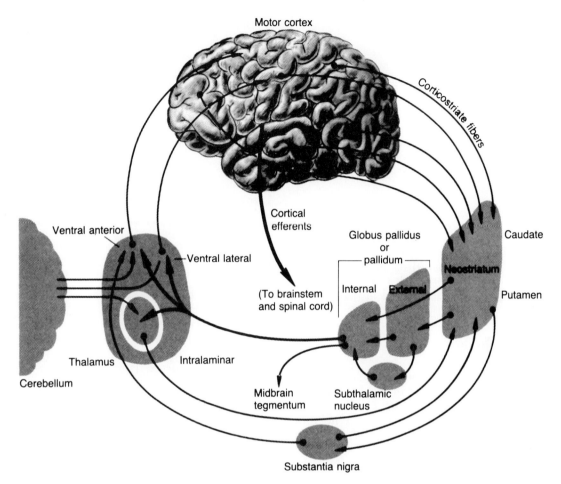

FIGURE 7–3.   Circuitry showing the relationship between the basal ganglia and cortex. Note that projections from all parts of the cortex enter the basal ganglia but that only the motor cortex receives projections from the basal ganglia. (After DeLong, 1974; from Kolb, B., Whishaw, I.Q.: Fundamentals of Human Neuropsychology, ed. 2. San Francisco, Freeman, 1985. Copyright © 1980, 1985 by W.H. Freeman and Company. Reprinted by permission.)

3.   Short-term memory: lower part of temporal lobe
4.   Somatosensory: parietal lobe

Output Areas of Cortex

The output, or motor, part of the cerebral cortex controls various functions. The motor area is located on the posterior half of the frontal lobe. Three divisions are recognized, each controlling different functions:

1.   Primary motor cortex: specific muscle movements
2.   Premotor cortex: coordinated muscle movements
3.   Broca's area: speech

Basal Ganglia

Deep within the brain are paired (right and left) areas of gray matter (groupings of nerve cell bodies) called nuclei. The basal ganglia are a group of nuclei that generally control background gross body movements, such as stance. The following five nuclei are usually grouped together as the basal ganglia (Fig. 7–3):

1.   Caudate nucleus
2.   Putamen
3.   Globus pallidus
4.   Claustrum
5.   Amygdala

DIENCEPHALON

The diencephalon connects the cerebrum with the lower brain parts. In humans, there is no strict boundary between it and the cerebrum. The diencephalic structures of importance are groups of nuclei surrounding the third ventricle (a cavity filled with fluid called cerebrospinal fluid). The thalamus and hypothalamus are the most important of these groups.

Thalamus

Almost all messages between cerebral structures and other parts of the brain are relayed through the egg-shaped thalamus. First awareness of crude sensations such as touch, temperature, and pain probably occurs at this level.

Hypothalamus

The hypothalamus lies below the anterior end of the thalamus. It is one of the brain's main control centers for homeostasis, affecting internal body functions and the autonomic nervous system.

One way in which the hypothalamus exerts its control over bodily functions is through its influences on the endocrine system. This control is achieved through two main mechanisms: (1) direct release of neuroendocrine products into general circulation and (2) indirect control through the pituitary gland. Several indirect control circuits have been identified, one of which is the hypothalamic-pituitary-adrenal axis.

Limbic System

The limbic (border) system consists of cerebral and diencephalic structures adjacent to the hypothalamus (Fig. 7–4). This system controls emotional and behavioral activities and includes the following parts:

1. Amygdala
2. Hippocampus
3. Mammillary body
4. Septum pellucidum
5. Limbic cortex (cingulate gyrus, cingulum, insula, parahippocampal gyrus)

The Papez circuit, which encompasses a number of limbic system structures (cingulate cortex, hippocampus, septum, hypothalamus, mammil-

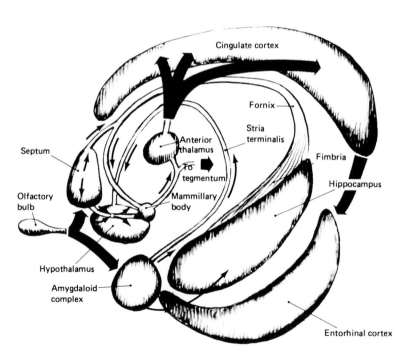

FIGURE 7–4. Simplified schematic representation of the limbic system. (From Neil R. Carlson, Physiology of Behavior. Copyright ©1977 by Allyn & Bacon. Reprinted with permission.)

lary body, and anterior thalamus), has been proposed to underlie many aspects of motivation and emotion. Under various formulations and reformulations of the original proposal, different structures within this circuit are thought to be involved in aggression, pleasure, sexuality, social behavior, and emotionality.

MESENCEPHALON

The mesencephalon, or midbrain, is part of the brain stem, along with the pons and medulla (Fig. 7–5). The brain stem connects the forebrain with the spinal cord. Nuclei and fiber tracts are the structures of importance in the mesencephalon. The cerebral peduncles account for most of the mesencephalon, except for the posterior tectum:

1. Cerebral peduncles
   a. Corticospinal and corticopontine fibers
   b. Substantia nigra
   c. Tegmentum (medial lemniscus, medial longitudinal fasciculus, cranial nerve nuclei, red nucleus, periaqueductal gray, reticular formation)
2. Tectum
   a. Superior colliculi
   b. Inferior colliculi

PONS

Containing nuclei and fiber tracts, the pons is in many ways an extension of the mesencephalon. Some mesencephalon structures extend into it. The pons is divided into ventral and dorsal parts; the dorsal part is also called the tegmentum of the pons, being an extension of the tegmentum of the mesencephalon. The dorsal pons contains the cranial nerve nuclei and descending and ascending fiber tracts. The ventral pons is a large structure consisting of large collections of fiber bundles interspersed with pontine nuclei.

MEDULLA

The medulla, short for medulla oblongata, forms the lower end of the brain stem and tapers into the spinal cord. Like the mesencephalon and pons, it contains nuclei and fiber tracts. On the anterior medulla, two protruding longitudinal columns known as *pyramids* carry fibers originating in the motor and somatosensory aspects of the cerebral cortex to the spinal cord. These fibers cross before entering the spinal cord, which is the reason that the right cerebral cortex controls the left side of the body, and the left cortex the right side. A swelling on each side of the medulla is called the olive; to the interior

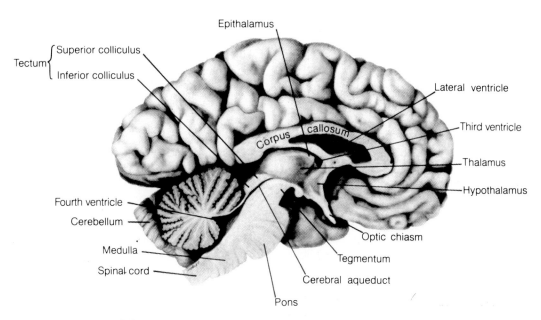

FIGURE 7–5. Medial view through the center of the brain, showing structures of the brain stem. (From Kolb, B., Whishaw, I.Q.: Fundamentals of Human Neuropsychology, ed. 2. San Francisco, Freeman, 1985. Copyright © 1980, 1985 by W.H. Freeman and Company. Reprinted by permission.)

of each olive, lies the *inferior olivary nucleus.* The medulla also contains parts of the reticular formation, including nuclei that control vegetative functions such as respiration, skeletal muscle tonus, and cardiovascular function.

CEREBELLUM

The cerebellum, located posterior to the brain stem, is structured like the cerebrum in that it has two hemispheres which contain the *cerebellar cortex* (made up of nerve cell bodies), the *subcortical white matter* (made up of nerve fibers), and the *deep nuclei* (comparable to the basal ganglia). The largest of the deep nuclei is the *dentate nucleus.* The cerebellum modulates movement, delicately coordinating and smoothing out the ongoing actions of opposing muscle groups.

The *cerebellar peduncles* constitute the input and output pathways of the cerebellum. The *superior cerebellar peduncle* connects the cerebellum with the mesencephalon; the *middle cerebellar peduncle* connects it with the pons; and the *inferior cerebellar peduncle* connects it with the medulla.

OVERVIEW OF NEUROCHEMICAL PATHWAYS

For the most part, communication between different neurons is achieved by chemical means. Neurotransmitters are synthesized within each neuron and are stored in vesicles in the nerve terminal. Action potentials reaching the nerve terminal release the neurotransmitter into the synaptic cleft. The neurotransmitter then defuses across the synaptic cleft and acts on postsynaptic receptors, causing a conductance change. Conductance changes of sufficient magnitude lead to the generation of action potentials by the postsynaptic neuron and the propagation of the signal from one neuron to the next. The effects of neurotransmitters on postsynaptic cells can be either excitatory or inhibitory. Neurons can be classified in terms of the specific neurotransmitter used.

Many different neurotransmitters have been identified in the nervous system. The most studied neurotransmitters are the following:

- Acetylcholine
- Norepinephrine
- Dopamine
- Serotonin

In addition, a number of neuropeptides and amino acids have been shown to possess neurotransmitter-like activity. In general, the various neuropeptides have been found to be colocalized with other neurotransmitters. From a strictly quantitative point of view, the amino acid transmitters are much more abundant in the mammalian nervous system than are the classic transmitters (acetylcholine, norepinephrine, dopamine, and serotonin); however, the functions and distribution of the amino acid transmitters are not as well understood.

For a more detailed discussion, see Chapter 8: Neurophysiological and Neurochemical Basis of Behavior; Chapter 9: Neurotransmitter Receptor Function; and Chapter 10: Neuropeptides.

Neuroanatomic Tracts

The advent of advanced histochemical and immunohistochemical techniques has allowed the visualization of the neuroanatomic tracts associated with different neurotransmitters. Some neurotransmitter systems, such as the noradrenergic and serotonergic systems, are widely distributed within the brain. Others, such as the cholinergic and dopaminergic systems, are more discrete. The cell bodies of serotonergic, noradrenergic, and dopaminergic neurons are located in the midbrain and hindbrain (raphe nuclei, locus coeruleus, and substantia nigra, respectively), whereas their axons travel long distances to terminate on forebrain and spinal cord structures.

The distribution of neuropeptides and amino acid transmitters is less well understood. Many neuropeptides are associated with hypothalamic structures, and amino acid transmitters are more highly concentrated in diencephalic areas. It should be noted that although neuropeptides and amino acid transmitters are more plentiful in these areas, their distribution within the brain is ubiquitous.

Chapter 8

Neurophysiological and Neurochemical Basis of Behavior

Michael Murphy, M.D., Ph.D., and
Stephen I. Deutsch, M.D., Ph.D.

The first part of this chapter emphasizes neurophysiology, and the second, neurochemistry. Neurophysiological descriptions revolve around the neuron and its immediate environment and emphasize communication plasticity (capacity for change). Neurochemical data are presented on a system-wide or multiple-neuron level. Both presentations emphasize an integrated approach to brain function.

NEUROTRANSMISSION

How Can Behavior Change?

Three seemingly unrelated clinical phenomena underscore the apparent paradox that alterations in central nervous system function may occur without changes in anatomical reorganization. Each example implies a malleability in neuronal communication that may not be captured during discussions of cellular morphological characteristics.

Example 1 ▬▬▬▬▬▬▬▬▬

The first example involves the recovery of the nervous system after accidental or intentional lesions. Clinicians realize that physical damage to the spinal cord or brain does not always produce functional losses that are irreversible. The extent and rapidity of recovery of function after certain massive brain lesions in children, for example, can be impressive. Functions return or escape damage when they apparently should not, particularly if one adheres to a rigid ultra-localizationist view of brain organization.

Example 2 ▬▬▬▬▬▬▬▬▬

The second clinical example involves the stages seen in recovery from hemiplegia in adults after stroke; these stages parallel the normal development of voluntary control of grasping in newborn infants. In the infant, there is progression from traction response through a grasp reflex to an instinctive grasp reaction and ultimately voluntary grasp control. The traditional interpretation for this observation in children is that myelinization or some other anatomical neurological alteration takes place. Yet, in adults, myelinization and neuronal regeneration cannot be easily invoked as a mechanism of recovery. Because a parallel between recovery after stroke and infantile development exists, a functional reorganization is partially implied. The functional reorganization of existing neuronal elements in adults allows simple reflexes to become incorporated and transformed into more elaborate behavioral patterns.

Example 3

The third example by way of introduction to the concept of malleable neuronal communication can be borrowed from everyday experience. A variety of organisms, endless in diversity of form and function, modify behavior in response to the environment. Information is channeled along neuronal pathways, is modified by past experience, and is then acted on in an integrated fashion. Various paradigms used in psychopharmacological research are based on this assumption, as are many clinical techniques employed during psychotherapy.

These three examples offer interesting and related paradoxes. The development of connections between most neurons within the central nervous system is largely determined by genetic processes. How does a largely predetermined nervous system allow for recovery of function in some patients with massive central nervous system damage? How does a predetermined nervous system allow for the obvious ability to modify behavior based on experience? Because learning and other behavioral modifications are characteristically of long duration (years), how can a relatively brief pattern of neural activity produce a long-term modification of function in a group of structurally invariant neurons and their connections?

Among a number of proposed solutions, the most interesting demand an appreciation of the communication modalities available to individual neurons and neuronal clusters. This particular orientation relegates to secondary importance an impressive literature describing the regeneration of nervous tissue and morphological changes in neurons that may result from environmental demands.

Neuronal Communication: Broad Concepts

Much of what is assumed about the behavior of individual neurons in mammals has been extrapolated from work in invertebrate systems. There are several reasons for this. In contrast to vertebrates, invertebrates do much less, and behavioral patterns are repetitive and stereotyped. Complex, higher-order behavior in invertebrates, although involving choice and decision, can be broken down into simple units of activity. Invertebrates thus offer an opportunity to study behavioral sequences within a relatively simple nervous system, and the chain of cellular interactions that then results in very complex behavior can be delineated. Moreover, the operating characteristics of each neuronal element can be described in great detail (for example, location, synaptic connections, function).

Dendrites and Soma

Regardless of location, every neuron can be morphologically characterized as having receptive (dendrites, soma), conductive (axon), and transmissive (presynaptic terminal) components (Figs. 8–1 and 8–2).

The receptive elements of the neuron are classically considered to be dendrites and soma, although axoaxonic input is commonly encountered in many species. The number of potential inputs onto the receptive components of a single neuron can be extremely large (8000 to 20,000 in the case of the human cerebral cortex, for example), and an integrative function is required. Indeed, an averaging of many thousands of small graded potentials seems to be prerequisite before information transfer along conductive elements takes place. When dendritic structures are in close approximation, dendrodendritic electrical interactions can also occur; these interactions alter the net electrical bias existing on an adjacent neuronal membrane to increase or decrease overall cell excitability. Thus a receptive element in the classical sense can become a conductive element when viewed from a larger perspective.

Axon

The conductive element of a neuron is its axon, which for illustrative purposes is often assigned the properties of a cable. The cable, or passive, properties include membrane resis-

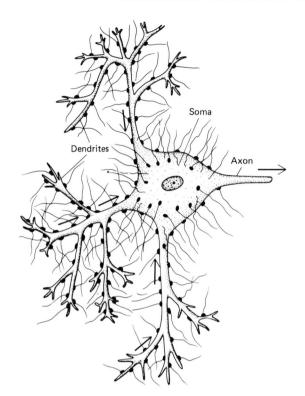

FIGURE 8–1. A typical motor neuron, showing presynaptic terminals on the neuronal soma and dendrites. Note also the single axon. (From Guyton, A.C.: Basic Neuroscience: Anatomy and Physiology. Philadelphia, W.B. Saunders, 1987.)

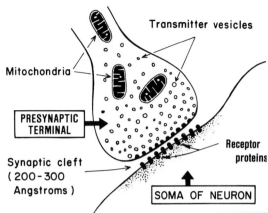

FIGURE 8–2. Physiological anatomy of the synapse. (From Guyton, A.C.: Basic Neuroscience: Anatomy and Physiology. Philadelphia, W.B. Saunders, 1987.)

tance and capacitance, which do not change value as a function of membrane voltage. Active responses, depending on ionic flux, also occur within the conductive element in the form of either action potentials or small graded electrical signals from synaptic input. This interplay of passive and active properties characterizes the axon as an "electrical bridge" between receptive and transmissive components of the neuron.

The passive properties of the neuron are more than abstractions; tangible, measurable changes occur in the ability of an axon to transmit a signal when cable properties are altered. For example, the *time constant* measures the rate at which the potential of an axon can be varied. An average time constant is 100 ms in invertebrates, but a range from 1 ms to hundreds of milliseconds can be demonstrated. The shorter the time constant, the more easily stimulated (or inhibited) will be the neuron and the faster will be that neuron's response to any given input.

Likewise, a *space or length constant* can be defined: it is a measure of distance over which subthreshold signals can be effectively propa-

gated. Since the space constant increases with diameter and membrane resistance, a small-diameter, low-resistance axon will rarely efficiently couple receptive and transmissive elements electronically.

The axon is remarkably nonhomogeneous in its excitability and in the ionic mechanisms that subtend it. Regardless of the method of stimulation employed, an axonal trigger zone near the cell body reaches threshold first and then initiates a rapid, regenerative change in current and voltage, termed an *action potential*. Each action potential propagates in an antidromic (toward receptive elements) and an orthodromic (toward transmissive elements) direction, and a change in axon diameter accompanied by small local magnetic fields have been shown to accompany the movement of this current.

As the action potential propagates orthodromically, it can encounter one or more branch points before its termination within the presynaptic terminal of the axon. As a rule, each branch is smaller than the trunk from which it originates, and branching is often asymmetrical. Because of this morphological "mismatch" at each branch point, further impulse conduction becomes problematic. From a communication viewpoint, a number of interesting possibilities may arise distal to the branch in which a whole section of an axonal tree is activated, while another section remains quiescent. The more rapidly action potentials are generated, in fact, the more probable are axon conduction blocks and the more directional a neuron's electrical output may become. In essence, simple cable properties of an axon can now become the most important factor in the transformation of temporal events (for example, action potential frequency) into a spatial pattern of output. The more complicated its morphological features, the more important the axon becomes as a factor in neuronal communication.

Presynaptic Terminal

A transmissive structure called the presynaptic terminal is the last element in the classic three-compartment model of a mammalian neuron (dendrites and soma; axon; presynaptic terminal). Chemical, electrical, and chemical-electrical synapses have been described. The biochemistry of the presynaptic region of the chemical synapse has assumed an unparalleled importance in neurophysiology and pharmacology; yet, for all its complexities, the function of this synapse is fairly concise. The presynaptic terminal has the ability to convert one form of energy into another; that is, the action potential generates an electrical field that results in mechanical movement of large proteins and the eventual liberation of a chemical (rather than an electrical) signal to postsynaptic elements (Fig. 8–3).

The presynaptic terminal is thus part of a functional contact between cells, called a synapse. A chemical synapse has two remarkable properties: (1) input-output relationships are distinctly nonlinear, with small presynaptic potentials above a threshold level producing a tenfold postsynaptic response, and (2) coupling between presynaptic and postsynaptic elements is contingent on that synapse's recent experience. Simply stated, even though neurons and their connections develop by a fixed plan, the strength or effectiveness of each connection between neurons is not predetermined. The history of a chemical synapse alters the effectiveness of neuronal communication, and it is this structure that embodies the concept of neuronal plasticity.

Plasticity and Chemical Synapse

The plastic capabilities of neurons can be demonstrated in many ways. Perhaps the simplest and most illustrative example is to monitor the effects of usage on a neuronal pathway obtained through repetitive electrical stimulation. The stellate ganglion of the cat has preganglionic and postganglionic neurons connected at a single synapse. After repetitive stimulation of the presynaptic fibers (tetanic stimulation), the number of postsynaptic cells that are discharged when a *single* electrical stimulus is later applied is greatly enhanced. Because the enhancement of chemical transmission persists after the period of tetanization, the phenomenon is termed post-tetanic facilitation or potentiation. Although the facilitation may last only minutes in the example provided, facilitation can last hours through the use of longer tetanizations or the stimulation of other synapses. Enhanced discharge rates of these and other postsynaptic neurons have been shown to result from an augmentation of neurotransmitter release from presynaptic elements. Each action potential that invades the presynaptic terminal after tetanic facilitation produces a larger release of neurotransmitter and thus a bigger postsynaptic response.

In addition to chemical synapses, electrical synapses, characterized by unique synaptic structures called gap junctions, have been demonstrated for invertebrates and in structures such as the retina, cortex, hippocampus, and hypothalamus of vertebrates. These electrical synapses have the advantage of speed and reliable information transfer but do not share the plastic properties of the chemical synapse. The chick ciliary ganglion, for example, contains a dual chemical-electrical synapse between preganglion and postganglion fibers. After tetanization, only the chemical synapse demonstrates facilitated transmission, while the electrical syn-

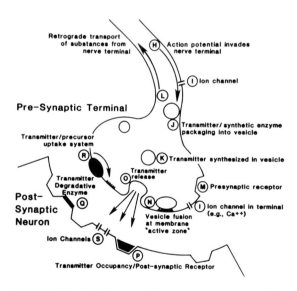

FIGURE 8–3. Diagram of the presynaptic terminal. (From Uhl, G.R.: Transmitters and receptors, in Diseases of the Nervous System: Clinical Neurobiology, A.K. Asbury, G.M. McKhann, and W.I. McDonald (eds.). Philadelphia, W.B. Saunders, 1986.)

TABLE 8–1.   Mechanisms Modifying Information Transfer and Encoding Within a Single Neuron

Receptive elements	Dendrodendritic interactions
	Dendritic-soma interactions
	Soma-trigger zone electrotonic effects, including autoactive rhythms
Conductive elements	Changes in passive electrical properties
	Selective modification of ionic processes for action potentials
	Changes in number of remote trigger sites
	Axon conduction blocks
Transmissive elements	Homosynaptic and heterosynaptic changes in presynaptic membrane potential
	Presynaptic and postsynaptic receptor regulation (number and possible affinity)
	Changes in functional neurotransmitter pools (dynamics, number, transmitter concentration)
	Use of "comodulators"
	Joint electrical and chemical synapses

aptic potential remains unaffected. Humans, therefore, have sacrificed speed by having a tremendous preponderance of chemical synapses within the brain but have gained an enormous potential for adaptability.

Mechanisms modifying information transfer within a single neuron are listed in Table 8–1.

Small-System Operating Characteristics

Mechanisms of posttetanic facilitation and depression at chemical synapses suggest that environmental requirements can alter very fundamental properties of neurotransmission. Other phenomena exist in systems of multiple neurons; for example, repetitive use of one pathway may change transmission characteristics in another. These interacting systems are anatomically related through presynaptic contacts that may be chemical or electrical in nature or both. Either presynaptic inhibition or augmentation of transmitter release thus can occur by a graded hyperpolarization or depolarization of the membrane. When depolarization is noted, the phenomenon is termed heterosynaptic facilitation.

Chemical synapses, electrical synapses, and geometric effects on electrotonic spread suggest that the neuron can be an extraordinarily reliable and sophisticated communication device. Reliable and efficient communication can be ensured when the rate of information flow is reduced to a point below total channel capacity. The most obvious way that humans reduce information flow in speech, for example, is simply by speaking slower. But there is a second technique to reduce information rate and yet maintain high reliability. This technique may actually saturate channel capacity, but it generally reduces information uncertainty by creating context and deliberately using redundancy. In es-

sence, it transmits the same information spread over different systems and symbols. For example, a didactic, compact verbal presentation is less effective than a rapid, redundant one with multiple examples, restatements, and illustrations. Misrepresentation of an important point (that is, an error) will not damage message integrity if context has been created. Within the nervous system, context and redundancy have also clearly been demonstrated. When events are transmitted over parallel neuronal pathways that have different biochemical and electrical representations, and when groups of such neurons are coupled, even complicated behaviors can be accurately represented.

Summary

Behavior is not predetermined, because neuronal communication has built-in plasticity. Even though genetic makeup produces an invariant structural basis for behavior, the relative importance of any connection is largely determined by experience. To predict the future operating characteristics of a synapse, one must understand its immediate history.

The neuron can be structurally and functionally compartmentalized. Each component contributes to an integrated output, which occurs through the use of chemical and electrical energy. The geometry of the neuron may be as important as its chemical composition, and this feature may help the central nervous system convert temporal events into spatial representations. Likewise, the importance of chemical transmission cannot be overemphasized. The chemical synapse amplifies presynaptic events and, in large measure, provides for adaptability. Finally, the properties of small populations of neurons may not be readily discernible from the behavior of individual elements. Groups of coupled neurons provide an enormous capability for information flow and create order in an unpredictable environment.

NEUROCHEMISTRY

General Concepts of Synapse

The neurochemistry of behavior is the chemistry of the synapse—the presynaptic terminal, the synaptic cleft, and the postsynaptic membrane. A brief review of the major morphological features of this functional connection is appropriate and is annotated with appropriate comments.

1. Presynaptic and postsynaptic membranes are fairly close together; there is no intervening cellular material.

The synaptic cleft is approximately 100 to 200 μm wide, although some preparations have demonstrated almost complete closure of the gap for resolutions of about 25 μm. A synaptic ground substance is present but is poorly organized. The material is a complex of highly hydrated molecules of mucopolysaccharides and protein in an ionic environment partially regulated by glia.

2. The presynaptic terminal and, to a lesser degree, the postsynaptic terminal contain vesicular structures 400 to 500 μm in diameter.

Vesicles may result from the breakup of an interconnected tubular system that is continuous with the surface membrane. The sarcoplasmic reticulum in muscle, for example, is continuous with the external environment but appears to be vesicular on section. Indeed, a statistical distribution of round to oval profiles similar to those seen in synaptic terminals can be obtained by sectioning spaghetti embedded in gelatin. Stereoscopic views of the synaptic terminal, however, definitely suggest round vesicular structures.

3. Within synaptic terminals, a large number of mitochondria are present, with specialized structures generally absent near presynaptic membranes.

Many morphological criteria for synapses are fulfilled in many regions that are nonsynaptic. A definition of the synapse must include both functional and anatomic criteria.

4. Presynaptic and postsynaptic membranes are inhomogeneous, highly fluid structures that contain specialized regions (receptors) to interact with chemical mediators.

Membrane fluidity is three dimensional (the surface layer and in and out) and can be greatly modified by exogenous substances such as drugs. The essential function of synaptic receptors is to add charge to (hyperpolarize), or remove charge from (depolarize), membranes. Hyperpolarization and depolarization are usually mediated by different receptors, but the direction of voltage change is contingent on both the receptor and the chemical mediator. Thus, in theory, the same chemical neurotransmitter may be excitatory in one brain region and inhibitory in another. Presynaptic receptors can modulate the firing rate of a neuron and thus change neurotransmitter release.

5. Neurotransmitters are synthesized in the presynaptic terminal cytoplasm, stored in vesicles, and subsequently released.

The cell body synthesizes the proteins and enzymes necessary to make chemical neuromodulators and transports this material down the axon by fast and slow processes. Within the presynaptic terminal, neurotransmitters may be stored in vesicles bound to adenosine triphosphate (ATP) and protein in a definite stoichiometric relationship. Vesicular storage keeps the compound physiologically inactive and protects it from degradation by ubiquitous catabolic enzymes.

As an action potential invades the terminal, vesicles move toward the presynaptic membrane through a calcium-dependent mechanism. Vesicles fuse with the presynaptic membrane, release their contents into the synaptic cleft, and collectively produce miniature postsynaptic potentials. Some vesicles are more resistant to electromechanical coupling than others, and functional compartments, that is, "neurotransmitter pools," are usually described. Different pools are available for release and may be replenished from neurotransmitters within the cytoplasm. It is also probable that, in some systems, the releasable transmitter is in the cytoplasm rather than in a vesicle. More than one substance may be released as a chemical neurotransmitter (a violation of Dale's principle of biochemical specificity). In addition, "comodulators" have been described that both have a trophic function on postsynaptic elements and alter the input-output relationship of the synaptic transform.

6. The presynaptic terminal has a major role in the termination of a neurotransmitter effect.

After release, the action of a neurotransmitter can be terminated by three different events: (1) diffusion into the bloodstream (or glia), (2) enzymatic degradation within the synaptic cleft, or (3) reentry into the presynaptic terminal. Depending on the transmitter, certain mechanisms predominate. For example, the neurotransmitter acetylcholine is mainly destroyed by enzymatic hydrolysis within the cleft; very little diffuses away, and none reenters the presynaptic terminal. On the other hand, catecholamines and indoleamines (serotonin) are preferentially removed from the cleft by an uptake mechanism, with synaptic degradation playing a secondary role. Except under somewhat artificial circumstances, diffusion from the cleft is insignificant.

Neurotransmitter Criteria

Neurotransmitters are chemicals that convey information, contained within action potentials, across synaptic clefts to neighboring target cells. They are released into the synaptic cleft on depolarization at the presynaptic terminal. Subsequent to their release, they diffuse across the cleft to alter electrical and biochemical properties of postsynaptic elements.

A large number of substances within the brain can serve as a chemical neurotransmitter or neuromodulator. Only a fraction of these substances have met what are generally accepted as criteria in support of neurotransmission. These criteria are presented simply to emphasize that the degree of interest in any central nervous system transmitter may reflect ease of study rather than physiological importance.

1. The candidate neurotransmitter should be present in highest concentration within presynaptic terminals.
2. The substance should be released in a calcium-dependent manner on electrical and potassium-induced depolarization.
3. The candidate transmitter, when it is applied to the postsynaptic membrane, should mimic the effects of electrical stimulation of the presynaptic terminal.
4. The effects of presynaptic electrical stimulation and exogenous transmitter application should be altered in parallel by drugs known to change the natural synaptic potentials.
5. The candidate transmitter should bind to postsynaptic membranes in a stereoselective and saturable fashion with high affinity.
6. A mechanism of rapid synaptic inactivation of the electrical and biochemical effects of the neurotransmitter should exist.

Neurotransmitter Mechanisms

Despite the wide variety of chemically distinct neurotransmitter candidates, all mediate synaptic transmission through a common and finite number of effects on postsynaptic cells. Neurotransmitters affect the electrical excitability of postsynaptic membranes by changing transmembrane permeabilities to one or more ions, thus changing membrane resistance.

The resting membrane potential (RMP) of the postsynaptic membrane is negatively charged, inside with respect to outside, and removed from the equilibrium potential of the major ionic species. The resting membrane potential is maintained by the asymmetrical ionic concentration of various species because of selective membrane permeability to certain ions and the activity of energy-dependent ionic pumps. A neurotransmitter-induced increase in membrane permeability to a specific ion results in movement of the membrane potential toward the equilibrium potential for that ion. If permeability to either K^+ or Cl^- is increased, the net result is membrane hyperpolarization, whereas an increase in permeability to Na^+ results in depolarization. An increase in transmembrane permeability to any ion is associated with a decrease in transmembrane resistance. These postsynaptic responses to a neurotransmitter are termed "fast," require no energy, and are driven by electrochemical concentration gradients. The increases in ionic permeability are thought to be due to the transmitter-activated opening of specific ion channels. "Fast" channels are thought to exist for both Na^+ and K^+, and for Na^+ alone.

"Slower" transmitter-activated increases in postsynaptic membrane permeabilities to specific ions are also known to occur. These "slower" transmitter-activated ionic channels may be responsible for mediating a variety of sustained effects on the postsynaptic neuron, in addition to alterations in the electrical excitability of their membranes. For example, the "slower" transmitter-activated increase in calcium permeability discovered in invertebrates may influence a variety of calcium-dependent processes, besides immediate effects on transmembrane electrical potential.

A second mechanism by which neurotransmitters affect the electrical excitability of postsynaptic membranes is the structural alteration of membrane resistance. These effects are more prolonged, are energy dependent, and appear to be mediated by secondary messengers, for example, cyclic adenosine monophosphate (cAMP).

In general, relatively constant levels of neurotransmitter are maintained within presynaptic nerve terminals despite marked fluctuations in neural activity. The regulation and maintenance of a readily releasable pool of neurotransmitter molecules are controlled by a number of mechanisms. These regulatory mechanisms include effects on synthesis, storage, and release of neurotransmitter by the neuron. For example, the biosynthesis of active neurotransmitter can be influenced by product inhibition of the rate-controlling step, cofactor or precursor availability, hormonal factors, oxygen tension, and the number of synthetic enzyme molecules.

Complete information is available for only a few neurotransmitters and candidates. Table 8–2 shows one system of classifying neurotransmitters, neuromodulators, and neuroreceptors. The following are among those most studied: catecholamines (dopamine, norepinephrine), serotonin, acetylcholine, histamine, γ-aminobutyric acid (GABA), glycine, glutamate, and aspartate.

Catecholamines

Catecholamines are a group of neurotransmitters derived from a common metabolic step, the enzymatic hydroxylation of tyrosine (Fig. 8–4). Within the central nervous system, these compounds occur in distinct pathways and are involved in a wide variety of essential processes. Catecholamines include dopamine, norepinephrine (also called noradrenaline), and epinephrine (adrenaline). Since epinephrine is principally located in the adrenal medulla, its role in central

TABLE 8–2.   Representative Neurotransmitters, Neurotransmitter Candidates, and Receptors

Neurotransmitter		*Receptor(s)*
	I. Classic	
A. Cholinergic	1. Acetylcholine	1. Muscarinic cholinergic, M_1 and M_2
		2. Nicotinic cholinergic
B. Monoaminergic	1. Norepinephrine	1. Alpha adrenergic, $\alpha1$ and $\alpha2$
	2. Epinephrine	2. Beta adrenergic, $\beta1$ and $\beta2$
	3. Dopamine	3. Dopaminergic, D1 an D2
	4. Serotonin	4. Serotonin, 5-HT_1 and 5-HT_2
	5. Histamine	5. Histamine, H_1 and H_2
	II. Amino Acid	
	1. γ-Aminobutyric acid (GABA)	1. GABA
		1a. Coupled benzodiazepine
	2. Glutamate	2. Glutamate, several subtypes
	3. Glycine	3. Glycine
	4. Aspartate	4. Aspartate
	III. Cyclic Nucleotides	
	1. Adenosine	1. Adenosine A_1 and A_2
	IV. Peptide	
A. Opiate	1. Enkephalin (met-leu-)	μ opiate
		δ opiate
	2. β-Endorphin	κ opiate
	3. Dynorphin	σ opiate
B. Releasing inhibiting factors	1. Thyrotropin releasing hormone	1. TRH
	2. Somatostatin (14 to 28)	2. Somatostatin
	3. Corticotropin releasing hormone	3. CRF
	4. Gonadotropin releasing hormone	4. GnRH
C. Widely distributed	1. Cholecystokinin (8 and 33)	1. CCK
	2. Neurotensin	2. Neurotensin
	3. Vasoactive intestinal peptide	3. VIP
	4. Substance P/substance K	4. Substance P/substance K
	5. Motilin	5. Motilin
	6. Neuropeptide Y	6. NPY
D. Posterior pituitary	1. Vasopressin	1. Vasopressin
	2. Oxytocin	2. Oxytocin
E. Other	1. Bradykinin	1. Bradykinin
	2. α–Melanocyte-stimulating hormone	2. α-MSH
	3. Angiotensin	3. Angiotensin
	4. CGRP	4. Calcitonin/CGRP
	5. Glucagon-like	5. Glucagon-like
	6. Insulin	6. Insulin
	7. Carnosine	7. Carnosine
	8. Atrial enaturietic factor	8. AEF

CGRP = calcitonin gene-related peptide
From: Uhl, G.R.: in Diseases of the Nervous System: Clinical Neurobiology, A.K. Asbury, G.M. McKhann, and W.I. McDonald (eds.). Philadelphia, W.B. Saunders, 1986.

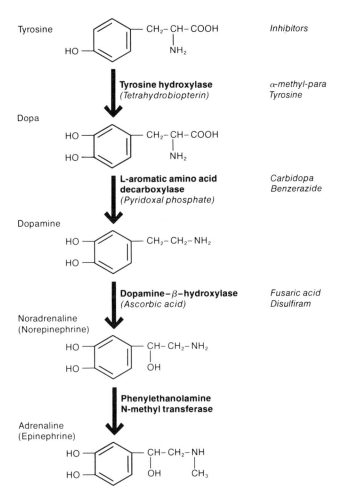

FIGURE 8–4.   Enzymatic hydroxylation of tyrosine in the sequential synthesis of catecholamines. (Courtesy Upjohn Company.)

neurotransmission is probably limited. Dopamine and norepinephrine will be reviewed.

Dopamine

Dopamine Neuroanatomy

Dopamine is located in well-defined tracts depicted in the longitudinal brain section shown in Figure 8–5. Five different pathways exist: three long tracts; one tract of intermediate length; and ultrashort tracts located in the retina (not shown). Dopaminergic tracts arise from three locations: long tracts sprout from the substantia nigra *(A9)* or ventral tegmental area *(A10)*, near the brain stem; intermediate tracts arise only from the hypothalamus. The innervation pattern of a tract naturally determines the effect of its activation. Figure 8–6 is a schematic representation of dopaminergic projections in the human forebrain.

Nigrostriatal Tract.   The long tract called the nigrostriatal tract regulates movement by innervation of the caudate nucleus, putamen, and globus pallidus. If dopaminergic transmission is altered in this area, a change occurs in the amount of movement and its coordination. The "pill rolling" hand movements and shuffling gait seen in persons with Parkinson's disease occur after reduction in dopaminergic transmission, whereas direct (apomorphine) and indirect (amphetamine) dopamine agonists increase the general level of movement and stereotypy.

Mesolimbic Tract.   The mesolimbic tract innervates the septum and related areas, suggesting a role in the motoric expression of emotional states.

Mesocortical Tract.   The mesocortical projection into the cortex may be partially respon-

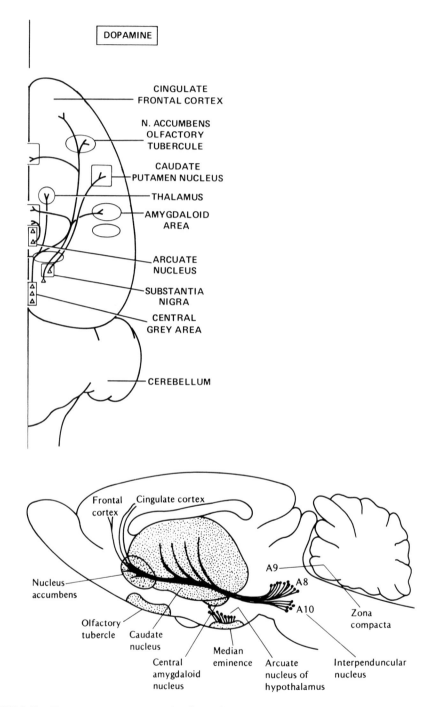

FIGURE 8–5.   Dopamine neuroanatomy of rat brain. (From Ciaranello, R.D., Patrick, R.L.: Catecholamine neuroregulators, in Psychopharmacology: From Theory to Practice, J.D. Barchas, et al. (eds.). New York, Oxford University Press, 1977.)

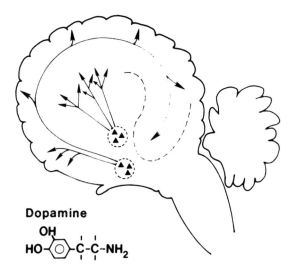

Dopamine

FIGURE 8–6. Schematic representation of dopaminergic projections in the human forebrain. (From Coyle, J.T.: Aminergic projections from the reticular core, in Diseases of the Nervous System: Clinical Neurobiology, A.K. Asbury, G.M. McKhann, and W.I. McDonald (eds.). Philadelphia, W.B. Saunders, 1986.)

sible for the experience of emotion and for the decision process that precedes the act of choice. The mesolimbic and mesocortical tracts hold the most interest for psychiatrists and yet are the least understood projections of the dopaminergic system.

Tuberoinfundibular Tract. The tuberoinfundibular tract connects the pituitary gland to the hypothalamus. This pathway influences the secretory activity of the anterior lobe of the pituitary gland and has poorly specified functions in heat loss, satiety, rage, and gastric acidity. Thus a direct dopamine agonist such as apomorphine produces hypothermia in humans and, in addition, elevates growth hormone and suppresses prolactin concentrations; dopamine antagonists, such as neuroleptics, can do the opposite. The tuberoinfundibular tract can be used as a rough monitor of dopaminergic activity for all of the tracts.

Dopamine Neurochemistry

All dopamine tracts employ identical synthetic and catabolic mechanisms in the utilization of neurotransmitters. Figure 8–4 presents the synthetic pathways for catecholamines, of which dopamine is an example. Tyrosine is the precursor taken into the presynaptic terminal by passive processes. The synthetic machinery first creates a catechol by adding a hydroxyl group to the ring; it then creates an amine by removal

of a carboxyl group from the side chain. Thus a two-step process is required to create a catecholamine. The addition of the hydroxyl group occurs through use of a very specific enzyme; the removal of the carboxyl group requires a nonspecific enzyme. Both reactions occur in the cytoplasm before vesicular uptake.

Of the two enzymes, the nonspecific one (L-aromatic acid decarboxylase) is of secondary importance. The specific enzyme, tyrosine hydroxylase, is the rate-limiting step in the synthetic process; it is a "choke point" that can be maximally saturated by precursor and regulated in part by the cofactor tetrahydrobiopterin. Tyrosine hydroxylase is also subject to regulation by the concentration of dopamine (end-product inhibition), which may be monitored through specialized autoreceptors on the presynaptic terminal.

Once dopamine is released from the presynaptic terminal, its action is generally terminated by uptake, although extraneuronal degradation and diffusion may occur. Enzymatic breakdown requires two major enzymes that convert dopamine to homovanillic acid (HVA) and, to a lesser extent, dihydroxyphenylacetic acid (DOPAC). The sequence in which the major enzymes react with dopamine largely determines intermediate reaction products (Fig. 8–7). HVA, mainly from the nigrostriatal tract, serves as a monitor of central nervous system dopaminergic activity.

See the discussion under the heading Dopamine, in Chapter 12: Hypothalamic Control. See also the discussion under the heading Dopaminergic System in Depression, in Chapter 26: Pathogenesis of Mood Disorders. For a discussion of the dopamine hypothesis of schizophrenia, see Chapter 28: Biology of Schizophrenia.

Norepinephrine

Norepinephrine Neuroanatomy

The anatomy and biochemistry of the norepinephrine (noradrenaline), or noradrenergic, system are similar to those of the dopaminergic system. All cell bodies are located in the hindbrain, principally the pons and medulla, and the most abundant number of cells arise in the locus coeruleus (Figs. 8–8 and 8–9). Although most of the innervation is unilateral, a substantial number of contralateral axons exist. Projections are widespread; pathways have been identified into the spinal cord, cerebellum, a number of limbic system structures, and the cortex. This

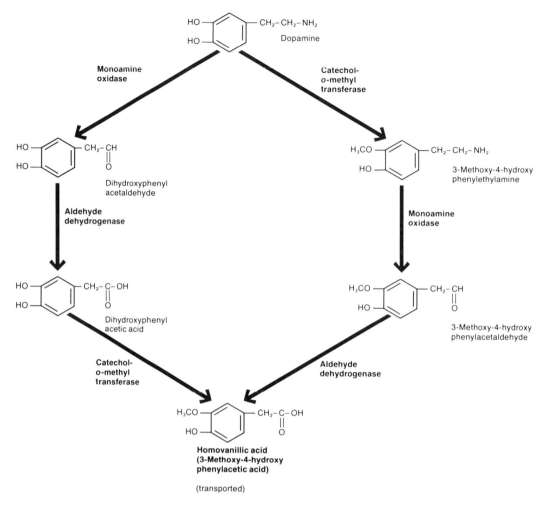

FIGURE 8–7. Dopamine catabolism. (Courtesy Upjohn Company.)

diffuse type of projection suggests a neuromodulatory role for norepinephrine, rather than discrete and easily delineated behavioral responsibilities. Indeed, the ability to modulate attention, perception, mood, locomotion, and cardiovascular phenomena has been demonstrated for noradrenergic projection systems. With such a broad range of functions, it is not surprising that modification of noradrenergic activity can be therapeutic in syndromes in which many physiological parameters are altered, such as narcotic abstinence.

Norepinephrine Neurochemistry

The synthesis of norepinephrine continues as an extension of the metabolic pathway for dopamine (Fig. 8–4). Norepinephrine is derived from dopamine by the addition of a hydroxyl group to the side chain. This reaction occurs in the storage vesicles, rather than the cytoplasm, of noradrenergic neurons after dopamine has been synthesized and transported into the vesicles. The enzyme responsible for the conversion is dopamine β-hydroxylase (DBH), which is not saturated by dopamine under normal physiological conditions.

As with dopamine, the noradrenergic neuron has self-regulating mechanisms, and an autoreceptor (α_2) has been characterized. Activation of the receptor (for example, by a drug such as clonidine) causes the cell to stop firing and norepinephrine is no longer released. Other regulating presynaptic receptors have different characteristics, and compounds such as opiates, prostaglandins, GABA, and dopamine can modify noradrenergic function through specific presynaptic loci of action.

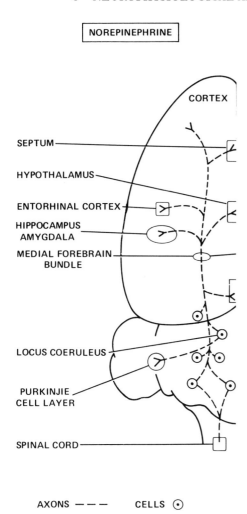

NOREPINEPHRINE

AXONS — — — CELLS ⊙

FIGURE 8–8. Noradrenergic pathways in the rat brain. (From Ciaranello, R.D., Patrick, R.L.: Catecholamine neuroregulators, in Psychopharmacology: From Theory to Practice, J.D. Barchas, et al. (eds.). New York, Oxford University Press, 1977.)

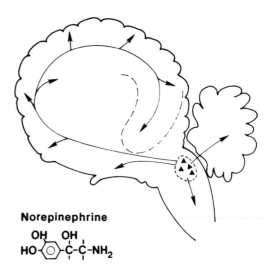

Norepinephrine

FIGURE 8–9. Schematic representation of the projections from the noradrenergic locus coeruleus in the pons. (From Coyle, J.T.: Aminergic projections from the reticular core, in Diseases of the Nervous System: Clinical Neurobiology, A.K. Asbury, G.M. McKhann, and W.I. McDonald (eds.). Philadelphia, W.B. Saunders, 1986.)

Norepinephrine catabolism is more complex than that of dopamine (Fig. 8–10). See the discussion under the heading Norepinephrine in Chapter 12: Hypothalamic Control. See also the discussions under the headings Noradrenergic System in Depression (Chapter 26: Pathogenesis of Mood Disorders) and Norepinephrine (Chapter 28: Biology of Schizophrenia).

Serotonin

Serotonin Neuroanatomy

Serotoninergic pathways emanate from cell bodies situated in midline raphe nuclei (Figs.

8–11 and 8–12). Projections are inadequately described, but innervation of the forebrain, lateral geniculate, superior colliculus, and especially limbic system structures occurs. Another important pathway extends into the spinal cord, is functionally connected to enkephalinergic and substance P neurons, and may have a significant role in pain perception. A striking quality of serotoninergic neurons is their tonic firing activity, invariably of an inhibitory quality, which may subserve a pacemaker function within the central nervous system. Serotoninergic neurons in general have a widespread behavioral suppressant quality; changes in arousal, sexual interest, aggression, and the ability to pursue goal-directed behavior are intimately contingent on the operating characteristics of this system.

Serotonin Neurochemistry

The indoleamine serotonin (5-hydroxytryptamine, 5-HT) is synthesized from the essential amino acid tryptophan (Fig. 8–13). Less than 2 percent of dietary tryptophan is eventually converted to 5-HT; the precursor must be taken up into the brain by an energy-dependent process, and very wide fluctuations in *plasma* tryptophan concentration do little to modify serotoninergic function (although clinical anecdotes suggest otherwise). Tryptophan is hydroxylated on the six-membered aromatic ring of the indole by

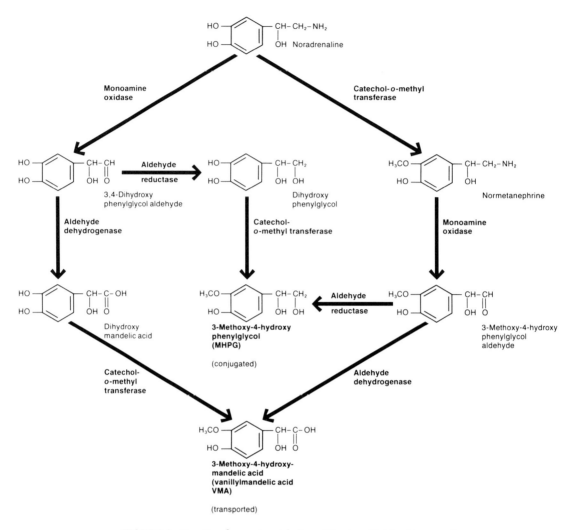

FIGURE 8–10.   Noradrenergic catabolism. (Courtesy Upjohn Company.)

tryptophan hydroxylase, with tetrahydrobio-pterin as a cofactor. As in the case of tyrosine hydroxylase, this enzyme is the rate-limiting step of the synthetic pathway.

Tryptophan hydroxylase, however, is apparently not subject to end-product inhibition; under normal conditions, substrate concentrations are below enzyme capacity. 5-Hydroxy-tryptophan, the product of ring hydroxylation, is decarboxylated (the indole side chain) by *L*-aromatic acid decarboxylase to create serotonin.

5-HT is stored in presynaptic vesicles and in a mobile extragranular pool. Its action is terminated by an energy-dependent uptake process that may be inhibited by the presence of certain antidepressants. Three enzymes account for the principal catabolic pathway with the initial event, aldehyde formation, through mito-

chondrial monoamine oxidase (MAO). The aldehyde is then reduced (minor path) or dehydrogenated (major path). The dehydrogenated product, 5-hydroxyindoleacetic acid (5-HIAA) can be used as a monitor of 5-HT metabolism in the brain.

Acetylcholine

Acetylcholine Neuroanatomy

Acetylcholine (or cholinergic) pathways have been defined only recently, and much of the evidence for their existence has been indirect. The best technique has employed immunohistochemical staining of the enzyme choline acetyltransferase (CAT) as a fairly specific marker for cholinergic neurons (acetylcholinesterase is

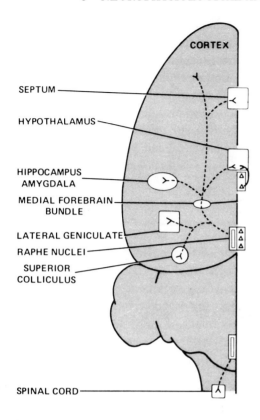

CORTEX

SEPTUM

HYPOTHALAMUS

HIPPOCAMPUS
AMYGDALA

MEDIAL FOREBRAIN
BUNDLE

LATERAL GENICULATE

RAPHE NUCLEI

SUPERIOR
COLLICULUS

SPINAL CORD

AXONS ----- CELLS

FIGURE 8-11. Serotoninergic pathways in the rat brain. (From Elliott, G.R., et al.: Indoleamines and other neuroregulators, in Psychopharmacology: From Theory to Practice, J.D. Barchas et al. (eds.). New York, Oxford University Press, 1977.)

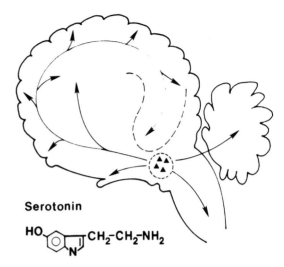

Serotonin

HO⟨⟩CH$_2$-CH$_2$-NH$_2$

FIGURE 8-12. Schematic representation of the projections from the serotoninergic raphe nuclei in the midbrain. (From Coyle, J.T.: Aminergic projections from the reticular core, in Diseases of the Nervous System: Clinical Neurobiology, A.K. Asbury, G.M. McKhann, and W.I. McDonald (eds.). Philadelphia, W.B. Saunders, 1986.)

not). Cholinergic pathways broadly include ventral horn cells to all muscles, striatal interneurons, and cortical and hippocampal projections from an area medial to the globus pallidus and the septum (Fig. 8-14). Projections from near the globus pallidus arise in a phylogenetically old area of the septum containing three nuclei: the nucleus basalis, the nucleus diagonal band of Broca, and the preoptic nucleus. Of these three nuclei, the diagonal band and the basalis have the most input from the hippocampus and have generated the most clinical interest. It should be noted that all cholinergic pathways may be interconnected by a major ascending tegmental-mesencephalic-cortical system. In addition, cholinergic synapses are mainly muscarinic within the cerebrum and nicotinic within the brain stem. Functions of acetylcholine are manifold and include sleep, arousal, nociception, the modulation and coordination

of movement, and memory acquisition and retention.

Acetylcholine Neurochemistry

In contrast to the uncertainties of cholinergic neuroanatomy, the synthetic and catabolic pathways for acetylcholine are thoroughly characterized (Fig. 8-15). Acetylcholine synthesis occurs within the presynaptic cytoplasm through the combination of choline with an acetyl radical. Choline is available from the diet or is synthesized in the liver and enters the neuron by both passive and energy-dependent processes. There is evidence that the active process is a high-affinity choline uptake mechanism that is directly coupled to transmitter synthesis. The acetyl radical is provided by acetyl coenzyme A derived from general metabolic function. The enzyme CAT catalyzes this reaction, which is not saturated with precursor under normal physiological conditions. It is impossible to deplete a physiologically normal cholinergic neuron of neurotransmitter, without the addition of specific pharmacological toxins; there is no end-product inhibition.

After release, acetylcholine is subjected to hydrolysis by specific cholinesterases associated with presynaptic and postsynaptic membranes, as well as with the synaptic cleft. Cholinesterase has the distinction of being one of the faster enzymes within the body.

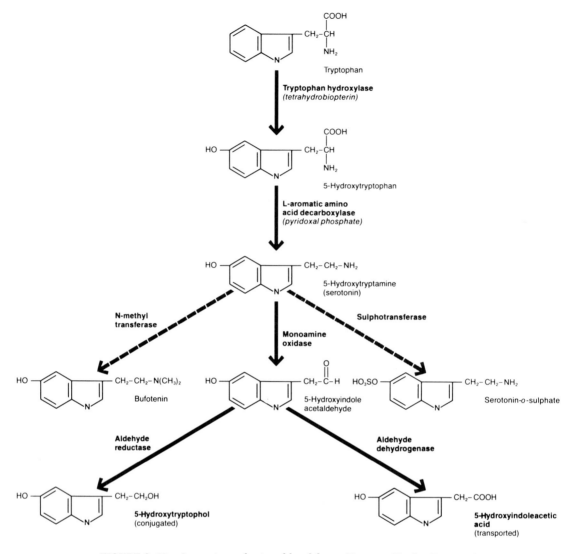

FIGURE 8–13.   Serotonin synthesis and breakdown. (Courtesy Upjohn Company.)

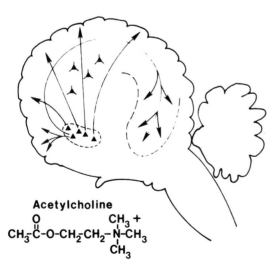

FIGURE 8–14.   Schematic representation of basal forebrain cholinergic projections. (From Coyle, J.T.: Aminergic projections from the reticular core, in Diseases of the Nervous System: Clinical Neurobiology. A.K. Asbury, G.M. McKhann, and W.I. McDonald (eds.). Philadelphia, W.B. Saunders, 1986.)

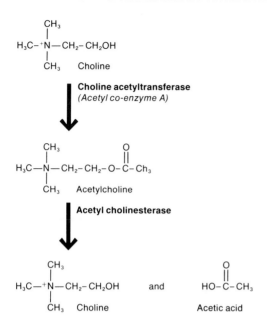

FIGURE 8–15. Acetylcholine synthesis and breakdown. (Courtesy Upjohn Company.)

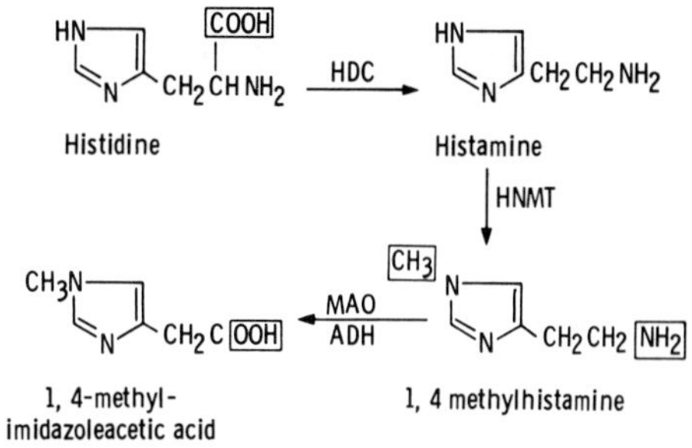

FIGURE 8–16. Synthesis and metabolism of histamine.

After acetylcholine is hydrolyzed, up to half the choline produced reenters the presynaptic terminal for resynthesis. The rate of acetylcholine synthesis is contingent on the firing rate of the neuron and the saturation of the high-affinity choline transport process. Thus, at face value, precursor loading with dietary choline to increase neurotransmitter synthesis has merit; that is, choline is nontoxic, there is no blood-brain barrier, choline is definitely taken into nerve terminals, and, in experimental manipulations, loading increases acetylcholine levels in specific brain regions with releasable neurotransmitter. Although possibly effective in many clinical disease states resulting from decreases in cholinergic transmission, precursor loading has proved to be of benefit in tardive dyskinesia. On the other hand, disorders of cognition such as Alzheimer's disease have generally proved to be more responsive to the alternative strategy of cholinesterase inhibition. For a discussion of precursor loading strategy, see Chapter 22: Delirium and Dementia.

See the discussion under the heading Dopaminergic System in Depression in Chapter 26: Pathogenesis of Mood Disorders. See also the discussion under the heading Acetylcholine-Dopamine Interaction in Chapter 28: Biology of Schizophrenia.

Histamine

Histamine is formed in a one-step decarboxylation of the amino acid histidine. Histidine is widely distributed in plants and animals and is a constituent of many venoms. The peripheral role of histamine in mediating allergic and inflammatory reactions has been known for well over five decades. Evidence strongly suggests that histamine also is a neurotransmitter within the central nervous system. Figure 8–16 shows the synthesis and metabolism of histamine.

Although the exact processes mediated by histamine within the central nervous system are uncertain, data suggest that histamine may play a role in depressive illness. A series of clinically effective antidepressant medications have been shown to selectively bind to histamine receptors within the central nervous system. The binding of these drugs to histamine receptors may, in part, be involved in some aspect of the therapeutic mechanism of action. The availability of potent, centrally active histamine antagonists should help to clarify the role of this neurotransmitter in the central nervous system.

See the discussion under the heading Histamine in Chapter 12: Hypothalamic Control.

GABA

γ-Aminobutyric acid (GABA) is an inhibitory neurotransmitter widely distributed throughout invertebrate and vertebrate nervous systems. Pharmacological interest in this neurotransmitter has intensified as a result of studies showing that (1) saturable and stereoselective receptor binding of GABA exists within a well-defined "supramolecular" receptor complex; (2) the anticonvulsant and anxiolytic properties of benzodiazepines may be mediated, in part, through

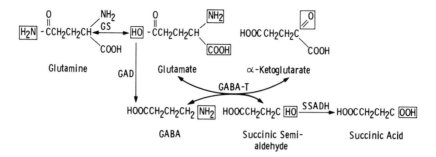

FIGURE 8–17.   Synthesis and metabolism of GABA.

GABA-mimetic properties; (3) interference with GABA catabolism may be beneficial in the treatment of certain seizure disorders; and (4) deficiency of GABA and its synthetic enzyme occur in the basal ganglia of patients with Huntington's chorea.

Figure 8–17 shows the synthesis and metabolism of GABA. Figure 8–18 shows some putative inhibitory and excitatory interrelationships and pathways of GABA and other neurotransmitters.

See the discussion under the heading GABA in Chapter 12: Hypothalamic Control. For a possible role of GABA in schizophrenia, see the discussion under the heading GABA in Chapter 28: Biology of Schizophrenia.

Glycine

Glycine, the prototypic amino acid neurotransmitter, has been implicated in the pathogenesis of certain types of spastic disorders. Structurally, it is the simplest known amino acid, consisting of only two carbon atoms and being devoid of any distinctive chemical group. Glycine is released from spinal cord inhibitory interneurons and, within the spinal cord, has a proven role in mediating postsynaptic inhibition. More recent data suggest that glycine also serves a limited neurotransmitter role within supraspinal regions of the neuroaxis. Glycine, despite its structural simplicity, is an important molecule that is involved in a diversity of neurobiological processes. Glycine's localization and biochemistry are the most fully studied of all the potential amino acid neurotransmitters.

Glycine is a nonessential amino acid supplied by dietary protein and is readily transported across the blood-brain barrier into the central nervous system. It can be rapidly synthesized in an enzymatic interconversion with serine,

which can serve as an immediate source of glycine.

A "glycine encephalopathy" is known to occur with toxic accumulations of this neurotransmitter amino acid in the brain and cerebrospinal fluid. This accumulation arises as a result of diminished or absent mitochondrial decarboxylation of this amino acid. The pathogenesis of this

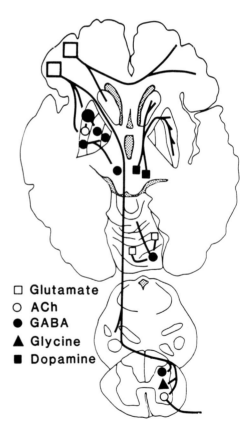

□ **Glutamate**
○ **ACh**
● **GABA**
▲ **Glycine**
■ **Dopamine**

FIGURE 8–18.   Putative inhibitory and excitatory relationships and the pathway of GABA. (From Young, A.B., Penney, J.B., Jr.: Pharmacologic aspects of motor dysfunction, in Diseases of the Nervous System: Clinical Neurobiology, A.K. Asbury, G.M. McKhann, and W.I. McDonald (eds.). Philadelphia, W.B. Saunders, 1986.)

syndrome, also known as nonketotic hypergly-cinemia, is thought to be due to both elevated levels of this neurotransmitter and diminution of the one-carbon pool.

Glutamate and Aspartate

Glutamate and aspartate are two additional putative amino acid neurotransmitters within the central nervous system. The absence of specific antagonists to their synaptic action has delayed identification of glutamate and aspartate transmitter tracts and characterization of receptors.

Pharmacological Implications

On the basis of the neurochemistry and neurophysiology of central nervous system neurons, at least six mechanisms of action may be available to pharmacological agents that disturb synaptic function.

1. Drugs can alter neurotransmitter synthesis.

2. Drugs can affect vesicular storage mechanisms and can selectively increase or decrease discharge.

3. Drugs can alter the rate of neurotransmitter degradation.

4. Drugs can block uptake mechanisms that terminate a transmitter's action. Antidepressants provide compounds that classically exert this effect.

5. Drugs can modify presynaptic regulatory responses through specific receptor interactions or change postsynaptic responsivity.

6. Drugs can alter the physical properties of synaptic membranes and change the rate of ionic flux. General anesthetics and alcohols are notorious membrane detergents at all dosage levels.

BIBLIOGRAPHY

Neurophysiological Basis of Behavior

Adey, W.R.: Neural information processing: Windows without and the citadel within, in Biocybernetics of the Central Nervous System, L.D. Proctor (ed.). Boston, Little, Brown, 1969.

Atwood, H.L., Wojtowicz, J.M.: Short-term and long-term plasticity and physiological differentiation of crustacean motor synapses. Int. Rev. Neurobiol. 28:275-362, 1986.

Bras, H., et al.: The dendrites of single brain-stem motoneurons intracellularly labelled with horseradish peroxidase in the cat: An ultrastructural analysis of the synaptic covering and the microenvironment. Neuroscience 22(3):971-981, 1987.

Burke, R.E.: Synaptic efficacy and the control of neuronal input-output relations. Trends Neurosci. 10:42-45, 1987.

Dunant, Y.: On the mechanism of acetylcholine release. Prog. Neurobiol. 26(1):55-92, 1986.

Grossman, Y., Kendig, J.J.: Modulation of impulse conduction through axonal branchpoint by physiological, chemical and physical factors. Israel J. Med. Sci. 23(1-2):107-114, 1987.

Gu, X.N., Macagno, E.R., Muller, K.J.: Laser microbeam axotomy and conduction block show that electrical transmission at a central synapse is distributed at multiple contacts. J. Neurobiol. (United States) 20(5):422-434, 1989.

Herkenham, M.: Mismatches between neurotransmitter and receptor localizations in brain: Observations and implications. Neuroscience 23(1):1-38, 1987.

Hughes, J.R., Evarts, E.V., Marshall, W.H.: Post-tetanic potentiation in the visual system of cats. Am. J. Physiol. 186:483-487, 1956.

Kandell, E.: Cellular Basis of Behavior: An Introduction to Behavioral Neurobiology. San Francisco, Freeman, 1976.

Kempinsky, W.H.: Experimental study of distant effects of acute focal brain injury—a study of diaschisis. Arch. Neurol. Psychiatry 79:376-389, 1958.

Kennedy, M.B.: Regulation of synaptic transmission in the central nervous system: long-term potentiation. Cell 59(5):777-787, 1989.

Knight, D.E., Baker, P.F.: Exocytosis from the vesicle viewpoint: An overview. Ann. N.Y. Acad. Sci. 493:504-525, 1987.

Landis, D.M.: Membrane and cytoplasmic structure at synaptic junctions in the mammalian central nervous system. J. Electron. Microsc. Tech. 10(2):129-151, 1988.

Larrabee, M.G., Bronk, D.W.: Prolonged facilitation of synaptic excitation in sympathetic ganglia. J. Neurophysiol. 10:139-154, 1947.

Luria, A.R.: Restoration of function after brain injury. New York, Macmillan, 1963.

Martin, A.R., Pilar, G.: Pre-synaptic and post-synaptic events during post-tetanic potentiation and facilitation in the avian ciliary ganglion. J. Physiol. (Lond.) 175:17-30, 1964.

Massey, J.L.: Information, machines and men, in Philosophy and Cybernetics, F.J. Crosson and K.M. Sayre (eds.). New York, Simon & Schuster, 1967.

Parnas, I.: Differential block at high frequency of branches of a single axon innervating two muscles. J. Neurophysiol. 35:903-914, 1972.

Parnas, I., Hochstein, S., Parnas, H.: Theoretical analysis of parameters leading to frequency modulation along an inhomogeneous axon. J. Neurophysiol. 39(4):909-923, 1976.

Roney, K.J., Scheibel, A.B., Shaw, G.L.: Dendritic bundles: Survey of anatomical experiments and physiological theories. Brain Res. Rev. 1:225-271, 1979.

Shaw, G.L., Harth, E., Scheibel, A.B.: Cooperativity in brain function: Assemblies of approximately 30 neurons. Exp. Neurol. 77(2):324-358, 1982.

Silinsky, E.M.: The biophysical pharmacology of calcium-dependent acetylcholine secretion. Pharmacol. Rev. 37(1):81-132, 1985.

Standaert, F.G.: Release of transmitter at the neuromuscular junction. Br. J. Anaesth. 54(2):131-145, 1982.

Tasaki, T.: A macromolecular approach to excitation phenomena: mechanical and thermal changes in nerve during excitation. Physiol Chem Phys Med NMR. 20(4):251-268, 1988.

Tauc, L.: Transmission in invertebrate and vertebrate ganglia. Physiol. Rev. 47:522-593, 1967.

Tauc, L.: Nonvesicular release of neurotransmitter. Physiol. Rev. 62(3):857-893, 1982.

Teyler, T.J., DiScenna, P.: Long-term potentiation. Ann. Rev. Neurosci. 10:131-161, 1987.

Thesleff, S.: Different kinds of acetylcholine release from the motor nerve. Int. Rev. Neurobiol. 28:59-88, 1986.

Vanderkloot, W.: Acetylcholine quanta are released from vesicles by exocytosis (and why some think not). Neuroscience 24(1):1-7, 1988.

Waxman, S.G.: Regional differentiation of the axon: A review with special reference to the concept of the multiplex neuron. Brain Res. 47:269-288, 1972.

Wilson, C.J.: Cellular mechanisms controlling the strength of synapses. J. Electron. Microsc. Tech. 10(3):293-313, 1988.

Wilson, H.R., Conan, J.D.: Excitatory and inhibitory interactions in localized populations of model neurons. Biophys. J. 12:1-22, 1972.

Neurochemical Basis of Behavior

Boarder, M.R.: Presynaptic aspects of cotransmission: relationship between vesicles and neurotransmitters. J. Neurochem. 53(1):1-11, 1989.

Elliott, G.R., et al.: Indoleamines and other neuroregulators, in Psychopharmacology: From Theory to Practice, J.D. Barchas et al. (eds.). New York: Oxford University Press, 1977, pp. 33-50.

Emson, P.C., Lindvall, O.: Distribution of putative neurotransmitters in the neocortex. Neuroscience 4:1-30, 1979.

Hornykiewicz, O.: Improvement of dopamine and dopamine receptors in brain disorders, in Frontiers in Cellular Surface Research. Westbury, New York, PJD Publications, 1982.

Jope, R.S.: High-affinity choline transport and acetyl CoA production in brain and their roles in the regulation of acetylcholine synthesis. Brain Res. Rev. 1:313-344, 1979.

Kandel, E.R., Schwartz, J.H.: Molecular biology of learning: Modulation of transmitter release. Science 218:433-443, 1982.

Levine, R.A., Miller, L.P., Lovenberg, W.: Tetrahydrobiopterin in striatum: Localization in dopamine nerve terminals and role in catecholamine synthesis. Science 214:919-921, 1981.

Malenka, R.C., Kauer, J.A., Perkel, D.J., Nicoll, R.A.: The impact of post synaptic calcium on synaptic transmission—its role in long-term potentiation. Trends Neurosci. 12(11):444-450, 1989.

McNaughton, N., Mason, S.T.: The neurophysiology and neuropharmacology of the dorsal ascending noradrenergic bundle—a review. Prog. Neurobiol. 14(213):157-219, 1980.

Nicoll, R.A.: The coupling of neurotransmitter receptors to ion channels in the brain. Science 241(4865):545-551, 1988.

Saper, C.B.: Function of the locus coeruleus. Trends Neurosci. 10(9):343-344, 1987.

Starke, K., Giothert, M., Kilbinger, H.: Modulation of neurotransmitter release by presynaptic autoreceptors. Physiol. Rev. 69(3):864 989, 1989.

Chapter 9

Neurotransmitter Receptor Function

Philip Kanof, M.D., Ph.D.

Neurons convey information to other neurons and other cell types in the body by the release of neurotransmitters. Neurotransmitters, acting on target organs, may induce changes in membrane potential, open ion channels, cause muscle contraction, induce secretion in glands, and have delayed effects such as regulation of protein synthesis. Molecules of neurotransmitter induce changes in postsynaptic cells by interacting with specific proteins, called receptors, located on the postsynaptic cell surface. The receptors present on these target organs are the biochemical transducers through which neurotransmitters, acting on the surface of the cell, influence physiological processes that occur in the interior of the cell.

The pharmacologic properties of receptors are defined by their interaction with different drugs. Compounds that mimic the physiologic effects of the neurotransmitter by activating the receptor are called agonists. Compounds that prevent the physiological effects of the neurotransmitter by binding to the receptor without activating it are called antagonists.

During synaptic transmission in the nervous system, activation of postsynaptic receptors by the neurotransmitter results in changes in the electrical properties of the neuronal membrane. These changes may include the alteration of membrane resistance or potential, the opening of specific ion channels, the activation of electrogenic pumps, and the generation of an action potential. The postsynaptic neuron may also have other delayed effects of receptor activation that occur as a result of biochemical effects of ion fluxes or of "second messengers." These delayed actions may include regulation of various enzymes involved in neurotransmitter synthesis and intermediary metabolism, as well as long-term regulation of the synthesis of specific proteins by the postsynaptic neuron.

Presynaptic neurons also often possess receptors for the neurotransmitter used by that neuron. These "autoreceptors" are located on the neuronal cell body and on synaptic terminals. Activation of autoreceptors on the cell body results in a decrease in the firing rate of the cell; activation of autoreceptors on the synaptic nerve terminals results in a decrease in the amount of neurotransmitter released per nerve impulse. These processes represent an inhibitory feedback mechanism that regulates the functional activity of the neuron.

LIGAND BINDING TECHNIQUE

The ligand binding technique has been widely used to study neurotransmitter receptors quantitatively. Ligands are radiolabeled drugs (usually antagonists) that bind with high affinity to the neurotransmitter receptor. Membrane fractions from the brain are incubated in the presence of various concentrations of the radiolabeled ligand. The ligand bound to the membrane is subsequently separated from the ligand not bound to the membrane by means of rapid filtration through a glass fiber filter. The radioactivity bound to the membrane fraction (and filter) is called the "total" binding.

Under these conditions, the radiolabeled ligand may bind not only to the receptor of interest but also to other membrane proteins, as well as to membrane lipids. To determine how much binding occurs specifically to the receptor, parallel incubations are done in the presence of a nonradioactive "displacing" ligand that prevents binding of the radiolabeled ligand to the receptor. This residual radioactivity bound to the membrane (and filter) under these conditions represents binding of the ligand to membrane lipid and to other nonreceptor membrane protein and is called the "nonspecific" binding. The difference between "total" and "nonspecific" binding represents the binding of the ligand to the receptor and is called the "specific" binding.

The pharmacological properties of receptors may be studied with this technique by measuring the capacity of different agonists and antagonists to displace bound ligand. The ability of various neurotransmitter receptor agonists and antagonists to displace specific ligand binding parallels their abilities to mimic or block the physiological effects of receptor activation. In addition, the ligand binding technique has been widely used to give quantitative information on the number of receptors present in different tissues.

RECEPTOR TYPES

Different biochemical mechanisms are involved in the function of different types of receptors. Three representative types of receptors are considered here: (1) a receptor directly coupled to an ionophore—the nicotinic cholinergic receptor; (2) a receptor coupled to adenylate cyclase—the β-adrenergic receptor; and (3) a receptor coupled to phosphatidylinositol turnover—the muscarinic cholinergic receptor.

Nicotinic Cholinergic Receptor

The nicotinic cholinergic receptor for acetylcholine is present at the neuromuscular junction. In muscle, acetylcholine induces the opening of an ion channel (ionophore). This causes an increase in the permeability of the membrane to sodium and potassium ions, leading to depolarization of the membrane and to the generation of an action potential in the muscle. The action of acetylcholine at the nicotinic receptor is mimicked by agonists such as carbamylcholine and is blocked by antagonists such as curare and certain snake venoms (for example, α-bungarotoxin).

The nicotinic receptor found in certain electrical fish (such as the marine electric ray *Torpedo marmorata*) has been studied extensively. The electric organ of *Torpedo*, containing an array of cholinergic terminals arranged in series, is highly enriched in nicotinic receptors. In the receptor from the nerve cell membranes of *Torpedo electroplax*, the purified receptor appears to exist as a dimer of two identical subunits, linked together by disulfide bridges and each a pentamer containing four peptides with the structure $\alpha_2\beta\gamma\delta$ (where each Greek letter denotes a distinct peptide).

Drugs that act at the nicotinic receptor, including agonists such as nicotine and antagonists such as curare and α-bungarotoxin, compete with acetylcholine for binding to the α subunit. (Each nicotinic receptor dimer is capable of binding four molecules of acetylcholine.) Each of the subunits is an integral membrane protein and traverses the entire cell membrane.

When *Torpedo* membranes or purified receptors reconstituted into lipid vesicles are examined by electron microscopy, each monomer of the nicotinic receptor appears as a hollow cylinder traversing the cell membrane along its length. The binding of acetylcholine to its recognition site on the external surface of the α subunit of the receptor is believed to cause a conformational change in the receptor, opening up the inner hole to allow an increased flux of cations through the membrane.

The physiological consequences of nicotinic receptor activation by acetylcholine can also be prevented by other classes of drugs that directly block the flow of cations through the ion channel. These drugs include some local anesthetics: quinacrine, phencyclidine, and chlorpromazine. Since these drugs exert their effects at a site separate from the acetylcholine recognition site of the receptor, they do not displace the binding of cholinergic drugs. However, by causing conformational changes in the receptor, these ion-channel blockers do alter the kinetics of drug binding to the acetylcholine recognition site.

With prolonged exposure (seconds to minutes) to acetylcholine, the nicotinic receptor "desensitizes," and the ion channel closes despite the continued presence of acetylcholine. This desensitization process, which renders the receptor refractory to further stimulation by acetylcholine, is thought to be due to a further conformational change in the receptor.

β-Adrenergic Receptor

Certain neurotransmitters exert their physiological effects by altering the activity of the enzyme adenylate cyclase (Fig. 9–1). This enzyme catalyzes the synthesis of cyclic adenosine monophosphate (cAMP) from adenosine triphosphate (ATP). cAMP, formed in the inside of the cell, initiates a series of biochemical reactions, most notably the phosphorylation of specific proteins by activation of a protein kinase. Many neurotransmitters and hormones act by increasing adenylate cyclase activity; some neurotransmitters and hormones act by decreasing adenylate cyclase activity.

The neuronal system providing the most convincing evidence for mediation of the electrophysiological effects of a neurotransmitter by cAMP is the noradrenergic projection to the Purkinje cells of the rat cerebellum. Stimulation of the noradrenergic pathway arising from the locus coeruleus reduces the firing rate of cerebellar Purkinje cells. Norepinephrine released from presynaptic nerve terminals activates a β-adrenergic receptor coupled to adenylate cyclase in the postsynaptic cell.

Convincing evidence exists that the β-adrenergic receptor and adenylate cyclase are two distinct proteins that are functionally coupled with one another in the cell membrane. The actual coupling of receptors to adenylate cyclase is mediated by a third set of proteins, called "G" proteins because their requirement for guanine nucleotide binding for biological activity. The G_s protein is the coupling protein that mediates the stimulation of adenylate cyclase activity; the G_i protein is the coupling protein that mediates the inhibition of adenylate cyclase activity. Figure 9–2 shows the proposed model for the actions of the G_s protein.

Muscarinic Cholinergic Receptor

The muscarinic cholinergic receptor is one example of a class of receptors linked to biochemical mechanisms involved in phosphatidylinositol (PI) turnover (Fig. 9–3). Only a few percent of membrane phospholipids contain inositol. PI is the predominant species, but two phosphorylated derivatives, phosphatidylinositol-4-phosphate (PIP) and phosphatidylinositol-4,5-diphosphate (PIP2), are present in much smaller quantities. These two phospholipids are synthesized by sequential phosphorylations of PI. When the muscarinic receptor is activated by acetylcholine, a phospholipase C in the mem-

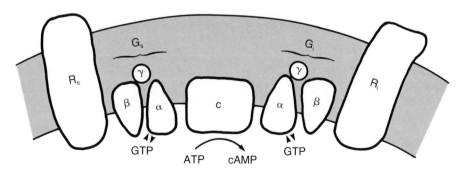

FIGURE 9–1. Components of the neurotransmitter-sensitive adenylate cyclase. The system is composed of stimulatory (R_s) and inhibitory (R_i) transmembrane receptors for a variety of extracellular signal molecules, stimulatory (G_s) and inhibitory (G_i) guanine nucleotide coupling proteins, each composed of α, β, and γ subunits, and a catalytic protein that, when activated, converts intracellular ATP to cAMP. GTP = guanosine triphosphate.

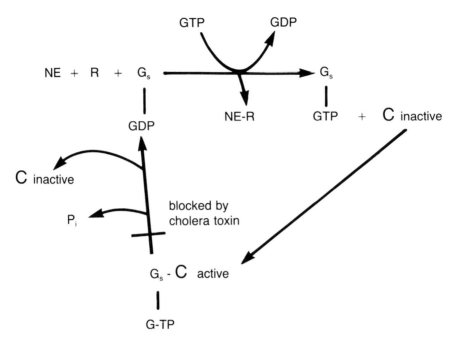

FIGURE 9–2.   Model proposed for the actions of the G_s protein. NE = norepinephrine; R = beta-adrenergic receptor; GDP = guanosine diphosphate; GTP = guanosine triphosphate; C = catalytic subunit of adenylate cyclase; P_i = inorganic phosphate.

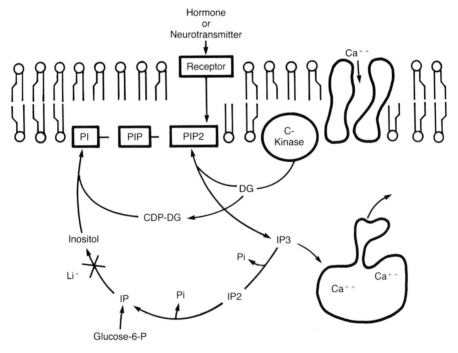

FIGURE 9–3.   Receptor-activated phosphatidylinositol hydrolysis. PI = phosphatidylinositol; PIP = phosphatidylinositol-4-phosphate; PIP2 = phosphatidylinositol-4,5-biphosphate; DG = diacylglycerol; CDP-DG = cytidine diphosphodiacylglycerol; IP = inositol-1-phosphate; IP2 = inositol-1,4-biphosphate; IP3 = inositol-1,4,5-triphosphate; Pi = inorganic phosphate; Glucose-6-P = glucose-6-phosphate; Li^+ = lithium.

brane is activated, cleaving PIP2 into the soluble compound inositol-1,4,5-triphosphate (IP3) and diacylglycerol (DG). IP3 and DG can be considered as two separate "second messengers" for the actions of acetylcholine.

IP3 acts to cause the release of Ca^{++} from internal stores, leading to the stimulation of many calcium-dependent enzymatic processes. DG activates a protein kinase termed kinase C, leading to the phosphorylation of a variety of substrate proteins on serine or threonine residues.

IP3 is subsequently metabolized to a variety of biologically less active compounds, including inositol-1,4-biphosphate (IP2), inositol-1-phosphate (IP), and free inositol, which are subsequently reused for new PI synthesis. Lithium ion is an extremely potent inhibitor of the enzyme that catalyzes the dephosphorylation of IP to free inositol. This biochemical action of lithium may be related to its therapeutic effects in the treatment of patients with bipolar disorder.

REGULATION OF RECEPTOR SENSITIVITY

The sensitivity of a target organ to a neurotransmitter is partially governed by its history of exposure to that transmitter. Thus, when a target organ is chronically deprived of its input by anatomical or pharmacological denervation, the exposure of the organ to small amounts of neurotransmitter often results in an enhanced physiological response. This has been termed *denervation supersensitivity*. When a target organ is exposed to more transmitter than usual, subsequent challenge with a small amount of neurotransmitter often results in a diminished physiological response. This process is called *subsensitization*.

BIBLIOGRAPHY

Benovic, J.L., Bouvier, M., Caron, M.G., Lefkowitz, R.J.: Regulation of adenyl cyclase-coupled beta-adrenergic receptors. Annu. Rev. Cell Biol. 4:405-429, 1988.

Berridge, M.J., Irvine, R.F.: Inositol triphosphate, a novel second messenger in cellular signal transduction. Nature 312:315, 1984.

Changeaux, J.P., Devillers-Thiery, A., Chemouilli, P.: Acetylcholine receptor: An allosteric protein. Science 225:1335, 1984.

Chuang, D.M.: Neurotransmitter receptors and phosphoinositide turnover. Annu. Rev. Pharmacol. Toxicol. 29:71-110, 1989.

Clark, R.B.: Desensitization of hormonal stimuli coupled to regulation of cyclic AMP levels. Adv. Cyclic Nucleotide Res. 20:151, 1986.

Drummond, A.M.: Lithium and inositol lipid-linked signalling mechanisms. Trends in Pharmacological Sciences 8:129, 1987.

Fisher, S.K., Agraroff, B.W.: Receptor activation and inositol lipid hydrolysis in neural tissues. J. Neurochem. 48:999, 1987.

Kikkawa, U., Kishimoto, A., Nishizuka, Y.: The protein kinase C family: Heterogeneity and its implications. Annu. Rev. Biochem. 58:31-44, 1989.

Lefkowitz, R.J., Caron, M.G., Stiles, G.: Mechanisms of membrane receptor regulation. N. Engl. J. Med. 310:1570, 1984.

Nishizuka, Y.: Turnover of inositol phospholipids and signal transduction. Science 225:1365, 1984.

O'Dowd, B.F., Lefkowitz, R.J., Caron, M.G.: Structure of the adrenergic and related receptors. Annu. Rev. Neurosci. 12:67-84, 1989.

Schramm, M., Selinger, Z.O.: Message transmission: Receptor controlled adenylate cyclase system. Science 225:1350, 1984.

Spiegel, A.M., et al.: Clinical implications of guanine nucleotide-binding proteins as receptor-effector couplers. N. Engl. J. Med. 312:26, 1985.

Chapter 10
Neuropeptides

Michael Davidson, M.D.

Until recently, the monoamines, acetylcholine, and the amino acids were thought to be the only mediators of neural transmission. The demonstration that "classical neurotransmitters" account for only 40 percent of the synapses in the central nervous system, and the recognition that conversion of some neural signals into physiological responses is mediated by peptidergic compounds, have led to the discovery and investigation of the neuropeptides. Most neuropeptides were found first in the periphery; the earliest report was in 1931, for substance P. That peptides affect complex behaviors was suggested only 30 years later by experiments demonstrating that removal of the pituitary gland, or parts of it, reduced the ability of rodents to acquire a conditioned avoidance response, and that this deficit could be corrected by exogenously replacing some of the peptides produced by the removed gland.

Peptides, like proteins, are encoded in the genome by specific DNA sequences. A sequence is transcribed into RNA only in those cells that express the particular gene. RNA directly copied from DNA is spliced to produce messenger RNA (mRNA), which is translated into proteins by ribosomes. The resulting inactive precursor peptides are then cleaved by endoproteolytic enzymes into biologically active peptides. Using molecular biology tools, neuroscientists can investigate the cascade of events regulating the expression of genetic information into biologically active neuropeptides.

Before the discovery of neuropeptides, one aspect of a neuron's phenotype was its unique secretory designation, that is, cholinergic, adrenergic, or dopaminergic. Advances in histochemical mapping techniques (retrograde tracing combined with immunochemistry) led to the identification of peptides in neurons already occupied by an amino acid or monoamine or even another neuropeptide. Although neuropeptides could be an alternative to the classical neurotransmitter, evidence suggests that neuropeptides exert a modulatory effect on neurotransmission. For example, neuropeptides have the capacity to increase or decrease the amount of classical neurotransmitter released by a given stimulus, or to alter the affinity of postsynaptic receptors for their respective transmitters.

CONTRASTS BETWEEN NEUROPEPTIDES AND NEUROTRANSMITTERS

Neuropeptides have some classical neurotransmitter properties: their release from nerve endings is calcium dependent; their postsynaptic action alters ion channel conductance or operates through second messengers. On the other hand, their metabolic pathways show marked differences of significant functional consequences. Monoamines are formed in the nerve terminals from dietary sources by one or two enzymatic steps and can be inactivated by neuronal reuptake. This process ensures rapid turnover and replacement of "used" neurotransmitter. In contrast, neuropeptide synthesis occurs in the neuronal cell and is directed by mRNA within the ribosomal machinery to be further processed into the active peptide by peptidase. At an estimated transport velocity of 5 mm/h throughout the axon, many hours elapse before a neuropeptide synthesized in the cell body of a peripheral neuron is transported to the nerve terminals to replace depleted pools. Theoretically, the availability of high neuropeptide reserve pools could have compensated for the slow synthesis and transport. However, this is not the case, since neuropeptides have low tissue concentrations (1/1000 pmol/g vs. 1/100 nmol/g for catecholamines).

Further support that classical neurotransmitters are more readily available to the synaptic cleft than neuropeptides derives from the difference in storage mechanisms within nerve terminals. Monoamines and acetylcholine are stored in both small and large vesicles, whereas neuropeptides are stored only in large vesicles. Low stimulation frequencies selectively activate small vesicles, which in turn release classical neurotransmitters. Neuropeptides, on the other hand, are released from the large vesicles only by high-frequency stimulation, which can also release classical neurotransmitters.

COEXISTENCE OF NEUROPEPTIDES AND NEUROTRANSMITTERS

Coexistence within the neuron of neuropeptides and classical neurotransmitters has been established primarily through immunohistochemical methods. However, in high concentrations, antibodies may react with peptides having similar amino acid sequences, suggesting that immunochemistry might represent a low-specificity research tool and that some "newly identified" peptides are not really new. On the other hand, the functional significance of many types of coexistence is unclear. It could be speculated that, in lower species, neuropeptides might have played a more important role but phylogenetically have been replaced by classical neurotransmitters. According to this speculation, at least some neuropeptides identified in aminergic neurons are "innocent bystanders."

NEUROPEPTIDE CLASSIFICATION

The classification of neuropeptides is somewhat arbitrary; names may depend on the original tissues in which the neuropeptides were localized (gastrointestinal tract peptides) or on some postulated pharmacological or functional aspects (opioid peptides). Therefore some peptides appear under more than one heading, whereas others do not fall into any given category. Moreover, the amount of information available on individual neuropeptides varies widely. For some neuropeptides, complex roles in behavior have been demonstrated; for others, only limited histochemical and pharmacological characteristics have been ascertained. This relatively scattered body of information prevents a truly comprehensive coverage of the subject. Only the most thoroughly investigated and behaviorally active neuropeptides are reviewed here. Table 10–1 lists some neuropeptides, along with some coexisting neurotransmitters. Figure 10–1 shows relative concentrations of some neuropeptides in central nervous system areas.

Opioid Peptides

Opioid peptides are endogenous substances that have in common some morphinelike pharmacological properties. Recombinant DNA techniques have demonstrated that all opioids presently identified derive from three different genes that produce three different biologically inactive precursor proteins: proopiomelanocortin (POMC), proenkephalin, and prodynorphin. Outside the ribosomal machinery, each precursor undergoes proteolytic cleavage and other posttranslational modifications to produce a plethora of bioactive peptides. The following

TABLE 10–1. Classification of Some Well-known Neuropeptides, with Some Classical Neurotransmitters that Coexist with Them in Central Nervous System Neurons

Neuropeptide	Classical Neurotransmitter
OPIOID PEPTIDES	
Dynorphin	
Met-enkephalin	
Leu-enkephalin	
β-Endorphin	γ-Aminobutyric acid (GABA)
GASTROINTESTINAL PEPTIDES	
Substance P	Acetylcholine, serotonin
Cholecystokinin (CCK)	Dopamine, GABA
Vasoactive intestinal polypeptide (VIP)	Acetylcholine
Neurotensin	Dopamine, glycine
Somatostatin	Acetylcholine, GABA
Thyrotropin releasing hormone (TRH)	Acetylcholine, GABA
Bombesin	
Gastrin	
Met-enkephalin	GABA
Leu-enkephalin	GABA
Insulin	
Glucagon, secretin	
Motilin	GABA
Pancreatic polypeptides	
HYPOTHALAMIC RELEASING HORMONES	
Thyrotropin releasing hormone (TRH)	
Growth hormone	
Somatostatin	
Corticotropin releasing factor (CRF)	
PITUITARY PEPTIDES	
Adrenocorticotropic hormone (ACTH)	
Melanocyte-stimulating hormone (MSH)	
Luteinizing hormone	
Thyrotropin	
NEUROHYPOPHYSEAL HORMONES	
Vasopressin	Norepinephrine
Oxytocin	
Neurophysin	
OTHERS	
Galanin	
Angiotensin	
Bradykinin	
Calcitonin	
Thymosin	
Neuropeptide Y	
Cardionatriuretic peptide	

products are derived from these three precursors:

Precursor	Product
POMC	Adrenocorticotropic hormone (ACTH)
	Melanocyte stimulating hormone (MSH)
	β-Endorphin
Proenkephalin	Met-enkephalin
	Leu-enkephalin
Prodynorphin	β-Neoendorphin
	Dynorphin

During the posttranslational maturation of opioid peptides, neuropeptides derived from the same precursor can acquire different bioactivities and be subjected to different regulatory mechanisms, depending on the tissue of expression.

Opioid peptides alter the release of dopamine and affect the spontaneous activity of the dopaminergic neurons. When administered to rats, opioid peptides produce a cataleptic-like syndrome, characterized by muscle rigidity, absence of spontaneous movements, and excessive grooming. These findings have made opioid peptide–dopamine interaction a focus of interest in schizophrenia research.

Substance P

Although substance P was the first neuropeptide to be discovered, it is one of the most obscure bioactive peptides; its physiological action in the brain is as yet unclear. Substance P is present in many parts of the central nervous system, being especially plentiful in neurons projecting from the dorsal root ganglia into the substantia gelatinosa of the spinal cord. Substance P is also present in the basal ganglia, amygdala, hypothalamus, and substantia nigra. Figure 10–2 shows a substance P immunoreactive axon. Substance P is stored in vesicles of nerve endings. When discharged to the synaptic cleft, it has potent depolarizing effects. The observation that substance P is especially concentrated in sensory fibers has led to the hypothesis that it may play a role in sensory transmission. Although an unlikely candidate to be a primary sensory neurotransmitter, substance P may still have a regulatory function in pain modulation, since it coexists with other neurotransmitters and prolongs and intensifies transmission within the cord. The only substantiated finding connecting substance P with central nervous system disorders is a reported decreased concentration in the substantia nigra of patients with Huntington's chorea; however, the pathophysiological implications of this abnormality are presently unclear.

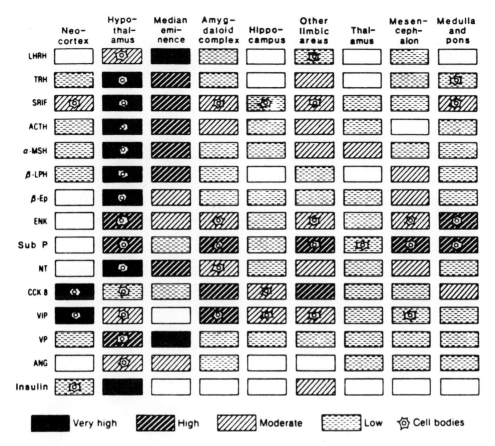

FIGURE 10–1. Relative concentrations of selected neuropeptides in selected central nervous system areas. The amygdaloid complex and hippocampus are considered as part of the limbic system. The median eminence refers to a specialized area of the hypothalamus located in the inferior portion of the third ventricle, containing endings of the hypophysiotropic and other neurons in the capillaries of the hypophyseal portal circulation. Also depicted are those areas in which cell bodies containing the designated peptides have been demonstrated immunocytochemically. Data are those of demonstration by various types or criteria. In the instances of the known neurotransmitters, releasing hormones, substance P, and enkephalin, their chemical identity has been established. The presence of the ACTH precursor molecule and other "pituitary" hormones contained therein has been established by immunocytochemical, immunoassay, biosynthetic, and complementary DNA hybridization techniques. The other peptides cited have thus far been characterized by immunoassay or immunocytochemistry. The data cited for vasopressin, long known to occur in the magnocellular nuclei and the tuberohypophyseal tract, represent that of the demonstration of its more widespread central nervous system distribution. Abbreviations used: SRIF = somatostatin; β-Ep = β-endorphin; ENK = enkephalin; NT = neurotensin; VIP = vasoactive intestinal polypeptide; VP = vasopressin; ANG = angiotensin; ACTH = adrencortociotropic hormone; α-MSH = α-melanocyte-stimulating hormone; Sub P = substance P. (From Krieger D.T.: Brain peptides: what, where and why? Science 222:975-985, 1983, with permission. Copyright 1983 by the AAAS.)

Cholecystokinin

Cholecystokinin (CCK) is a gastrointestinal tract hormonal peptide identified in the mammalian brain. The demonstration that CCK-like peptides and dopamine coexist within mesolimbic and mesocortical dopaminergic neurons has focused interest on the possible role of CCK in mental illnesses in which a dopaminergic abnormality has been invoked.

Vasoactive Intestinal Polypeptide

Vasoactive intestinal polypeptide (VIP) was initially isolated from the pig intestine and named after its biological vasodilator activity. Later, VIP immunoreactivity was demonstrated in the central nervous system. It seems that cyclic adenosine monophosphate (cAMP) is involved as a second messenger in the action of VIP in brain slices, and VIP's release is calcium

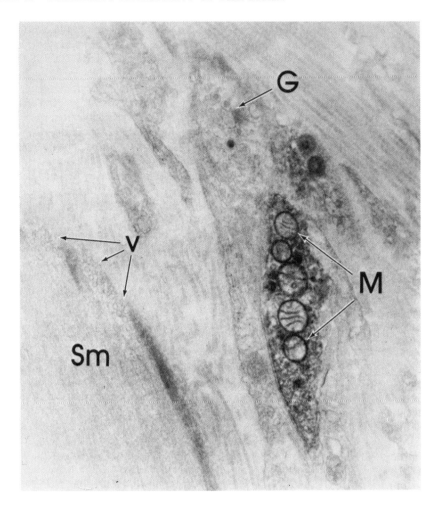

FIGURE 10–2.   An electron micrograph of a substance P immunoreactive axon in close proximity to a smooth muscle cell (Sm). Mitochondria (M) are abundant in this axon. Note the smooth-muscle-cell pinocytic vesicles (v). Often axons containing large granular vesicles (G) were seen contacting immunopositive fibers. ×25,760. (Reproduced with permission of Liu-Chen L.-Y., Liszczak T., King J., Moskowitz M.A. From Moskowitz, M.A., Beyerl, B.D., Hendrikson, B.M.: Approach to vascular head pain, in Diseases of the Nervous System: Clinical Neurobiology, A.K. Asbury, G.M. McKhann, and W.I. McDonald (eds.). Philadelphia, W.B. Saunders, 1986.)

dependent. A high concentration of VIP has been shown in the hypothalamus, where in vivo and in vitro studies suggested a stimulatory role of VIP in the secretion of prolactin (PRL) and possibly in luteinizing hormone and growth hormone. No specific behavioral effects have yet been demonstrated for VIP.

Neurotensin

Contrary to most other peptides, neurotensin was first isolated from the bovine hypothalamus and not from a peripheral organ. Later, neurotensin was also detected in the gastrointestinal tract of animals; therefore it is included in the gastrointestinal peptide group. Its name derives from its potent hypotensive effect. The central nervous system effects of neurotensin are increased turnover of dopamine, inhibition of hyperactivity produced by administration of dopamine, stimulation of growth hormone and prolactin release, and decrements in body temperature. In laboratory animals, neurotensin reduces locomotor activity, potentiates phenobarbital-induced sleep, and decreases muscular tone.

Some of these effects resemble neuroleptic-like effects; however, investigations have failed to implicate neurotensin in the pathophysiology of schizophrenia or to indicate a possible therapeutic role.

Somatostatin

Like neurotensin, somatostatin was initially identified in hypothalamic extracts. Its ability to inhibit growth hormone release was the first major biological activity to be described, and the peptide was named after it. The extra-hypothalamic area of the brain is also rich in somatostatin. Immunohistochemical studies have demonstrated complex systems of somato-statin-containing neurons in the cerebral cortex, hippocampus, thalamus, caudate, brain-stem nuclei, and spinal cord. The effects of somatostatin administration on the central nervous system are multiple. Electrophysiologically, it has a stimulatory effect on cortical cells. Biochemically, it has inhibitory effects on the release of adenylate cyclase, noradrenalin, and thyrotropin releasing hormone, and stimulatory effects on serotonin. Somatostatin stimulates the turnover and release of dopamine in the striatum, and of acetylcholine in the brain stem and hippocampus. Induction of sleep or tonic-clonic seizures, or both, has been reported in laboratory animals after administration of somatostatin. However, the net behavioral effects of this peptide are far from being elucidated.

The possibility that somatostatin might be secreted by cholinergic neurons made it an attractive candidate in the investigation of mental disorders in which a cholinergic abnormality has been invoked. In patients with Alzheimer's disease, Parkinson's disease, depression, and multiple sclerosis, somatostatin levels in the cerebrospinal fluid were found to be lower than in control subjects, but levels are higher after cortical and spinal cord injuries. High concentrations of somatostatin have been reported in brain specimens from patients with Huntington's chorea, and low concentrations in patients with Alzheimer's disease. See discussions under the headings Somatostatin and Somatostatin-Acetylcholine Relationship in Chapter 22: Delirium and Dementia.

Thyrotropin Releasing Hormone

Thyrotropin releasing hormone (TRH), a small tripeptide, was found to be widely distributed in the brain and in the gastrointestinal tract, pancreas, and body fluids, including amniotic fluid, cerebrospinal fluid, breast milk, urine, and blood. TRH stimulates release of thyroid-stimulating hormone (TSH), prolactin, growth hormone, oxytocin, and vasopressin. TRH receptors were demonstrated in the brain,

pituitary gland, retina, and spinal cord. Behaviorally, TRH attenuates the sedative effects of ethanol, diazepam, and barbiturates in laboratory animals. It also increases locomotor activity and muscle tremor and causes hyperthermia. Peripherally, TRH potentiates colonic and duodenal activity.

For more about TRH and other hormones, see Chapter 13: Biological Rhythms and the Neuroendocrine System. For the role of hormones in affective disorders, see Chapter 26: Pathogenesis of Mood Disorders.

Bombesin

Bombesin, another small (14-amino-acid) peptide, is found mainly in the hypothalamus, cortex, and midbrain. Bombesin releases prolactin and growth hormone and causes hypothermic effects that are reversed by naloxone, suggesting an interaction with endorphins. It has been proposed that bombesin, by increasing the blood sugar level and decreasing body temperature, may play a role in the organism's attempt to conserve energy. In laboratory animals, bombesin promotes satiety, leading to the speculation that it also plays a role as a satiety signal. Peripherally, bombesin increases the blood pressure and induces antidiuresis. In the gastrointestinal system, it stimulates gastric and pancreatic secretion, gastrointestinal tract motility, gallbladder contraction, and smooth muscle contraction.

Corticotropin Releasing Factor

A major step in a 30-year-long search for the agent of brain control over the pituitary gland was reached in 1981 with the purification and sequence analysis of corticotropin releasing factor (CRF). CRF is a potent stimulator of ACTH release, and this effect can be further augmented by vasopressin, norepinephrine, and angiotensin. In vitro CRF increases the frequency of action potential in hippocampal pyramidal cells. At small doses in the rodent's brain ventricle, CRF is a potent activator of spontaneous locomotion and can also produce an axiogenic-like response in different behavior paradigms. Because of its effects on the hypothalamic-pituitary-adrenal (HPA) axis and its involvement in cortisol secretion, the physiological effects of CRF might be aimed at mobilization of the bodily systems during stress. Low CRF immunoreactivity was reported in brain specimens from patients with Alzheimer's disease and from the cerebrospinal fluid of depressed patients.

Oxytocin and Vasopressin

Oxytocin and vasopressin are two neuropeptides, highly similar in structure, that are synthesized in the hypothalamus and stored in its axonal projection to the neurohypophysis. Each peptide is synthesized and stored as part of a larger propeptide, from which it is cleaved during the release process. Both vasopressin and oxytocin were found in extrahypothalamic neuronal tissue, projecting to the diencephalon, pons, and spinal cord. They appear to exert inhibitory effects on neurons projecting to the hypophysis. When given to humans (usually in the form of nasal spray), the peptides induce enhanced performance of attention-related memory tasks. It is of interest that the behavioral effects persist long after peripheral effects (such as blood pressure elevation) return to normal; moreover, they persist longer than any detectable circulating peptide.

Galanin

Galanin, a peptide isolated from the pig's small intestine, was later identified in the stria terminalis and the amygdala. Some galanin neurons contain choline acetyltransferase, indicating that this neuropeptide might be involved in modulating central cholinergic transmission and suggesting that it could play a role in memory processes and Alzheimer's disease.

Angiotensin

Angiotensin is not classified in any particular group of peptides. Until recently, the role of angiotensin was thought to be mainly the peripheral regulation of blood pressure. It was then discovered that all the peripheral precursors and enzymes needed for angiotensin II production are also found in the brain. Angiotensin was identified in the periventricular zone. In laboratory animals, angiotensin injected into the third ventricle enhances drinking.

NEUROPEPTIDES IN PSYCHIATRIC DISORDERS

Information regarding the behavioral activities of neuropeptides is primarily obtained by observing their effects after intracerebral administration to laboratory animals. Since intracerebral administration to humans is impractical, the behavioral effects of a particular neuropeptide are evaluated after peripheral administration, which, in turn, is dependent on the peptide's ability to penetrate the blood-brain barrier. The blood-brain barrier, a specialized vasculature in which nonfenestrated, enzymatically active endothelial cells are bound together, allows only for limited peptide penetration. Peptides that penetrate the blood-brain barrier do so by direct diffusion through the membranes as a result of their lipid solubility or via carrier-mediated systems. For most peptides, administration of very large peripheral doses produces increments in cerebrospinal fluid concentrations, suggesting that their blood-brain barrier penetration is possible. However, since most neuropeptides have peripheral effects as well as central effects, it is not inconceivable that their central effects are mediated by the interaction between the peptide and the peripheral nervous system. For example, the vagal afferents could mediate some of the central effects of neuropeptides acting on the gastrointestinal tract. On the other hand, the peripheral effects and adverse effects of the neuropeptides on the gastrointestinal tract limit the doses that can be safely administered to humans and that could otherwise penetrate the blood-brain barrier.

An additional objection to the peripheral administration of neuropeptides in behavioral studies is the uncertainty concerning whether the material enters the cerebrospinal fluid in the intact form or only as an immunoreactive fragment after being inactivated by peripheral peptidases. Consequently, if any neuropeptide proves to have therapeutic effects on the central nervous system, adequate delivery systems and specific peptidase inhibitors must be developed.

The growing interest in the role that neuropeptides may play in psychiatric disorders was stirred by the evidence that these peptides have a neuroregulatory role in the central nervous system. However, evidence implicating neuropeptide abnormality in the pathophysiology or treatment of psychiatric disorders is at best circumstantial.

Chapter 11
Integrative Brain Mechanisms

Thomas B. Horvath, M.D.

The central nervous system is organized on a hierarchical basis: the lowest level regulates tone or waking; the middle level deals with the obtaining, processing, and storing of information; and the highest level is involved with the programming and regulating of mental activities. This was described by A.R. Luria (1975), who also distinguished between posterior input-processing areas and anterior action-synthesizing ones.

More detailed neurophysiological work on perception and motor control, and more cognitive work on memory, revealed hierarchical complexities in each area. An important general principle emerged: older, simpler functions are not superseded nor inhibited, but are coopted in the service of higher-level functions. Hence clues to higher mental functions can be found in the simpler processes of input analysis and output organization.

- The neural circuits used in perceiving logical relationships may be the same as those used for seeing spatial arrangements.
- The neural structures involved in action sequences may be used for verbal reasoning.
- Anatomic areas involved in the temporal ordering of events may control evaluations of the past (memory) and plans for the future (motivation).
- The lateralization of language functions to one hemisphere may be related to small advantages one side has in the perception of phonemes.
- The function of attention, which spotlights the active areas of the brain, is superimposed on the core reticular centers that facilitate responsiveness to external and internal stimuli and that regulate arousal.

Thus the study of the simpler input, output, and control centers of the brain and their intercommunications can give clues to the understanding of higher mental functions.

SENSORY INPUT SYSTEMS

Olfactory System: Chemical Input

Interesting contrasts exist between the olfactory system, which has remained simple, and the visual system, which has superimposed a hierarchy of complex modifications over the early system.

In the olfactory system, the distance receptor is modeled on ordinary chemical neurotransmission. Stereospecific receptors for molecules make close identifications possible. The number of receptors activated (intensity of stimulus) is proportional to the slow potential and thus to the firing rate. The locations of neurons and their central connections code the quality and identity of the stimulus. Preprocessing is minimal, and almost direct connections are made to the earliest goal-defining system: the mesial temporal cortex and the underlying amygdala. Olfaction has a role not only in approach to food and avoidance of harm but also in territorial recognition and sexual attraction.

Visual System: Electromagnetic Input

The visual system in primates codes an extremely complex world. Stereoscopic color vision, with fine-grained central acuity, coupled with sensitive peripheral movement detection, requires a great deal of processing. Before this mass of data enters the brain, the retina actually preprocesses much of the visual information. The rods and cones communicate with the bipolar cells, the dendrites of which are interconnected by the horizontal cells (Fig. 11–1). Amacrine cells appear to modulate the transfer of information from bipolar cells to the ganglion cells, the output neurons of the retina. Efferents in the optic nerve control the rate of firing of the retinal ganglion cells.

A pattern analytic pathway leads from the retina to the geniculate body, on to the primary and secondary visual cortex, and then to the inferior temporal cortex. While information is processed sequentially from stage to stage, aspects of the original "raw data" are also made available to each succeeding stage, as well as to extravisual areas. Thus the visual response system does not have to proceed in lockstep. A response can be made to a fast-moving object on the basis of its position, which is extracted early, without detailed analysis of its surface markings.

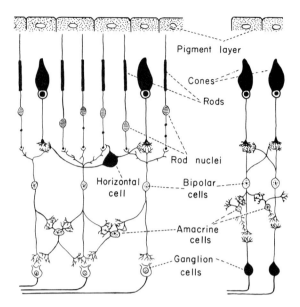

FIGURE 11–1. Neural organization of the retina: peripheral area to the left, foveal area to the right. (From Guyton, A.C.: Basic Neuroscience: Anatomy and Physiology. Philadelphia, W.B. Saunders, 1987.)

Movement detectors appear to have a somewhat separate pathway. Their retinal ganglion cells respond better to transient stimulation, and they conduct through larger, fast axons.

These eventually connect to a subcortical pathway (Fig. 11–2), which goes from the retinal ganglion cells to the mesencephalic optic tectum, that is, the superior colliculus. Not only does this pathway connect to oculomotor and neck movement centers; it projects upward to another hypothalamic nucleus, the pulvinar nucleus, and it sends a projection to the inferotemporal cortex, bypassing the main route of visual input. (The superior colliculus, in turn, receives input from the visual cortex and sends projections to the secondary visual cortex.) This subcortical detour to the inferotemporal cortex may be responsible for the analysis of location in visual space, whereas the main path deals with analysis and categorization of the objects in that space. Independent operation of this accessory system may account for the possibility of "blind sight" in cases of cortical blindness.

As the central visual field scans an object, it receives a series of code elements in time. These elements can be reintegrated into a spatially coherent form. However, if the central attentional function that controls scanning eye movements is disturbed, perceptual distortions can occur, as in delirium and schizophrenia.

The posterior part of the inferotemporal cortex receives inputs from the higher visual as-

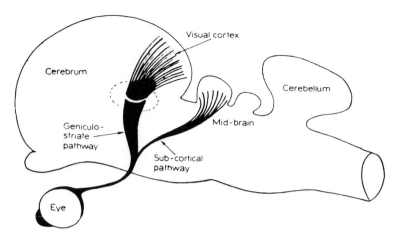

FIGURE 11–2. Schematic diagram showing central visual pathways. (From Humphrey, N.: Seeing and nothingness. New Scientist 53(789):682-684, 1972.)

sociation areas. The posterior part projects to the anterior part, which in turn connects to limbic areas and forebrain structures. Damage to the posterior part of the inferotemporal cortex disturbs discrimination between similar objects. In humans, the most complex objects of the social environment are faces, and the clinical disorder of prosopagnosia (the failure to recognize faces) is associated with lesions in the inferotemporal area. Lesions in the anterior part of the inferotemporal cortex, on the other hand, lead to problems with classification of objects into groups.

Damage to high visual associative areas may cause an inability to synthesize parts of a picture into a coherent whole or may lead to a dissociation between pattern and location.

The visual system has a set of intricately and topographically connected elements that carry several feature analyses in parallel, through selective convergence and lateral inhibition. This specific "wiring" is partly the result of embryological, epigenetic development, through chemical identification of target cells and loss of unconnected cells; the wiring is also partly sculpted by experience.

Somatosensory System: Proximate Mechanical Input

The special interest that the somatosensory system has for the study of brain function is its close interface with movement and action. The basal ganglia feed back a large amount of information to the somatosensory cortex. The sensory strip has a close connection to the motor strip.

Purely sensory, object-perceiving functions of the somatosensory cortex are organized in a similar, although simpler, manner to vision. There is the same progression from primary to secondary areas, and it is likely that the two systems "meet" in the central parietal-occipital-temporal area.

Auditory System: Distant Mechanical Input

Auditory processing of temporal patterns of frequency and amplitude also show an underlying similarity to vision. Pitch as frequency is translated to a place code on the membrane in the cochlea, and intensity is coded by the frequency of neuronal firing. A number of neuronal relays introduce delays that are important in the analysis of temporal information. In the brain stem, interactions between the two sides encode phase differences important to auditory localization. In the brain stem, compound excitatory-inhibitory tuning mechanisms provide for a sharp frequency response. Some cells in the inferior colliculus are sensitive to spatial location of the sound source. Thus the auditory cortex receives coded pitch, amplitude, and phase information.

In humans, lateralizing differences appear and may be very important for language development. The left hemisphere treats certain auditory stimuli differently from the way the right hemisphere treats them. Certain phonemes, called formant transitions, occur during speech pronunciation; when they are presented to the left auditory cortex, a consonant is heard, and

when to the right, only a chirping noise. If the
frequency spectrum is changed, the right side
hears a changing complex tone while the left side
hears a constant consonant to a point when,
abruptly, another consonant is heard. Some lin-
guists, including Noam Chomsky, believe that
the left hemisphere is biologically specialized in
applying grammatical translation rules to a variety of neuronal languages.

Higher levels of auditory analysis in the secondary and tertiary association areas involve the
translation from the phonetic to the phonemic
code; these phonemes are integrated into words
through a semantic translation. Words are
grouped into phrases through symbolic, grammatical rules. In long-term memory, semantic
but not phonemic groups are stored and are
acted on by innate translation rules. Chomsky
argued that this language *capacity* is inborn in
humans, whereas the language *content* is culturally acquired.

The left hemisphere perceives sounds categorically; despite distortions, given words are
heard until they change abruptly to a different
word or a meaningless sound. Musical sounds
are perceived continuously and noncategorically
(to which functions the right hemisphere seems
better suited). Recent evidence suggests, however, that musicians may categorically perceive
whole musical phrases and relationships and
may employ their left hemisphere in this
process.

The posterior aspect of the auditory area of
the left hemisphere, on the parietotemporal
junction, is perhaps the highest auditory association area. Damage to it causes an inability to
associate meaning with words and an inability
to relate words to each other grammatically or
semantically (Wernicke's aphasia).

Highest Association Areas: The Integration of Input

The highest association areas of the three main
sensory modalities—visual, auditory, and somatosensory—seem to converge on the central
parietal-occipital-temporal area. It is tempting
to locate here the site for the construction of a
multimodal model of the external world. This
area is larger in humans than in apes; it myelinates late in development—in adolescence—as
does the prefrontal cortex. Intermodal transfer
of information is a surprisingly late phylogenetic
development. Only apes approximate the human capacity to identify complex objects by sight
and touch, and even apes are unable to associate

words with specific objects with a high degree
of reliability.

Once equivalency is detected between objects
perceived by different sensory modalities, further analysis can proceed in a nonmodality-
specific way. In particular, the relationship of
objects to one another can be analyzed. Lesions
in this "highest associative area" impair skills
such as dressing, telling the time from nondigital
watches, and copying figures with many parts.
Such patients can understand the meaning of
words such as "in front of" or "to the left of," but
they cannot attach significance to them in a concrete situation. These patients also have difficulty in comprehending the meaning of complex
sentences or of sentences in which the order of
the transaction can be reversed.

The ability to analyze the relationship of objects to one another leads to a fundamental property of this central parietal area, emphasized by
Luria: the spatial relationship between objects
in the multidimensional world space is the substrate from which static logical and grammatical
relationships emerge. The logical relationships
of algebra are at first associated with concrete
object relationships in space. The concept of
number itself precedes these operations. For
people with acalculia, the concept of number is
not lost, but mathematical operations and the
comprehension of complex numbers are lost.
However, dynamic reasoning is not lost. These
patients can indicate appropriate goals and plans
of action, even if they cannot perform all the
operations, and they can clearly see cause-and-
effect chains.

The preceding discussion tracked the processing of input from simple sensory qualities in
peripheral receptors through increasingly complex, integrated sense impressions to high-level
abstract logical relationships in the posterior associative areas. The following sections turn to
the reverse process of translating abstract plans
of action into specific motor behavior. Goal setting and motivational and affective mechanisms
are also considered. Behaviors are built up from
simple motor output at a spinal level and
are elaborated progressively further up the
neuraxis.

MOTOR OUTPUT SYSTEMS

Lower Motor Neurons: The Final Common Motor Pathway

It is better to speak of a hierarchically organized lower motor neuron *system* than to think

of specific neurons. This system controls the number and sequence of motor units that need to be brought into action and determines the mix of fast, rapidly firing and slow but persistent muscle fibers. (Persons with schizophrenia may have an abnormality in the neuronal control of fast and slow fibers.) The system adjusts for local conditions through negative feedback. Descending influences act on the system by resetting its bias, or "thermostat," rather than by starting the neuron itself.

The output of a lower motor neuron system travels up the neuraxis as information for high centers and also enters the output of other lower motor neuron systems. Thus the lower motor neurons function as a set of interactive, parallel "intelligent terminals." By processing the bulk of data about movements locally, they allow the upper levels to act in a more general way and to coordinate movements into complex behaviors. This is similar to the use of nested subroutines, controlled by a master program, in data processing. It is even more powerful, however, because the cord carries out the computation in parallel, whereas computer subroutines have to be run sequentially.

Several specialized systems can interact with this hierarchy of lower motor neuron systems. A control system may calculate the details of the planned action in detail and then execute it, or a control system may continuously monitor the results of the movements and apply corrections if they deviate from the goal. The cerebellum appears to act on the first principle (feedforward), and the basal nuclei on the second (feedback).

Cerebellum: A Feed-forward Processor

The cerebellum receives its input from the parallel climbing fibers of the olivary cells and from the mossy fibers of vestibular and other afferent cells (Fig. 11–3). The parallel fibers make contact with a row of output elements, the Purkinje cells. These are probably activated in sequence, so that a progressive delay is set up. The Purkinje cells are inhibited by γ-aminobutyric acid (GABA) terminals from Golgi cells that synapse close to the Purkinje cell body. Noradrenergic terminals from cells in the locus coeruleus also synapse close to the soma. They have a long-lasting effect on the membrane; they have little effect by themselves. When locus coeruleus activity is coupled with climbing fiber stimulation, the Purkinje cell is excited; when locus

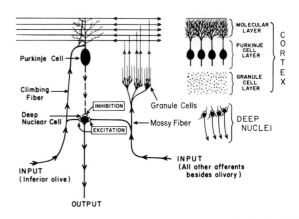

FIGURE 11–3. Basic neuronal circuit of the cerebellum, showing excitatory pathways. At right are the three major layers of the cerebellar cortex and also the deep nuclei. (From Guyton, A.C.: Basic Neuroscience: Anatomy and Physiology. Philadelphia, W.B. Saunders, 1987.)

coeruleus stimulation is coupled with Golgi cell activation, the Purkinje cell is inhibited. Thus noradrenergic activity in the cerebellum *enables* rather than *stimulates* activities.

Other intermediary cells selectively inhibit individual Purkinje cells and control interactions between parallel row systems. These specific events sharpen the interactions between inputs from several different elements. The cerebellum, of course, receives inputs from the vestibular system, from lower motor neuron systems, and from the cortex. These mossy fibers synapse with granule cells in the cerebellar cortex. Sequences of planned motor actions generated in the lower motor neuron and other systems are sent to the cerebellum, where they interact through parallel and mossy fiber activity; the resultant modified command is put out through the cerebellar nuclei and is sent back to the motor output areas. The whole sequence of correction of action takes place *before* any muscle action needs to occur. Many rapid learned movements, such as piano playing, depend heavily on the cerebellum. Once learned, the sequence is too rapid for feedback guidance by the auditory or visual system.

Until recently, the cerebellum was thought to have functional relevance to movements but not to behaviors. It now seems that the anterior vermis of the cerebellum not only sequences truncal movements but has something to do with the sequencing of emotional states through its connection with the limbic system. The use of cerebellar pacemakers in violent patients and the behavioral effects of cerebellar atrophy in some persons with schizophrenia and in many persons with alcoholism indicate the clinical relevance of the cerebellum.

Basal Ganglia: Feedback Processors

The caudate nucleus, putamen, and globus pallidus constitute the true basal ganglia; because they act in coordination with the substantia nigra, subthalamus, and important parts of both the thalamus and reticular formation, all these organs are generally referred to as the basal ganglia system.

The basal ganglia differ from the cerebellum in not having an orderly structure. They have numerous interconnected local elements, most of which are inhibitory and self-inhibitory (Fig. 11–4). The main response of the basal ganglia to input is self-inhibitory. Thus behavior routed through the basal ganglia continues only if the command is either sustained or reinforced. The basal ganglia receive input through the striatum from the association cortex, with some topographic specificity and with glutamic acid as the transmitter. The basal ganglia receive input also from the thalamus. The striatum has excitatory cholinergic and inhibitory "GABAergic" neurons. Output from the basal ganglia is mostly inhibitory (GABA), with some excitatory substance P as well. The striatum projects to the pallidum, which in turn projects back to the ventroanterior and ventrolateral nuclei of the thalamus, using the inhibitory transmitter GABA (Fig. 11–5). The ventrolateral nuclei project back to the motor and premotor cortex, completing a loop.

The third input to the basal ganglia comes from the monoaminergic mesencephalic nuclei: the substantia nigra with dopamine, and the raphe nuclei with serotonin. These mesencephalic inputs make synaptic contacts with a very large number of neurons in the basal ganglia. The effect of these outputs may well be to "enable" the basal ganglia to proceed with motor action. It could well be that the basal ganglia induce the organism into action when these mesencephalic structures signal some regulatory interest. Normal operation of the basal ganglia is essential for approach to stimuli, for persistence of "homing" behavior, and for the use of sensory information to provide feedback about behavior. Thus not only movement problems but sensory deficiencies associated with active explorations of the environment can be expected in basal ganglia disorders. (In Parkinson's disease there are subtle sensory and motivational problems in

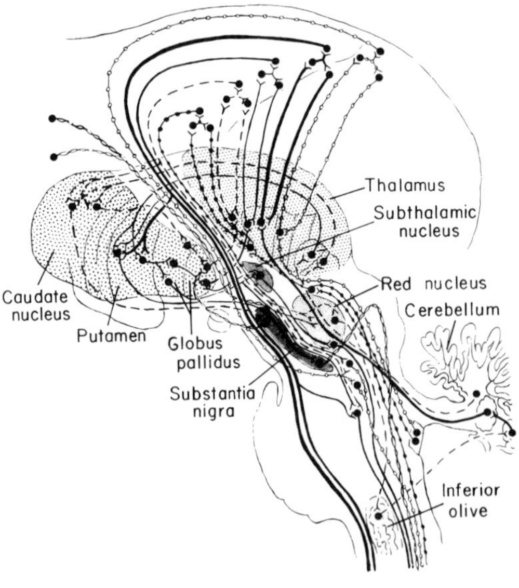

FIGURE 11–4.   Pathways through the basal ganglia and related structures of the brain stem, thalamus, and cerebral cortex. (From Jung, R., and Hassler, R.: The extrapyramidal motor system, in Handbook of Physiology, sec. 1, vol. II. Bethesda, Md., American Physiological Society, 1960, p. 870.)

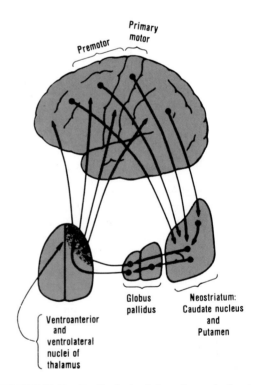

FIGURE 11–5.   Feedback circuit from the cerebral cortex to the basal ganglia, through the thalamus, and back to the cortex. (From Guyton, A.C.: Basic Neuroscience: Anatomy and Physiology. Philadelphia, W.B. Saunders, 1987.)

addition to the well-known motor disorders of rigidity, tremors, and bradykinesia.)

Sensorimotor Cortex: "Images of Action" (Pribram)

Both the basal ganglia and the cerebellum receive a substantial input from the neocortex. This output appears to be related not to the design of specific motor movements but, rather, to the planning of sequences of actions. It is notable that the somatosensory cortex provides much of this input. The somatosensory cortex also deals with exteroreceptive touch stimulation, but in the context of movements the focus is on the kinesthetic sense of body position. Without this postural sense, voluntary action becomes impossible; visual or vestibular feedback can compensate for it only to a limited extent. Thus, in a stroke affecting the anteroparietal area, disability is out of proportion to paralysis, and quick, skilled voluntary movements are severely affected even when gross motor power is spared.

Posterior to the sensory side of the rolandic fissure, the analysis of posture becomes progressively abstract and generalized. Moving forward from the motor side, an interesting mirror image increase is noted in the generality of the motor plan. Whole action subroutines are deleted in lesions of the premotor cortex. This is best illustrated in lesions of Broca's area. Such aphasic patients have problems in ordering a sequence of phonemes or words. Units may be spoken out of order, or one word may fail to lead to another. These problems are marked for newly synthesized sequences, whereas well-rehearsed patterns (such as prayers, curses, or cliches) are not affected. More anterior lesions may lead to mutism because the patient is unable to initiate the sequence. In languages in which writing depends on an association between visual symbols and sound symbols, writing is impaired in lesions of Broca's area; it is not impaired in languages that utilize pictorial ideogram writing.

In general, fragmentation of novel fine motor sequences can coexist with the retention of gross, overlearned movements.

Frontal Cortex: The Planning of Behavior

Patients with frontal lobe damage have a peculiar difficulty in shifting from one way of acquiring abstract information to another, related way. Patients with a prefrontal lesion often show no focal neurological signs and can execute sequential motor acts for most behaviors. They can also use words and concepts. They would appear neuropsychologically intact but for their obviously inappropriate behavior. Such a person is unable to work out a reasonable plan for reaching a desired or required goal.

Patients with frontal lesions have no difficulty with meanings of words or phrases or with logical or grammatical implications. On the other hand, they often show difficulty in acquiring or understanding complex and sequential verbal reasoning.

Luria pointed out that verbal reasoning, particularly the representation of an action schema by verbs, appears to use the same structures and programs used in the sequencing of motor acts into ensembles of behavior. It is at this level that verbal instruction can change behavior, whether the verbal sequences are internal self-instructions or come from another person, such as a parent, or from society. The frontal system is that part of the brain that matures and myelinates last. It is also the part that is peculiarly sensitive to certain chemical insults, especially alcohol. The deteriorated, amoral behavior of many persons with alcoholism may find its genesis in demonstrable frontal cerebral atrophy. The recent demonstration of reduced blood flow and reduced radioactive glucose uptake into the frontal lobes of some persons with schizophrenia may explain their poorly motivated, often verbally nonresponsive behavior.

Integration of Motor Responses into Behavior

A hierarchical reflex motor system handles much of the routine traffic and is instructed by higher systems. The basal ganglia system, using feedback principles, integrates input from cortical feature analyzers and from mesencephalic reward-reinforcement structures. The basal ganglia system controls the lower motor neuron systems partly directly and partly through the lower thalamus, where its effect is integrated with that of the cerebellum; it influences the motor cortex. The cerebellum performs rapid feedforward comparisons and coordinations between various action sequences. The motor cortex, in conjunction with the sensorimotor strip, can bypass most of these slow and somewhat archaic structures and instruct even specific lower motor neurons in voluntary movement! The frontal cortex establishes the goals and sequences of motor movements and integrates them into actions.

CONNECTIONS BETWEEN INPUT AND OUTPUT PROCESSES

Certain similarities have been noted between input and output processing: both have general abstract features that are connected to specific concrete events by a set of hierarchically arranged serial processors. The most abstract level of input processing takes place in the parietal-occipital-temporal cortex. On the left side, this involves verbal and mathematical implications; on the right side, it involves perception and perhaps the simultaneous apprehension of complex nonverbal variables such as facial expression and communicative body movement. The most abstract level of output processing is in the prefrontal region and includes not only action sequencing but also verbal reasoning and the verbal mediation of behavior. It is notable that there are reciprocal connections between brain regions of similar abstract levels. E. W. Kent (1981) observed that analysis of the most detailed level of input is made available directly to areas synthesizing the most detailed level of action and that conversely, information from the most abstract level of input analysis flows directly to the area responsible for the most general level of behavioral planning.

Similar interconnections between input and output functions are seen in the basal ganglia. The plan of action presented to the basal ganglia by the cortex must include the movements themselves and the predicted future sensory conditions that will signal the action's completion; at that point, the actual environmental state will be compared with the desired one, and behavior will continue until a "good enough" match is found. This seems to account for the large feedback loop from the globus pallidus through the thalamic nuclei to the cortex.

What is the difference between somatosensory cortex feedback and basal ganglia feedback? Basal ganglia behavior seems to have to take place in real time, is generally "hard-wired" and inflexible, and constitutes responses to species-specific stimuli. Somatosensory cortical mechanisms have a choice in both stimuli and responses and can employ plan-ahead, rehearsal-type calculations.

GOAL-SETTING MECHANISMS

At a very simple level of analysis, brains evolved to enable organisms to eat and to avoid being eaten; they seem to operate to maximize pleasure and to avoid pain. In addition to the anterior hypothalamic and septal areas that evoke self-stimulation (and, in humans, subjective pleasure), there are posterior regions where stimulation is avoided and dysphoria is experienced. Self-stimulation can be blocked by reducing monoaminergic transmission, and the aversive effects of posterior stimulation may be alleviated by anticholinergic and opioid agents. But it would be simplistic to refer to these areas as "pleasure" and "pain" centers.

The hypothalamus is the main center regulating homeostatic mechanisms that maintain the "milieu interior." Regulatory actions that are triggered may be internal as well as external and behavioral. The hypothalamus does not organize behavioral sequences directly; instead, it stimulates brain areas that synthesize actions by the means of "drives." The enkephalins and endorphins function here as neuromodulators, as does substance P and other peptide transmitters. See Chapter 12: Hypothalamic Control.

The anticipation of external stimuli signaling the drive systems is emotion. Primary goal stimuli (for example, food or pain) activate the emotional-motivational mechanisms directly. Stimuli that precede these events can acquire the ability to trigger the same physiological mechanisms. However, there is a difference between the operation of emotive and motivational mechanisms:

- Motivational processes impel the organism into direct action to satisfy a drive.
- Emotion initially arrests ongoing behavior that is irrelevant to the signaled drive. Emotion is an anticipatory response, and it affords the organism some time to prepare a plan of action.

The emergence of emotional and motivated behaviors is possible only if the organism takes into account past behaviors and their effects on drive state reduction. It is not altogether surprising that many of the structures and functions involved in emotional behaviors are also those involved in aspects of memory formation and retrieval. See Chapter 2: Learning and Memory.

BIBLIOGRAPHY

Carlson, N.R.: The Physiology of Behavior, ed. 3. Boston, Allyn and Bacon, 1986.

Ellis, C.H., Hunt, R.R.: Fundamentals of Human Memory and Cognition, ed. 4. Dubuque, William C. Brown, 1989.

Kandel, E.R., Schwartz, J.H.: Principles of Neural Science, ed. 2. New York, 1985.

Kent, E.W.: The Brains of Men and Machines. New York, BYTE/McGraw-Hill, 1981.

Luria, A.R.: The Working Brain. New York, Penguin Books, 1975.

McGeer, P.L., Eccles, J.C., McGeer, E.G.: Molecular Neurobiology of the Mammalian Brain. New York, Plenum Press, 1987.

Ottoson, D.: Physiology of the Nervous System. New York, Oxford University Press, 1983.

Pribram, K.H.: Languages of the Brain, ed. 2. Englewood Cliffs, N.J., Prentice-Hall, 1971.

Schmidt, R.F.: Fundamentals of Sensory Physiology, ed. 3. New York, Springer Verlag, 1986.

Chapter 12

Hypothalamic Control

Ronnie Halperin, Ph.D.

The hypothalamus is best viewed as an integrative mechanism in the control of behavior. It is unique among brain structures in the diversity of its connections. The hypothalamus contains specialized cells sensitive to chemical changes in cerebrospinal fluid and blood. It receives neural afferents from sensorimotor pathways, structures involved in cognitive processes, the limbic system, the retina, and a variety of midbrain and hindbrain structures involved in arousal and pain perception. The hypothalamus exerts a profound influence on both divisions of the autonomic nervous system, the endocrine system, the limbic and somatomotor systems, and the reticular formation. To understand the unique integrative role of the hypothalamus in controlling behavior, one must first understand its anatomic organization, its neural connections, and its control of the autonomic and endocrine systems.

NEUROANATOMY

The hypothalamus is a diencephalic structure that extends about 10 mm rostrocaudally along the ventral surface of the brain. It surrounds the third ventricle from the level of the optic chiasm rostrally, to the mamillary bodies caudally. It is bordered dorsally by the thalamus and the subthalamic region, laterally by the internal capsule and the optic tracts, and ventrally by the optic tracts and the pituitary gland.

The hypothalamus is composed of several nuclei. In addition, and of great anatomic and functional significance, the medial forebrain bundle, a large and diffusely organized fiber tract, courses through the lateral hypothalamus. The medial forebrain bundle is a conglomerate of several fiber tracts containing a large portion of the monoaminergic projections from the hindbrain and midbrain to the forebrain. More medially, the fornix, a smaller and more compact fiber tract, courses through the hypothalamus in its path from the hippocampal formation, where it originates, posteriorly and ventrally to the mamillary bodies. The fornix is generally considered to be the dividing line separating the lateral from the medial hypothalamic areas. Several organizational systems have been applied in systematically describing the neuroanatomy of the hypothalamus. The system adopted here is that of dividing the hypothalamus rostrocaudally into the supraoptic, tuberal, and mamillary regions.

Regions of the Hypothalamus

Supraoptic Region

The anterior portion of the supraoptic region is occupied by the lateral preoptic area and the medial preoptic area. Some anatomists have not included the preoptic area as part of the hypothalamus proper. Just caudal to the medial preoptic area is the paraventricular nucleus, which is a wing-shaped nucleus surrounding the dorsolateral edges of the third ventricle. Lateral to the paraventricular nucleus is the anterior hypothalamic nucleus. In the ventral portion of the supraoptic hypothalamic region, the suprachiasmatic nucleus occupies the area just dorsal to the optic chiasm. More posterolaterally, the supraoptic nucleus occupies the dorsolateral edge of the optic tracts.

Three structures, known collectively as the circumventricular organs, lie in close proximity to the third ventricle. They are the subfornical organ, the organ vasculum of the lamina terminalis (OVLT), and the subcommissural organ. These structures are highly vascularized and lie outside the blood-brain barrier. They are therefore responsive to blood-borne substances.

Tuberal Region

The dorsomedial nucleus and ventromedial nucleus occupy the medial portion of the tuberal region of the hypothalamus, and span its rostrocaudal extent. The lateral hypothalamus also spans the rostrocaudal extent of the tuberal region and extends posteriorly into the mamillary hypothalamic region. The lateral hypothalamus contains cell bodies and fiber tracts. It is the area through which the medial forebrain bundle passes. The rostral portion of the posterior hypothalamus extends into the posteromedial portion of the tuberal region, although, for the most part, this structure lies in the mamillary region of the hypothalamus. The arcuate nucleus and the median eminence lie on the ventral edge of the tuberal hypothalamic region. The arcuate nucleus contains cell bodies that project through the median eminence to the anterior lobe of the pituitary gland.

Mamillary Region

The posterior hypothalamus occupies the medial portion of the mamillary region. The lateral hypothalamus occupies the lateral mamillary region. Three mamillary nuclei lie along the ventral edge of this region. They are the medial mamillary nucleus, the intermediate mamillary nucleus, and the lateral mamillary nucleus.

Connections of the Hypothalamus

Major neuroanatomic pathways connect the hypothalamus with more caudal brain-stem structures (in the medulla, pons, and midbrain), limbic structures (the septum and amygdaloid complex), the thalamus, and phylogenetically older cortical structures (the hippocampus and the pyriform cortex). The hypothalamus, in addition to its connections with other brain structures, also possesses neural connections with the pituitary gland and the retina.

Pathways Connecting the Hypothalamus to More Caudal Brain-stem Structures

Medial Forebrain Bundle. The medial forebrain bundle contains both afferent pathways to and efferent pathways from the hypothalamus. The afferent contribution of the medial forebrain bundle to the hypothalamus originates mainly in the septum, but also in a variety of other limbic structures in the basal olfactory region. The efferent component of the medial forebrain bundle arises from the lateral hypothalamus and sends its fibers rostrally to the nuclei of the diagonal band and the septum.

Mamillotegmental Tract. The mamillotegmental tract, which arises from cells in the medial mamillary nucleus, projects to and terminates in the dorsal and ventral tegmental nuclei of the midbrain.

Dorsal Longitudinal Fasciculus. The dorsal longitudinal fasciculus provides the major neuroanatomic connection between the hypothalamus and the midbrain. The afferent component of this pathway arises from cells in the midbrain central gray matter and projects diffusely through periventricular regions of the hypothalamus.

Mamillary Peduncle. The mamillary peduncle, which originates from cells in the dorsal and ventral midbrain tegmental nuclei, terminates in the lateral mamillary nucleus.

Pathways Connecting the Hypothalamus to Limbic Structures

Fornix. The fornix, which originates in the hippocampal formation, and the septum project mainly to the medial mamillary nucleus.

Stria Terminalis. The stria terminalis is the major pathway connecting the hypothalamus with the amygdaloid complex. It is bidirectional.

Amygdalofugal Fibers. Amygdalofugal fibers form a more ventral pathway from the amygdala and pyriform cortex, and project to the lateral hypothalamus.

Pathways Connecting the Hypothalamus to the Thalamus

Thalamohypothalamic Fibers. Thalamohypothalamic fibers, arising from midline thalamic nuclei, project to the mamillary bodies.

Mamillothalamic Tract. The mamillothalamic tract, which arises from cells in the medial mamillary nucleus, projects to the anterior thalamic nuclei (including the anteroventral nucleus and the anteromedial nucleus).

Pathways Connecting the Hypothalamus to the Pituitary Gland and the Retina

Tuberohypophysial Tract. The tuberohypophysial (or tuberoinfundibular) tract arises from the cells of the arcuate nucleus and terminates in the capillary beds of the hypophysioportal system; it exerts neural control of the anterior lobe of the pituitary gland.

Supraoptic Hypophysial Tract. The supraoptic hypophysial tract originates from cells of the paraventricular and supraoptic nuclei and projects to the posterior lobe of the hypophysis.

Retinohypothalamic Fibers. Retinohypothalamic fibers, which arise from the retinal ganglion cells, terminate in the suprachiasmatic nucleus. Thus information about the light or dark condition of the environment can affect the hypothalamus. The transmission of this information to the hypothalamus is thought to be important in hypothalamic control of cyclic hormonal processes and behaviors.

NEUROTRANSMITTERS AND NEUROPEPTIDES

In the past 25 years the development of fluorescence histochemistry has enabled neuroanatomists to visualize neurotransmitters or specific neurotransmitter markers. As a result, great progress has been made in understanding the organization of neurotransmitter systems in the brain. The very complex organization of neurotransmitter systems emanating from, passing through, and terminating in the hypothalamus has begun to be understood. All of the biogenic amine neurotransmitters and several peptide neurotransmitters are found in the hypothalamus.

Norepinephrine

The norepinephrine in the hypothalamus arises from the projections of norepinephrine-containing neurons that lie in the medulla, the pons, and the midbrain. Most of the norepinephrine arises from neurons in the reticular or lateral tegmental areas of the medulla and pons and enters the hypothalamus through the medial forebrain bundle. A second source of norepinephrine comes from more medial-lying pontine and midbrain cells, including those of the locus coeruleus.

Dopamine

Of the five dopamine systems in the brain, two are contained largely within the hypothalamus, and three course through the hypothalamus.

The incertohypothalamic dopamine system lies medially and spans a large rostrocaudal extent. The cells of this system have short axons that terminate within the hypothalamus. The regional distribution of their terminals has not been thoroughly mapped.

The tuberohypophysial dopamine system consists of dopamine-containing cells in the arcuate nucleus that project through the medial eminence to the adenohypophysis, where they terminate on nonneural tissue.

The nigrostriatal pathway, which is the largest dopamine tract in the brain, courses through the lateral hypothalamus in its path to the striatum.

The mesocortical and mesolimbic dopamine systems course through the hypothalamus as part of the medial forebrain bundle in their path to more rostral limbic and cortical brain sites.

Serotonin

The serotonin-containing cells that project to the hypothalamus lie mainly in the dorsal raphe and the medial raphe nuclei of the midbrain. They enter the hypothalamus through either the medial forebrain bundle or more medial pathways. These cells innervate neurosecretory cells and appear to exert a modulatory influence over the hypothalamic control of pituitary functions, play an important role in regulating circadian rhythms, and may modulate sympathetic responses and sex hormone regulation.

Acetylcholine

Acetylcholine exists in small amounts in the hypothalamus. It is found mainly in the paraventricular and supraoptic nuclei, where it appears to exert a stimulatory influence on the release of vasopressin and oxytocin.

γ-Aminobutyric Acid

Large amounts of γ-aminobutyric acid (GABA) are found in the hypothalamus, mainly in the preoptic areas, the anterior nucleus, and the dorsomedial nucleus. These neurons have short axons that terminate within the hypothalamus.

Histamine

The highest concentrations of brain histamine are found in the hypothalamus. Within the hypothalamus, the mamillary region, ventromedial nucleus, and supraoptic nucleus are richest in histamine content. Since the neurotransmitter role of histamine in the brain has only recently been recognized, and techniques for studying histaminergic neural transmission are new, relatively little is known about the function of histamine in the brain.

Neuropeptides

In addition to the classical neurotransmitter systems just described, a plethora of neuropeptides, neurohormones, and neuropeptide fragments have been identified in hypothalamic brain tissue. Many of these substances are synthesized by neurons that lie outside the boundaries of the hypothalamus and send afferent projections to this structure. These peptides are almost always colocalized with one or more classical neurotransmitters in nerve terminals, where they perhaps modulate the action of the colocalized neuroactive substances.

Another rich source of neuropeptides and neurohormones originates from local synthesis in hypothalamic nerve cells. In the neurons of the paraventricular nucleus alone, as many as 30 neuropeptides and neurotransmitters are synthesized! Among these are neurons containing opiate peptides, some of which have intrinsic projections and are likely to be involved in modulating hypothalamic functions such as feeding. Others project to neural targets in other brain regions.

HYPOTHALAMIC CONTROL OF THE AUTONOMIC NERVOUS SYSTEM

The hypothalamus has been shown to exert an important influence on the viscera through the autonomic nervous system. The medioposterior hypothalamus activates the sympathetic nervous system, causing an increase in heart rate, respiration, and blood pressure (vasoconstriction), and causing pupillodilation. The septum, basal forebrain, preoptic area, anteromedial forebrain bundle, and medioanterior thalamus activate the parasympathetic nervous system, causing a decrease in heart rate and respiration and pupilloconstriction, defecation, eating automatisms, salivation, and vomiting. Many of the changes in cardiovascular functions controlled by the hypothalamus are correlates of emotional states such as anger, fear, and sexual arousal.

Another important hypothalamic function controlled by the autonomic nervous system is that of thermoregulation. The anterior and preoptic hypothalamic regions appear to be sensitive to changes in blood temperature, and to influence the dissipation of body heat through sweating and cutaneous vasodilation. Conversely, the posterior hypothalamus, through the sympathetic nervous system, controls mechanisms involved in the conservation of body heat, such as cutaneous vasoconstriction, increased visceral activity, and shivering.

The hypothalamus, in its control of the autonomic nervous system, influences physiological states (of preparedness) that are at times facilitatory and at other times a necessary substrate for the occurrence of particular behavioral responses. The autonomic nervous system has an important role in the regulation of feeding and drinking.

HYPOTHALAMIC CONTROL OF THE ENDOCRINE SYSTEM

The involvement of the endocrine system in the modulation of behavior and the responsiveness of the pituitary gland to psychological and physiological stressors have long been recognized. Immunocytochemical techniques have enabled investigators to identify and manipulate the neurohormonal substances in the hypothalamus that innervate the pituitary gland. Radioimmunoassay has made possible the measurement of very small but physiologically significant amounts of hormone in blood and brain. Through the use of these techniques, a picture of dynamic interaction between the brain and the endocrine system has emerged, with far-reaching implications that have revolutionized the view of the way the brain controls behavior. The unique and critically important integrative role of the hypothalamus in this dynamic brain-endocrine system interaction is the subject of the discussion that follows.

The hypothalamus controls the endocrine system through its direct influence on the pituitary gland, to which it is connected by the hypophysial stalk. The hypothalamus exerts control over the posterior lobe of the pituitary gland (neurohypophysis) through efferent neural pathways. It controls the anterior and intermediate lobes (adenohypophysis) through neural pathways that terminate in the hypophysioportal system. In addition to neural control by the hypothalamus, the adenohypophysis receives input from hormonal substances in the cerebrospinal fluid via specialized cells known as tanycytes. These cells line the third ventricle and appear to serve a transport function from the cerebrospinal fluid to the anterior pituitary.

Most of the hypothalamic neurons that project to the pituitary gland contain hormones or their precursors, rather than traditional neurotransmitter substances. The hormones are contained in the cell, in dense granules that bind to carrier proteins called neurophysins. Like other neurons, these secretory cells are activated by traditional neurotransmitter substances and have action potentials that cause release in the nerve terminals. Unlike other neurons, their thresholds of activation are regulated by local concentrations of glucose, electrolytes, and steroids. For the most part, it is through innervation of these neurosecretory cells that other brain cells exert control over endocrine function.

Neural Control of Neurohypophysis

Neural control of the posterior pituitary is through the supraoptic hypophysial tract, which originates in neurosecretory cells in the supraoptic and paraventricular nuclei (Fig. 12–1), passes through the median eminence, and terminates in a capillary bed in the neurohypophysis. The neurosecretory cells contain vasopressin (antidiuretic hormone [ADH]) and oxytocin. Both of these substances are nonapeptides. Blood-borne vasopressin stimulates water retention in the kidney and is part of a more complicated process of body fluid homeostasis that involves fluid intake (drinking) as well as output. For example, there are a number of conditions under which it is adaptive for an organism to conserve body fluid; these include conditions of severe hemorrhage and times when the plasma is hyperosmotic. Vasopressin-containing cells of the paraventricular nucleus are known to have specialized chcmorcccptors (known as osmoreceptors) and to receive input (autonomically mediated) from carotid baroreceptors that sense changes in blood pressure. Vasopressin can thus be released (and is released) during hyperosmotic and hypovolemic states, and exerts influence on the kidneys to inhibit the release of body fluid. Moreover, vasopressin has been found to be a potent vasoconstrictor in certain vascular beds such as those supplying the skeletal muscles, the kidneys, and the carotid artery.

Oxytocin is released on suckling and controls milk letdown. It is also released in response to stress and during sexual arousal.

Neural Control of Adenohypophysis

To understand hypothalamic control of the adenohypophysis, one must first understand how the hypophysioportal system functions. The superior and inferior hypophysial arteries, which arise from the internal carotid artery, form a capillary bed in the median eminence, or infundibulum. Portal vessels carry this venous blood from the hypothalamus to the adenohypophysis, where a secondary plexus is formed (Fig. 12–2). Venous blood from the secondary plexus is then pooled with the general venous circulation. It is important to note that the pituitary gland re-

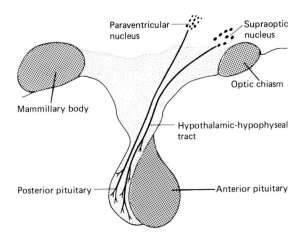

FIGURE 12–1. Hypothalamic control of the posterior pituitary. (From Guyton, A.C.: Basic Neuroscience: Anatomy and Physiology. Philadelphia, W.B. Saunders, 1987.)

ceives only venous blood from the hypothalamus. Because this blood has not, at that point, been mixed with the general circulation, any substances secreted into it by the hypothalamus reach the pituitary gland in undiluted concentrations.

A small circulatory system in which blood flows from the pituitary gland to the hypothalamus has an unknown function. It may provide the vehicle for a short feedback loop from the pituitary gland to the hypothalamus.

Hypothalamic control of the adenohypophysis is through the tuberoinfundibular tract, which originates in neurosecretory cells, mainly in the arcuate nucleus, and terminates in the primary capillary plexus in the median eminence. Although these neurosecretory cells are activated by traditional neurotransmitter substances, their thresholds are regulated by local concentrations of glucose, electrolytes, and steroids. The neurosecretory cells from which the tuberoinfundibular system arises contain releasing or inhibiting factors that control the release of pituitary hormones. Although these factors were believed for many years to exist, their actual purification and the characterization of their chemical structure are recent events. The releasing and inhibiting factors currently known through direct or indirect methods are discussed below.

Thyrotropin Releasing Hormone (TRH). This tripeptide was the first purified releasing factor. It causes the release of thyrotropin-stimulating hormone (TSH) and prolactin. TRH-containing cell bodies lie mainly in the median eminence, preoptic areas, and dorsomedial nucleus.

Gonadotropin Releasing Hormone (GnRH). Also referred to as luteinizing hormone releasing hormone (LHRH), this decapeptide is found in cells of the preoptic area, arcuate nucleus, and anterior hypothalamus. It stimulates the release of follicle-stimulating hormone (FSH) and luteinizing hormone (LH). GnRH-containing cells are also found in extrahypothalamic sites, where they are believed to control the execution of sexual behavior.

Growth Hormone Releasing Hormone (GHRH). This hormone has been only partially purified. It controls the release of growth hormone.

Corticotropin Releasing Factor (CRF). This 41–amino acid peptide has recently been characterized. Immunocytochemical investigations show that CRF is synthesized in hypothalamic neurons that send their terminals to the median eminence. It controls the release of adrenocorticotropic hormone (ACTH), which causes the release of corticosterone from the adrenal cortex.

Somatostatin. This tetradecapeptide has been purified. It inhibits the release of growth hormone. Somatostatin-containing neurons are found in the periventricular region from the anterior hypothalamus, extending caudally to the mamillary region. Somatostatin is also present in the periphery—importantly in the pancreas, where it modulates glucagon and insulin release.

Prolactin Inhibiting Factor (PIF). This factor has long been hypothesized to exist.

Vasopressin. Vasopressin-containing cells that project to the median eminence have been identified and are believed to inhibit prolactin release.

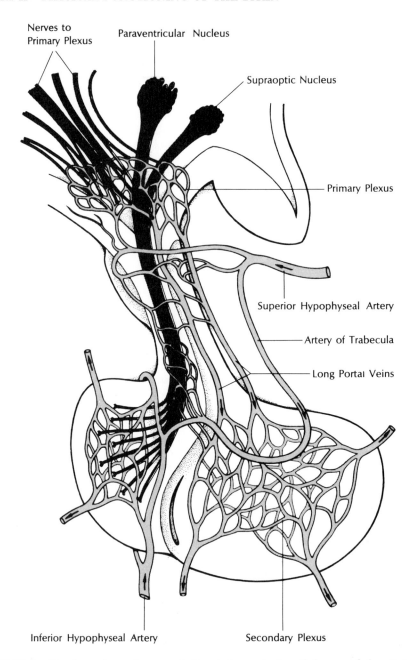

FIGURE 12–2. Vascular and neural communications between the hypothalamus and the pituitary gland. (Reprinted with permission from Krieger, D.T., Hughes, J.C. [eds.]: Neuroendocrinology. Sunderland, Mass., Sinauer Associates, 1980. Illustration by Neil O. Hardy.)

Dopamine. Dopamine in the median eminence is released into the portal system, where it also inhibits the release of prolactin. It is the only classical neurotransmitter known to have this kind of function. Dopamine receptors on LHRH nerve endings in the median eminence appear to cause the release of that substance. Dopamine is likely to be a physiological PIF.

GAP Peptide. A very potent PIF was recently identified as a component of the prohormone gene that encodes GnRH. This GnRH-associated peptide, or GAP peptide, is more than 1000 times more potent than dopamine in inhibiting prolactin release in anterior pituitary cell culture.

Feedback Loop to the Pituitary Gland

Hormones secreted by the pituitary gland and some target glands reach the hypothalamus, where they serve as part of a feedback loop in hypothalamic regulation of the pituitary. For example, estrogen and progesterone, most likely through their action on dopamine neurons in the arcuate nucleus and preoptic areas, inhibit the release of GnRH. Similarly, hormones secreted by target glands act directly (in a feedback capacity) on the pituitary gland.

The Brain as a Target Organ

Hormones released by the pituitary gland or by target glands concentrate in specific brain regions, where they have a variety of transient and permanent effects on behavior. Estrogen and testosterone concentrate in the hypothalamus. The presence of testosterone during a critical period of development (prenatally in primates and the first 5 postnatal days in the rat) exerts an organizing effect on the brain. In the rat, a sexually dimorphic nucleus has actually been identified in the preoptic area. The absence of testosterone (during the critical period in males) has immediate effects on development of the reproductive tract and delayed effects on sexual behavior. Similarly, in females the presence of testosterone during this critical period alters development of the reproductive tract and has the delayed effect of increasing aggressive behavior later in life. The immediate and more transient behavioral effects of estrogen and testosterone in the hypothalamus are discussed later.

The stress hormone corticosterone is released from the adrenal glands. Recently, corticosterone-concentrating cells have been identified in the hypothalamus and limbic system, and they most likely play a crucial role in the feedback inhibition of CRF release.

Neurotransmitter Control of Endocrine Function

Neurotransmitters in the hypothalamus alter endocrine function (1) by acting on receptor sites of the peptidergic neurons that contain the hypothalamic releasing factors, (2) by acting directly on the adenohypophysis, or (3) through polysynaptic connections to either the pituitary gland or the peptidergic neurosecretory cells of the hypothalamus. They can affect hormone release in any one of three ways: they can modulate basal levels of hormone release or cyclic aspects of hormone release, or they can be involved in linking hormonal release to an environmental or internal event. The only transmitter interactions that occur on pituitary cells themselves are those of dopamine and GABA, both of which exert an inhibitory influence on basal levels of prolactin. In addition, under certain pathological conditions, such as acromegaly, dopamine inhibits release of growth hormone.

Basal levels of ACTH are enhanced by acetylcholine and inhibited by GABA, norepinephrine (α-adrenergic receptors), and serotonin. Basal levels of FSH are increased by dopamine and inhibited by serotonin. Dopamine inhibits basal levels of LH.

The rhythmic, or cyclic, release of certain hormones (most commonly circadian cycles but also ultradian, or longer-than-circadian, cycles) appears to be under the control of serotonin. The suprachiasmatic nucleus of the hypothalamus has been identified as playing a major role in control of endogenous circadian rhythms.

Release of certain hormones is tied to environmental events. For example, stress induces an increased release of ACTH, and ovulation causes release of FSH and LH. Estrogen and suckling cause release of prolactin. Hypoglycemia causes release of growth hormone, and cold environment stimulates release of TSH.

Patients with a wide range of psychiatric illnesses exhibit abnormalities in basal, cyclic, and stimulated levels of pituitary hormone release. Biological psychiatrists have attempted to use pituitary hormone levels as indicators of the possible neurotransmitter dysfunctions that may underly these illnesses. Although in some cases this approach can be useful in shedding light on the brain neurotransmitter systems affected by the condition in question, the limitations of this approach should be recognized. To the extent that a psychiatric illness is associated with a *general* (brain-wide) neurotransmitter dysfunction, then abnormalities in pituitary hormone level may indicate abnormalities in the level of brain neurotransmitter that regulates it. However, another logical (and likely) possibility is that a neuroanatomically *specific* neurotransmitter system may function abnormally. In the latter case, pituitary hormones would not shed light on underlying brain pathology. Rather, abnormalities in hormone release could be secondary to the direct effects of the disorder. Finally, if the psychiatric illness under investigation is believed to result directly from a hypothalamic dysfunction, pituitary hormone levels might be expected to indicate an abnormal process underlying the illness.

HYPOTHALAMIC CONTROL OF BEHAVIOR

The hypothalamus plays an important role in the mediation of behaviors such as feeding, drinking, aggression, and maternal and sexual behavior. From an evolutionary vantage point, these behaviors are critically important for the survival of the individual or the species, or both. Therefore the involvement of an "older" brain area such as the hypothalamus should come as no surprise.

Most complex behaviors, including those just mentioned, are determined by many factors. For example, hunger is one factor that determines whether people eat, but certainly it is not the only one. Hedonic and cognitive factors also play a role. The presence of a tasty, aromatic dish would provoke most people to eat even if they were not hungry. On the contrary, sitting down to eat in a restaurant and noticing unclean conditions could cause some people to lose their appetite even if they had been hungry 5 minutes earlier! Being in a social situation tends to cause people to eat, as does the knowledge that it is dinnertime. Factors such as level of arousal, homeostatic conditions, hedonics, and cognition all play a role in determining whether a given behavior will occur. These determinants operate through separate and distinct brain mechanisms, and information about each must be integrated before a final "decision" can be made. In the example of feeding, all the information about hunger, time of day, dining atmosphere, and taste of food must ultimately be integrated. People and animals differ in the extent to which each of these factors influences their behavior. (Some people eat to live, whereas others live to eat.) In certain pathological conditions, the relative influences of some of these factors becomes unbalanced.

The mechanisms for determining homeostatic conditions lie, in large part, within the hypothalamus. Brain regions such as the pons, where arousal is controlled, and the cortex, where cognitive processes are mediated, have many neuroanatomic connections with the hypothalamus. Thus the hypothalamus is advantageously positioned to receive and integrate information about a variety of circumstances that determine behavior. Furthermore, the hypothalamus, because of its direct control of the endocrine system and the autonomic nervous system, as well as its recently discovered influence over the somatomotor system, is uniquely capable of synchronizing physiological and hormonal states of readiness with the execution of behavior.

Female Sexual Behavior

In most species the female sexual response occurs only when the animal is in the optimal hormonal condition for conception. This state, known as estrus, can vary seasonally or according to a season-free estrous cycle. The hypothalamus, through its control of the endocrine system, plays a critical role in controlling the hormonal events of the estrous cycle in animals and the menstrual cycle in humans. In humans, sexual behavior occurs throughout all points of the estrous cycle; however, transient motivational states may still be dependent on hormonal conditions. Moreover, changes in sexual behavior that are associated with certain forms of depression, and with anorexia nervosa, are probably mediated in part by hypothalamic dysfunction.

Hypothalamic GnRH control of the cyclic release of both LH and FSH from the anterior pituitary is governed by levels of circulating estrogens released by the ovaries. Estrogen also acts directly on the pituitary gland to control the release of these gonadotropic hormones. These "long negative feedback loops" through which estrogen exerts an inhibitory influence on those structures that regulate its release have long been believed to exist and are now well established.

Male Sexual Behavior

The role of the hypothalamus in controlling the production and secretion of testosterone and in controlling spermatogenesis is well understood; however, as in the female, the precise relationship of these hormonal processes to sexual behavior is unclear. GnRH-containing neurons of the hypothalamus control pituitary release of LH and FSH. The Leydig cells of the testes secrete testosterone and small amounts of estradiol in response to LH release. Testosterone, released by the testes, and FSH are necessary for the induction of spermatogenesis.

Testosterone and estradiol, as well as inhibin (produced as a result of spermatogenesis), exert inhibitory influence on hypothalamic GnRH release, and also directly on gonadotropin release by the pituitary gland. Thus the negative feedback loops from the gonads to the brain and the pituitary gland parallel those which exist in females.

PATHOLOGICAL CONDITIONS ASSOCIATED WITH THE HYPOTHALAMUS

Depression

Major depressive episodes are characterized by a broad range of behavioral and experiential abnormalities, one of which always includes a profoundly dysphoric mood. In addition, depressed patients often report diminished ability to experience pleasure in normal activities. They frequently exhibit changes in behavior that suggest alterations in the level of motivation. For example, appetite disturbances or weight changes (due to actual changes in eating), or both, and decreases in both libido and sexual activity are often reported. Moreover, one often sees disturbances in cyclic behaviors such as sleep. Cognitive dysfunction, characterized by diminished ability to concentrate and a marked pessimism that colors all thought, is common during a major depressive episode. That patients who experience major depressive episodes constitute a heterogeneous group is suggested by the fact that this clinical syndrome alone does not predict the efficacy of any of a broad array of treatments available for depression.

Among patients who meet criteria for major depressive episodes, those with the subtype of melancholia constitute a more homogeneous group. Melancholia is highly predictive of the efficacy of tricyclic antidepressant drugs and electroconvulsive therapy. Patients with melancholia exhibit a *more* profound, *more* pervasive, and somewhat distinct mood disorder that is remarkably unresponsive to environmental events, in comparison with patients who meet the criteria for major depressive episodes but not the subtype of melancholia. Patients with melancholia exhibit more severe disturbances in appetite, eating, and the ability to experience pleasure, and they have specific disorders in circadian rhythmicity of sleep and mood. The nature of these disturbances suggests that melancholia may involve some specific disturbance in hypothalamic function. Among the more obvious links between these symptoms and disorders seen in animals after hypothalamic manipulations are those associated with appetite, eating, and sexual function. It should be remembered, too, that various hypothalamic preparations exhibit a disordered balance in response to internal versus external stimuli, that the suprachiasmatic nucleus is an important circadian pacemaker, and that hypothalamic catecholamines may play an important role in the mediation of reward. It is thus possible to associate every symptom distinguishing patients of the melancholia subtype with a hypothalamic dysfunction.

Obesity

It appears virtually certain that the term "obesity" encompasses a broad and heterogeneous group of disorders of behavior and metabolism, many of which remain elusive to clinical investigation and treatment. However, manipulations of the medial hypothalamic feeding system in the rat, and their effects on autonomic and behavioral processes, have provided a relevant model for at least one kind of human obesity. Both the behavioral and autonomic alterations exhibited by obese people parallel those observed in rats who have lesions of the ventromedial hypothalamic region. That is, obese people, in addition to overeating, appear to be less responsive to internal or biological "hunger" cues than their normal-weight counterparts. Rather, their eating behavior seems to be under the control of external or environmental factors. Although obese people tend to overeat good-tasting food, they actually eat less than their normal-weight counterparts when the taste or texture of the food is slightly adulterated. They may overeat in social situations, and yet they tend to eat less than normal when food is not readily available.

The treatment of obesity has been problematic, although some success has been reported with the use of behavior-modification techniques. However, the problems with treatments such as those using high-protein nutritional supplements (Sustacal; Metrical) become evident in light of what has just been discussed. Because obese people have less difficulty with inhibiting the eating of ill-textured foods, it is not surprising that their body weights drop when they are placed on a Metrical diet. It is the eating response to good-tasting foods that is aberrant, and this may explain the failure of this treatment to result in the maintenance of reduced body weight once patients return to "food" diets.

Anorexia Nervosa

Anorexia nervosa is an eating disorder that occurs most frequently in adolescent girls but can also occur in young women. Like depression, it is characterized by affective, cognitive, and behavioral abnormalities; however, the focus of these symptoms is on eating and body weight. This syndrome is characterized by active avoidance of food and feeding; an intense fear of becoming obese, which is marked by body weight loss; and a distorted body image. Young girls who are mildly overweight may have some predisposition to this illness. Recent studies report that the onset of anorexia nervosa occurs during dieting.

Patients with anorexia exhibit a wide range of symptoms associated with hypothalamic dysfunction. These include changes in a variety of hormonal functions, decreased libido, and temperature dysregulation. These patients often exhibit amenorrhea and decreased basal levels of LH and FSH in plasma. In addition, circadian patterns of LH secretion are immature. In many cases, abnormalities in endocrine function may be secondary to body weight loss; however, some are not. Notably, amenorrhea precedes any significant weight loss in 25 percent of these patients and may therefore be of etiologic significance. Growth hormone response to levodopa or apomorphine is abnormal in these patients before weight loss and after recovery from weight loss. Further, decreased pituitary storage of LH, which is associated with anorexia nervosa, appears to be a result of hypothalamic dysfunction. Like depressed patients, during the episode of illness, patients with anorexia do not show the typical suppression of cortisol release in response to a dexamethasone challenge.

In addition to aberrations in endocrine function, a number of processes under autonomic nervous system control appear disordered. Many of these patients are hypothermic and exhibit constipation, hypotension, and bradycardia. The extent to which these symptoms are secondary to starvation is unclear.

The facts that (1) the onset of anorexia nervosa occurs at adolescence and (2) the growth hormone response to dopaminergic challenges is abnormal suggest abnormality in hypothalamic dopamine and estrogen function. The fact that hypothalamic dopamine neurons contain estrogen receptors provides an interesting avenue for further investigation of the biological basis of anorexia nervosa.

Sexual Dysfunction

Surprisingly little data exist on the relationship of human sexual disorders to hormonal variables. Although many investigators claim that human sexual behavior is more loosely linked to hormonal states than in animals, comparable studies have not been conducted. In animals, hormonal variables are studied in relation to directly observed, quantified responses, such as number of intromissions, latency of ejaculation, and refractory period. These responses are studied under controlled conditions of sensory stimulation and availability. In humans, measures are usually based on questionnaires and examine response frequency or subjective ratings of experience under widely varying conditions of environmental stimulation.

In men with normal sexual functioning, there is no known correlation between sexual behavior and circulating levels of testosterone. However, in hypogonadal men, such a correlation does exist. Furthermore, castration in men results in a decline in erectile function and libido. However, the temporal course of the behavioral and motivational decline, in comparison with the almost immediate decline in testosterone levels, is extremely variable.

Although injection of testosterone enanthate appears to markedly increase the overall number of erections in hypogonadal men, it has not necessarily been shown to be effective in treatment, because the increase in the number of erections occurred for the most part during sleep. The effectiveness of testosterone enanthate in reversing erectile dysfunction during coitus or masturbation is questionable.

When hypogonadism is due to hypothalamic or pituitary dysfunction, LH and FSH levels are low. Kallmann's syndrome is a hypothalamic disorder resulting in hypogonadism. Patients with this disorder do not experience ejaculation (including nocturnally), are usually impotent, and usually have low libido. GnRH injection is an effective treatment in relieving some symptoms and, if administered at a young age, permits normal sexual maturation.

Oxytocin may play an important role in the regulation of male sexual behavior. It has recently been found that oxytocin is released during sexual arousal in males, and it increases the rate of flow of sperm from the epididymis. The relevance of these findings to clinical problems has not been determined.

In women, low estrogen levels are associated with decreases in vaginal lubrication. However, this condition does not result in sexual dysfunction because it can be reversed through the use of vaginal lubricants. Small amounts (0.5 mg daily) of testosterone are released by the ovaries and adrenals in women and can be associated with decreases in arousal.

BIBLIOGRAPHY

Fink, G., Harmer, A.J., McKerns, K.W.: Neuroendocrine Molecular Biology. New York, Plenum Press, 1986.

Hess, W.R., in The Functional Organization of the Diencephalon, J.R. Hughes (ed). New York, Grune & Stratton, 1957.

Hoebel, B.G., Novin, D.: The Neural Basis of Feeding and Reward. Brunswick, Me., Haer Institute for Electrophysiological Research, 1982.

McEwen, B.F., et al.: Adrenal steroid receptors and actions in the nervous system. Physiol. Rev. 66:1121-1188, 1986.

McEwen, B.S., et al.: The brain as a target organ for steroid hormone action. Ann. Rev. Neurosci. 2:65-112, 1979.

Pfaff, W.D.: Estrogens and Brain Function: Neural Analysis of a Hormone-Controlled Mammalian Reproductive Behavior. New York, Springer-Verlag, 1980.

Targum, S.D.: Neuroendocrine challenge studies in clinical psychiatry. Psychiatr. Ann. 13:385-395, 1983.

Chapter 13

Biological Rhythms and the Neuroendocrine System

Larry J. Siever, M.D.

Biological rhythms, that is, regular periodicities in biologic functions, may be observed in organisms ranging in complexity from the simplest single cells to humans. Probably the best understood and most familiar period for such rhythms is the 24-hour day-night cycle. Regular rhythms with approximately this period are termed circadian rhythms. In fact, circadian periodicities may be observed in specific enzyme systems and thus seem to represent a general property of biologic systems. These rhythms may be observed in the absence of external driving cycles, such as environmental fluctuations in temperature and illumination, with a free-running period that is usually close to 24 hours. This intrinsic periodicity implies the presence of internal oscillators that drive the circadian cycles. Under normal circumstances, the circadian cycles are entrained by environmental cycles of light, temperature, or even, in some cases, social cues. These rhythms are apparently inherent, genetically determined functions of the organism that coordinate its internal environment with its external environment in the service of maximal adaptation.

In this chapter, some general properties of biological rhythms in humans are reviewed, with a particular focus on the regulation of sleep and the neuroendocrine system, two systems with circadian periodicities. Abnormalities of these systems in depression are highlighted.

BIOLOGICAL RHYTHMS IN HUMANS

Circadian rhythms in humans may be observed in neuroendocrine secretory cycles, temperature, sleep-wakefulness cycles, motor activity, and neurotransmitter metabolite excretion. These rhythms may be internally coupled to each other; however, with specific environmental manipulations, the rhythms may become uncoupled, with the different variables exhibiting different periodicities.

Humans kept in isolation from external time cues show circadian rhythms of slightly greater than 24 hours, which may spontaneously undergo a desynchronization to bicircadian rhythms of approximately 48 hours' duration. In these bicircadian rhythms, ratios between activity and rapid-eye-movement sleep remain unchanged from the circadian cycle.

In humans, light-dark cycles play a crucial role in the entrainment of circadian rhythms. The suprachiasmatic nucleus of the hypothalamus receives projections from the retina and, on the basis of ablation studies, seems to play a pivotal role in this entrainment process in mammals. For example, when a lesion is created in the suprachiasmatic nucleus, individual components of the sleep-wakefulness cycle or estrous cycle remain intact but the normal rhythmicity is lost. However, the suprachiasmatic nucleus is not the only endogenous pacemaker in humans; a number of hierarchically organized oscillators may be synchronously entrained or dissociated. It is likely that there are at least two oscillators: one regulating temperature and the other regulating the sleep-wakefulness cycle.

BIOLOGICAL RHYTHMS IN PSYCHOPATHOLOGY

Circadian rhythms may be abnormal in psychiatric patients, particularly those wth affective disorders. Temperature and sleep cycles may be phase advanced (that is, may occur earlier in the day-night cycle) or desynchronized (that is, lacking in normal periodicities) in depressed patients. Urinary 3-methoxy-4-hydroxyphenylglycol (MHPG) excretion also shows an earlier daytime peak and an erratic pattern in depressed patients compared with normal subjects. Electroencephalographic sleep patterns in depressed patients are similar to those in normal subjects whose circadian rhythms have been shifted several hours earlier than normal relative to their sleep period. Antidepressant medications alter circadian rhythms. Experimental manipulations of the light-dark cycle and isolation from external time cues seem to have important, often beneficial effects on mood disorders. Seasonal affective disorder may represent a specific type of depression that emerges in the winter, is dependent on the timing and duration of daylight, and may be treated with bright lights.

SLEEP

The sleep-wakefulness cycle is perhaps one of the most fundamental of the biological period-

icities in humans. Under usual physiologic conditions, it is synchronized with other biological rhythms. The function of sleep is not well understood but may be related to the consolidation of learning and memory from the previous day. Its disturbance is a central feature of the depressive disorders.

Sleep Stages

The architecture of sleep has now been well characterized by the use of techniques that utilize simultaneous electroencephalogram (EEG), electromyogram (EMG), and electrooculogram (EOG) detection of changes in electrical potential deriving from central nervous system activity, muscle activity, and eye movements, respectively. Sleep may be divided into rapid-eye-movement (REM) periods and non-REM periods. There are four stages of non-REM sleep based on their EEG characteristics.

- *Stage 1:* non-REM sleep is characterized by decreased alpha activity (8 to 14 cycles per second), mixed beta activity (15 to 35 cycles per second), and slower theta activity (4 to 7 cycles per second).
- *Stage 2:* non-REM sleep is characterized by a theta background with superimposed spindles of rhythmic waves (12 to 14 cycles per second) and k-complexes composed of a high-amplitude negative wave, followed by a positive wave.
- *Stages 3 and 4:* non-REM sleeps are characterized by delta waves, which have high amplitude and low frequency (0.5 to 3 cycles per second).

During REM sleep, the EEG frequencies correspond approximately to those observed in stage 1 non-REM sleep but are also marked by the appearance of conjugate eye movements on the EOG. The non-REM sleep preceding the first REM period is called the REM latency period, normally 70 to 90 minutes. The sequence of stages during the REM latency is usually as follows:

Waking, stage 1, stage 2, stage 3, stage 4, stage 3, and stage 2; REM, stage 2, stage 3, stage 4, stage 3, and stage 2; REM . . .

The interval between REM periods constitutes the sleep cycle, usually 70 to 120 minutes.

Total sleep time declines in old age, while the number of awakenings increase. Circadian effects and duration of wakefulness before sleep contribute to the time required to fall asleep (sleep latency).

Neurotransmitter Regulation of Sleep

Although the mechanisms of neurotransmitter regulation of sleep are not fully understood, pharmacologic studies suggest that serotonin, norepinephrine, and acetylcholine are important in the initiation and maintenance of REM sleep in particular. The activity of the serotoninergic systems seems to be directly correlated with REM sleep, whereas the activity of the noradrenergic system seems to be negatively correlated with REM sleep. Cholinergic mechanisms are likely to be important in the initiation of REM sleep. In contrast, manipulations of the dopaminergic and histaminergic systems have had little effect in modifying sleep.

Neuroendocrine Mechanisms and Sleep

Growth hormone secretion is particularly tied to sleep, with increases observed during the early part of sleep, and may be associated with slow-wave sleep. Adrenocorticotropic hormone (ACTH) secretion is less closely tied to sleep, with alterations in the sleep-waking cycle having little effect on the circadian pattern of cortisol secretion. An increase in prolactin secretion occurs after the onset of sleep, and there is evidence that the secretory peak may be stimulated by serotoninergic activity.

Secretion of luteinizing hormone, follicle-stimulating hormone (FSH), and thyroid-stimulating hormone (TSH) has a weaker association with sleep. Melatonin is normally secreted during sleep, but its release is associated more closely with darkness and the nighttime period of the circadian cycle than with the state of sleep.

Sleep and Psychopathology

Insomnia may derive from a variety of causes and should not be presumed to be psychogenic without a careful clinical assessment. Sleep disorders can now be specifically clinically diagnosed and, in some cases, successfully treated. Sleep disturbances may be observed with both acute ethanol ingestion and chronic alcohol use, even in "dry" chronic alcoholics.

Compared with control subjects, depressed patients show delayed sleep onset, reduced REM latency, shallower sleep, a slower sleep cycle, more wakefulness, and increased variability from night to night. While ill or in remission, depressed patients show a greater decrease in REM latency after challenge with arecoline, a cholinergic agonist, than do control subjects. Experimental sleep deprivation has been reported to improve depression. Slow-wave sleep is reduced in patients with schizophrenia, and REM sleep may be reduced during periods of psychic turmoil. Some studies show a reduced REM latency and a decreased REM rebound after REM deprivation in subjects with schizophrenia. Altered circadian rhythms in the sleep-wakefulness cycle have also been reported in psychiatric patients, particularly those with affective disorders.

NEUROENDOCRINE MECHANISMS

The neuroendocrine system comprises those areas of the central nervous system, particularly the hypothalamus, that contribute to the regulation of secretion of the endocrine system and the endocrine system itself, including the pituitary, adrenal, thyroid, and pineal glands. Most endocrine hormones are secreted in a circadian rhythm, with more punctuated pulsatile release under specific conditions. The different elements of the neuroendocrine system are related by complex reciprocal feedback interactions in such a way that central nervous system structures may modulate endocrine secretion of hormones, which in turn act on the brain to influence various central nervous system functions, including the regulation of the endocrine system itself. The mutual interdependence of the central nervous system and endocrine function may reflect the role of hormones as neuromodulators, which transmit information by activating biologic receptors, as do neurotransmitters. However, circulatory hormones have a more diffuse impact, reaching more anatomically distant target organs after their release. The central regulation of the secretion of the major hormones, and the implications of this central regulation for human behavior, will be reviewed, with particular emphasis on neuroendocrine abnormalities observed in psychiatric patients.

Corticotropin Releasing Factor, ACTH, and Cortisol

Cortisol (hydrocortisone) is the principal natural glucocorticoid in humans. It is secreted by the adrenal gland, under the immediate regulatory control of ACTH, which is secreted from the anterior lobe of the pituitary gland (Fig. 13–1). ACTH derives from the larger peptide precursor proopiomelanocortin, which is also a precursor to β-lipotropin, which is a precursor to β-endorphin. ACTH is inhibited at the pituitary level by cortisol in a feedback inhibitory loop and is stimulated by corticotropin releasing factor (CRF) from the hypothalamus. Central amines modulate CRF-ACTH, probably at the hypothalamic level, with cholinergic influences playing a role in the stress activation of this axis. Serotonin may increase CRF-ACTH activity, whereas norepinephrine may have either a stimulatory or an inhibitory influence on this axis.

Plasma cortisol follows a diurnal rhythm, with maximum values between 4 AM and 8 AM and minimum values in late afternoon and evening (Fig. 13–2).

The role of cortisol in human behaviors is not well understood, although it seems to be secreted under stressful conditions. Exogenously administered steroids may cause mood disorders and psychosis. Animal studies suggest that ACTH may play a role in conditioned avoidance learning.

Thyrotropin Releasing Hormone, TSH, and Thyroid Hormones

Hypothalamic thyrotropin releasing hormone (TRH) stimulates the synthesis and release of thyrotropin or TSH by the pituitary gland (Fig. 13–3). TSH, in turn, stimulates the thyroid to secrete thyroxine (T_4) and triiodothyronine (T_3) by activating iodide uptake, hormone synthesis, and release (Fig. 13–4). The circulating thyroid hormones exert a negative feedback control on TSH secretion from the pituitary gland. Somatostatin secreted from the hypothalamus may also modulate thyroid release. Norepinephrine and perhaps dopamine appear to play a facilitatory role in TRH release, whereas serotonin

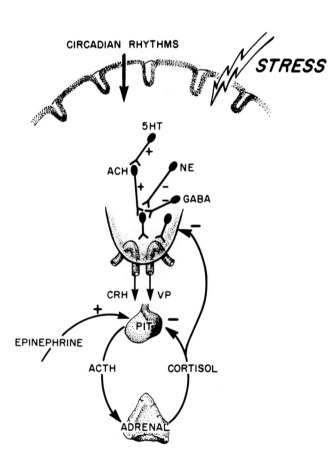

FIGURE 13–1. Elements of the hypothalamic-pituitary-adrenal cortical system for regulation of cortisol secretion are illustrated here. Secretion of ACTH is stimulated by corticotropin releasing factor, whose secretion is regulated by a complex set of neurotransmitter neurons that includes two stimulatory components (cholinergic and serotoninergic) and an adrenergic inhibitory pathway. These pathways mediate stress-induced and circadian ACTH secretory changes. Feedback effects of cortisol may be exerted on the nervous sytem as well as on the pituitary gland. This model is based on studies in rats and dogs. In human beings there appears to be an α-adrenergic stimulating pathway. Abbreviations: NE, norepinephrine; ACH, acetylcholine; GABA, γ-aminobutyric acid; CRH, corticotropin releasing hormone; VP, vasopressin; PIT, pituitary gland. (From Martin, J.B., Reichlin, S.: Clinical Neuroendocrinology, ed. 2. Philadelphia, F.A. Davis, 1987.)

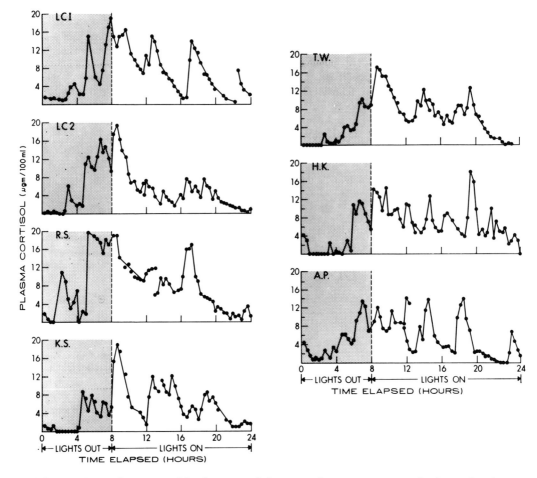

FIGURE 13–2. Plasma cortisol levels are sampled at intervals in seven unstressed subjects. Levels are highest between 4 and 9 AM, are lowest around midnight, and fluctuate during the day without obvious relationship to external events. (From Weitzman, E.D., et al: Twenty-four-hour pattern of the episodic secretion of cortisol in normal subjects. J. Clin. Endocrinol. Metab. 33:16, 1971. © by the Endocrine Society).

seems to have an inhibitory effect. However, the role of central monoamines in the regulation of TRH is not yet clear.

TSH and thyroid hormones are secreted in a pulsatile fashion, with highest levels usually occurring during the early morning hours.

Growth Hormone

Growth hormone is released from the pituitary gland in a pulsatile fashion, with secretory bursts throughout the day and particularly during the first part of the sleep cycle (Fig. 13–5). Growth hormone secretion is stimulated by growth hormone releasing hormone (GH-RH) and inhibited by growth hormone release inhibiting hormone (GH-RIH), or somatostatin, both

of which are synthesized in and released from the medial basal hypothalamus. Under certain conditions, growth hormone may inhibit its own release, perhaps via some lower-molecular-weight intermediaries, the somatomedins, which are synthesized by the liver. Growth hormone release may be associated with stress.

Norepinephrine, dopamine, and serotonin are all implicated in the stimulation of growth hormone release in primates and humans. Electric stimulation studies have shown that direct stimulation of monoaminergic neurons in the brain stem cause growth hormone release.

Neuroendocrine challenges such as insulin-induced hypoglycemia, L-dopa, amphetamine, 5-hydroxytryptophan (5-HTP), and clonidine have been reported to result in a deficient growth hormone response in depressed patients

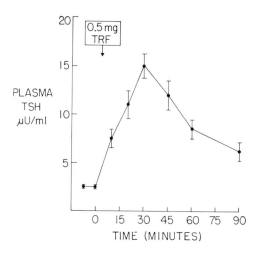

FIGURE 13–3. Plasma TSH response to 0.5 mg TRF in normal subjects. The peak of the response occurs at 30 minutes. (From Fleischer, N., et al.: Synthetic thyrotropin: recent factors—a test of pituitary thyrotropin reserve. J. Clin. Endocrinol. Metab. 34:617, 1972. © by The Endocrine Society.)

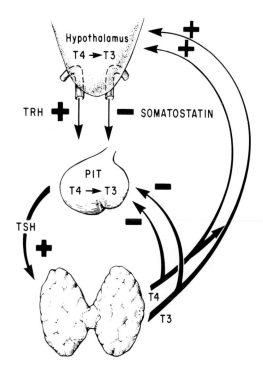

FIGURE 13–4. This is a diagram of regulation of the hypothalamic-pituitary-thyroid axis. Pituitary TSH secretion is stimulated by TRH and inhibited by somatostatin. The release of the hypothalamic hormones from peptidergic neurons are in turn regulated by bioaminergic neurons. Higher brain centers are involved in relay of stress- and temperature-mediated influences on hypothalamic centers. Thyroid hormones (T_3, T_4) feed back predominantly at the pituitary level but may have effects on hypothalamus. Estrogen facilitates, and growth hormone and glucocorticoids inhibit, pituitary responsiveness to TRH. The dopamine inhibitory component (conveyed by the tuberoinfundibular system) is not illustrated on this figure. (From Martin, J.B., Reichlin, S.: Clinical Neuroendocrinology, ed. 2. Philadelphia, F.A. Davis, 1987.)

(Fig. 13–6). The most consistent abnormalities have been observed with challenges specifically acting on the noradrenergic system.

Prolactin

Prolactin (PRL) is secreted by the anterior pituitary in an episodic pattern, with evidence for a circadian rhythm. It is released in response to suckling, physical and emotional stress, arginine infusion, hypoglycemia, and estrogen administration. Prolactin inhibitory factors (PIF) and prolactin releasing factors (PRF) are secreted at the hypothalamic level. Dopamine stimulates PRL secretion, whereas serotonin inhibits it. Dopamine antagonists, such as the neuroleptic drugs, increase prolactin secretion. Studies of PRL secretion in response to monoaminergic challenges have been used to explore the pathophysiology of the affective disorders and schizophrenia.

Gonadotropins and Gonadal Hormones

FSH and luteinizing hormone regulate reproductive function, including the secretion of sex steroids: the estrogens, progestins, and androgens. FSH and luteinizing hormone are stimulated by luteinizing hormone releasing hormone (LH-RH). The sex steroids regulate gonadotropic hormones through a negative feedback mechanism at the hypothalamic or pituitary level. FSH and luteinizing hormone are released in secretory bursts; in females, their secretion varies with the period of the menstrual cycle. Biogenic amines may influence the secretion of luteinizing hormone, with limited evidence of norepinephrine and dopamine playing a stimulatory role in luteinizing hormone release. Luteinizing hormone secretion may be altered in some psychiatric syndromes, and luteinizing hormone responses to LH-RH stimulation have been reported to be blunted in anorexia nervosa or exaggerated in persons with secondary depression.

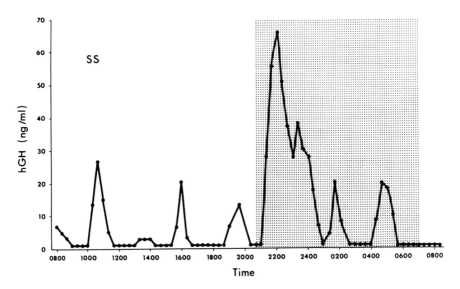

FIGURE 13–5. Episodic secretion of human growth hormone (hGH) in a normal male adolescent. Eight distinct secretory episodes are evident, with a large surge of secretion shortly after onset of sleep (shaded area). (Adapted from Finkelstein, J.W., et al.: Age-related change in the 24-hour spontaneous secretion of growth hormone. J. Clin. Endocrinol. Metab. 35:665, 1972. From Martin, J.B., Reichlin, S.: Clinical Neuroendocrinology, ed. 2. Philadelphia, F.A. Davis, 1987.)

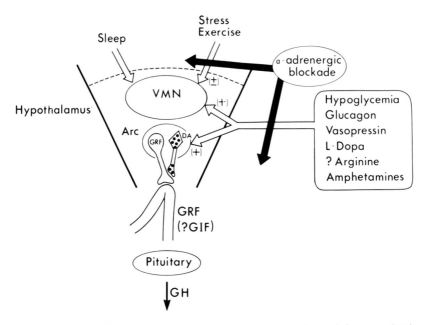

FIGURE 13–6. Diagram of hypothalamic mechanisms for regulation of growth hormone (GH) secretion. Adrenergic blockade (with phentolamine) partially or completely blocks growth hormone release to the stimuli shown. Sleep release of growth hormone is not affected. Abbreviations: VMN, ventromedial nucleus; DA, dopamine; GRF, growth hormone releasing factor; GIF, growth hormone–inhibiting factor. (Adapted from Martin, J.B.: Neural regulation of growth hormone secretion. N. Engl. J. Med. 228:1384, 1973. From Martin, J.B., and Reichlin, S.: Clinical Neuroendocrinology, ed. 2. Philadelphia, F.A. Davis, 1987.)

Arginine Vasopressin

Arginine vasopressin (AVP) interacts with kidney receptors to contribute to the regulation of fluid and electrolyte balance. It is released from the posterior pituitary and is sensitively regulated by inputs from local osmoreceptor and cardiovascular volume receptors. Acetylcholine plays an excitatory role in its release, whereas norepinephrine plays an inhibitory role.

Endorphins

The endorphins are released from the pituitary gland in the form of a common precursor for both ACTH and β-lipotropin, and immediate precursor for β-endorphin. They are involved in analgesia and perhaps affective states. The role of endorphins in psychiatric syndromes is unclear, although variations in endorphin levels and altered responses to opioid agonists and antagonists have been reported in populations of schizophrenic patients and those with affective disorder.

MSH and MIF-I

Melanocyte-stimulating hormone (MSH) is secreted from the pars distalis of the anterior pituitary. MSH-inhibiting factor (MIF-I) inhibits the release of MSH and has been used in pilot studies to treat depression.

Melatonin

Melatonin is secreted by the pineal gland during the nighttime hours; its release seems to depend on the onset of darkness, rather than on sleep. This hormone may modulate subcortical activity and other endocrine systems; its function is not well understood. Because of its close entrainment to the light-dark cycle and its fairly well defined neurotransmitter control, melatonin has become a valuable marker for studies of circadian-rhythm, neuroendocrine, and neurotransmitter alterations in psychiatric disorders.

BIBLIOGRAPHY

Brown, G.M., Seggie, J.: Neuroendocrine mechanisms and their implication for psychiatric research. Psychiatric Clin. North Am. 3:205-221, 1980.

Gwirtsman, H.E., Halaris, A.Z., Wolf, A.W., et al.: Apparent phase advance in diurnal MHPG rhythm in depression. Am. J. Psychiatry 146:1427-1433, 1989.

Hobson, J.A., McCarly, R.W.: The brain as a dream state generator: An activation-synthesis hypothesis of the dream process. Am. J. Psychiatry 134:1335-1348, 1977.

Jouvet, M., et al.: Toward 48-hour day: Experimental bicircadian rhythm in man, in The Neurosciences: Third Study Program, F.O. Schmitt and F.G. Worden (eds.) Cambridge, Mass., MIT Press, 1974.

Lewy, A.J., Sack, R.L.: Phase typing and bright light therapy of chronobiologic sleep and mood disorders, in Chronobiology and Psychiatric Disorders, A. Halaris (ed.). New York, Elsevier, 1987.

Martin, J.B., Reichlin, S.: Clinical Neuroendocrinology, ed. 2. Philadelphia, F.A. Davis, 1987.

Mendelson, W.B.: Human Sleep: Research and Clinical Care. New York, Plenum Press, 1987.

Moore, R.Y.: Central neural control of circadian rhythms, in Frontiers in Neuroendocrinology, vol. 5, W.F. Ganong and I. Martin (eds.). New York, Raven Press, 1978.

Muller, E.E., Nistico, G., Scapagnini, U.: Neurotransmitters and Anterior Pituitary Function. New York, Academic Press, 1977.

Pittendrigh, C.S.: Circadian oscillations in cells and circadian organization of multicellular systems, in The Neurosciences: Third Study Program, F.O. Schmitt and F.G. Worden (eds.). Cambridge, Mass., MIT Press, 1974.

Reynolds, C.F., III, Gillin, J.C., Kupfer, D.J.: Sleep and Affective Disorders. Psychopharmacology: The Third Generation of Progress. New York, Raven Press, 1987.

Sachar, E.J., et al.: Recent studies of the neuroendocrinology of major depressive disorders. Psychiatric Clin. North Am. 3:313-326, 1980.

Siever, L.J., Coccaro, E.F., Davis, K.L.: Chronobiologic instability of the noradrenergic system in depression, in Chronobiology and Psychiatric Disorders, A. Halaris (ed.). New York, Elsevier, 1987.

Wehr, R.A., Muscettola, G., Goodwin, F.K.: Urinary 3-methoxy-4-hydroxyphenylglycol circadian rhythm. Arch. Gen. Psychiatry 37:257-263, 1980.

Wever, R., Ütger, A.: The circadian system of man: Results of experiments under temporal isolation. New York, Springer Verlag, 1979.

Part III
CHILD PSYCHIATRY

INTRODUCTION

Child psychiatry is the only subspecialty in psychiatry that requires separate accreditation. It stands in relationship to general psychiatry as pediatric medicine relates to internal medicine. Thus it not only is concerned with the diagnosis and treatment of children and adolescents with psychiatric disorders but also is increasingly involved with early identification and preventive interventions for psychiatric disorders that more typically have their onset later in life.

Historically, child psychiatry evolved from a different tradition and quite independently of general psychiatry in the United States. The roots of child psychiatry were nurtured by the child guidance movement in the early part of the twentieth century. Out of concern over the exploitation by industry and the neglect of youth as a result of disadvantaged economic circumstances, freestanding clinics were established in various cities of the United States. The conceptual approaches of these clinics were largely oriented toward the social, psychological, and educational interventions. With the development of psychoanalytical theory, with its heavy emphasis on the important role of developmental life experiences in the etiology of psychiatric disorders, psychiatry assumed an increasing presence in the child guidance clinics, and specialty training in the diagnosis and treatment of psychiatric disorders of children came into being. In addition, the pioneering research of Jean Piaget laid the foundation for rigorous studies on the developmental aspects of cognitive functions and moral behavior that have grown immensely over the last three decades.

With few exceptions, such as the program started by Leo Kanner at the Johns Hopkins Hospital in 1933, most clinical training programs in child psychiatry developed independently of academic medical institutions. As a consequence, there has been a lag in the incorporation of biological concepts into the theories of the pathophysiological basis for childhood psychiatric disorders. However, over the last 15 years, as most programs of child psychiatry have become affiliated with academic departments of psychiatry, research into the biological basis of childhood psychiatric disorders has been advancing at an ever-increasing pace. And recent years have witnessed a refinement in diagnostic concepts and a more rigorous assessment of treatment strategies. In this context, a multidisciplinary approach toward the treatment of children and adolescents with psychiatric disorders that encompasses biological, psychological, familial, and educational strategies has gained ascendance.

Advances, especially in the realm of psychiatric genetics, will have considerable impact on the practice of child psychiatry. Thus the rapidly increasing pace of identification of gene loci responsible for major psychiatric disorders will soon lead to the feasibility of identifying children, and even fetuses, at risk for an expanding number of these disorders based on their occurrence in first-degree relatives. It is important to point out that many of these disorders, such as major depression, schizophrenia, anxiety disorders, and alcoholism, do not appear to have complete penetrance, and so it will become possible to more rigorously define those factors that protect the genetically vulnerable individual from manifesting the symptoms of the disorder. This will present child psychiatry with exciting new challenges to develop early interventions that prevent or considerably reduce the symptomatic manifestations of inherited psychiatric disorders. The strategy is analogous to the increasing use of genetic markers in pediatric medicine to identify children at high risk for cardiovascular disease, for example, and the early implementation of dietary restrictions to reduce this risk.

The following chapters introduce the student to the theories and practices of child psychiatry. In order to appreciate psychopathological conditions of childhood and adolescence, it is necessary to first understand the normal development of cognitive abilities, motor and language skills, interpersonal relationships, and moral capacities. For many psychiatric disorders of childhood and adolescence, the symptomatic features represent an inability to master or pass through one or more of these developmental stages, thereby bringing the child to the attention of the parents, teachers, or primary physician. For other more serious psychiatric disturbances, the developmental life stage at which they become apparent markedly affects the symptomatic features of the disorder as well as its course and treatment. Finally, mental retardation represents a group of disorders involving a severe deviation from normal development, for which there is a high risk of behavioral and psychiatric disturbance. Since the effective management of the mentally retarded child involves close interactions among the child psychiatrist, pediatric neurologist, and developmental pediatrician, a chapter has been devoted to this topic.

Child psychiatry is the most severely underpopulated specialty in medicine at present. The rapid advances in developmental and molecular neurobiology, as well as in human genetics, are increasingly strengthening the scientific foundations of child psychiatry. At the same time, research in developmental cognitive psychology, ego psychology, and family therapy is providing better methods for understanding the psychological consequences of psychiatric disorders of children and adolescents and nonmedical strategies for addressing them. Thus, for those who enjoy working with children and families and who can accept the challenge of developing new and interdisciplinary strategies for reducing psychiatric morbidity, child psychiatry is a specialty that has much to offer.

JOSEPH T. COYLE, M.D.

Chapter 14
Developmental Perspective*

James C. Harris, M.D.

The developmental perspective is essential for psychiatry. It emphasizes the capacity for change throughout life, an approach now referred to as the life span view of human development. The child is seen as an active, socially oriented, and developing person rather than either a passive respondent to the environment or an individual developing independently from psychosocial experiences. Development occurs in phases of progressive change as the individual child masters new developmental tasks. Early experiences are important in personality development, but there is a remarkable resilience to stress; and as new abilities emerge, the child often compensates for past difficulties.

Growth refers to changes in size of the body as a whole, and development addresses the differentiation of form, that is, changes in function resulting from interaction with the external environment. Development is an interactive pro-

cess and refers, particularly in psychiatry, to emotional and social development. The opportunity to attain one's full biological and psychological potential is a result of many interacting factors. Genetic factors are important in establishing the limits of potential, but they are interwoven with environmental experience. Physical trauma, particularly brain injury, and nutritional factors affect growth, development, and behavior.

A developmental perspective focuses on both growth and differentiation and addresses changing contexts and patterns of behavior over time rather than behavioral stability. It recognizes that younger children have considerable developmental plasticity in the nervous system but that, with the pruning of synapses that occurs with maturation, the brain's capacity to adapt to injury becomes more circumscribed. It acknowledges discontinuity in development but also connectedness in development exemplified by the persistence of temperamental traits over time. A developmental perspective asks how it is that certain behaviors first appear at one age

*This chapter adapted from *Principles and Practice of Pediatrics*, Frank A. Oski, M.D., Editor-in-Chief. Adapted and used by permission of J.B. Lippincott Co.

and not another. It addresses age-related vulnerability to stress and its mastery, recognizing that experiences that are debilitating for one individual may be strengthening for another. Through the study of developmental psychopathology, a developmental perspective asks how a major mental illness manifests at different ages, influences developmental tasks, and presents clinically. The psychiatric interview, the diagnostic system, and treatment approaches are then better informed by an appreciation of developmental processes, experiences, and task mastery. Finally, the developmental view suggests an opportunity for prevention through interventions within the developmental period.

From a social and emotional perspective, multiple factors affect personality development. These include the quality of the interaction of the infant and child with parents, siblings, and others, the child's position in the family, specific concerns and needs of the parents, and the type of child-rearing practices that are carried out. Child rearing is influenced by cultural as well as personal experiences in the family. The psychiatrist addresses the full spectrum of behavior from the molecular level—as seen in enzyme activation in the course of differentiation and interaction of metabolic and physical changes associated with the development of neurotransmitter and hormonal systems—to the development of cognition, intelligence, emotions, and reciprocal social interactions in the development of personal, family, and community relations.

BRAIN MATURATION

The growth of the brain, in contrast to other organ systems, occurs primarily in the infant and toddler years. By 6 months of age, the brain has reached half of its mature weight, and by 5 years, 90 percent of its adult weight. The rapid growth of the brain in contrast to the rest of the body has important implications from the developmental perspective. This rapid development has been linked to a maturational view which argues that abilities are little influenced by outside circumstances and will gradually unfold as long as two primary conditions are met: adequate nutrition and an opportunity to interact in a normal expectable environment (that is, an opportunity to practice behavior). Maturation would occur in an orderly sequence if there is no deprivation, and the extent of brain growth would determine the impact of specific training. This idea has been investigated through twin studies in which one twin was given early training and the other

was not, demonstrating that the early training did not generally enhance skills. It has also been investigated in classic studies of salamanders where motor activity was present in the early phase of development. When activity was prevented until a particular age, the salamanders could swim despite the lack of experience. However, there are marked *individual differences* in brain development, so that although there are average ages for maturational events, it is more appropriate to talk about a range over months when development will occur, for example, walking from 10 to 18 months.

One internal factor that apparently plays a part in brain growth is rapid-eye-movement (REM) sleep. Studies of infant sleep suggest that developmental changes in infancy do not indicate a unitary process but, rather, a change in organization, a reorganization, of brain structure. The development of neurotransmitter systems is of particular interest in this regard. The reticular core neurons—the noradrenergic, dopaminergic, serotonergic, and cholinergic neuronal systems—are located in the brainstem and are formed early in fetal development. The gamma-aminobutyric acid (GABAergic) intraneurons within the cortex are formed much later in development, during the genesis of the cerebral cortex. Some parts of the brain mature earlier than others, that is, the brainstem and limbic system mature before the cerebellum and higher cortical areas. Hearing and seeing are present early, but interpretation and understanding of what is heard take place later. These usual sequences of development may be relevant in children with developmental delays. Some children do not speak until 3 or 4 years of age, suggesting a potential delay in development. Delays are more common in boys than girls, suggesting a difference in their brain development. However, the association of developmental delay with maturation is hypothetical at this time. Much more needs to be learned about brain development, particularly in mental retardation.

Developing parts of the brain are the most susceptible to damage, which may be greatest at times of most rapid brain growth. However, the young brain is also more capable of adapting to damage, so that the practical consequences of damage may be less; for example, damage to a structure may be compensated for by redundancy of synaptic connections if it occurs sufficiently early in life. This is probably because brain functions are not specifically localized to one area; brain functions involve multiple connections that go throughout the brain, involving several regions, as demonstrated by 2-deoxyglucose positron emission tomography (PET) scan studies. However, some regions are vital to function, for example, the speech area in the left hemisphere, which, if damaged in the adult, results in severe damage. Yet, compensation may be possible in the infant or young child by increased activity in the other hemisphere, and recovery in young children may be more complete than expected because of this neuronal plasticity.

ENVIRONMENTAL INTERFACE WITH BRAIN

Development is not just a gradual unfolding; social experience is important, and learning requires brain growth and both physical and social stimulation. The timing of development also is not entirely genetically controlled, since external environmental stimulation is needed to initiate it. The term *plasticity* is used to signify the fact that the organism can be modified by the external environment. When behavior in response to stimulus is measured, plasticity is being measured. For example, if infant kittens are raised with one eyelid sutured closed, vision is impaired in that eye; but the loss is partially functional and plasticity is demonstrated, since vision can be substantially restored by GABA agonists after the sutures are removed.

W. T. Greenough designated experience-expectant neuronal information processes that have evolved in preparation for incorporating specific information into the brain. In many sensory systems, synapses are produced in excess and subsequent experiences determine the final pattern of connections. Experience-dependent storage allows incorporation of unique experiences and involves new synaptic connections. These terms have been introduced instead of the terms *critical* or *sensitive period*. Greenough's work on "super enriched environments" suggests that the effects of early enrichment may persist over time.

The chemistry of brain development is also affected by deprivation, so that lack of stimulation may retard growth; however, extra stimulation does not enhance it if adequate maturation has not occurred. Stimulation may influence particular infant behaviors as well; for example, babbling in infants is influenced by parents talking to them and by accommodating the prosody or rhythm of their voices to those of the infants. Children who receive specific language training in a day-care center are enhanced in their abilities by daily language training in comparison to those who are involved in free play. However, stress may interfere with development, as demonstrated by the persistence of enuresis in children with severe burns and the return to bed-wetting in children who have been stressed.

DEVELOPMENTAL MODELS OF BEHAVIORAL AND EMOTIONAL DEVELOPMENT

To understand the complex interaction between children and the biological and environmental influences on them, the child's development has been approached through use of several models. A focus on biological endowment is emphasized in the maturational and ethological approaches. The individual's interpersonal experience in mastering the environment is emphasized in the psychodynamic and systems theory approaches, and an emphasis on the environment as shaping the person is emphasized in the approach of behaviorism.

Maturational and Ethological Approaches

The *maturational model* has been popularized by A. Gesell and focuses on the development as occurring through orderly, nonrandom, patterned sequences determined by biological and evolutionary history. The rate of development, however, is influenced by the individual genetic endowment. Although the rate of development may be altered, despite illness, malnutrition, or stressful experience, fundamental biological factors direct development. A favorable environment facilitates, and an unfavorable one inhibits; neither circumstance changes the basic biological potential. Gesell sought to describe the form of both morphological or structural growth and psychological growth. He indicated that development has direction (cephalocaudal and proximodistal) and is organized through reciprocal relationships or interweavings; for example, flexors and extensors develop in a sequence that allows coordinated movement but may demonstrate functional asymmetry, an unbalanced development that occurs so that the individual can achieve mastery at a later stage of development, such as development of handedness. In its basic form, development is not changed by the environment, suggesting that environmental influence is limited in this area (individuating maturation). Finally, there is a self-regulatory fluctuation, with periods of instability followed by stability and consolidation; cycles of development exist, with equilibrium following disequilibrium.

Taking this approach, Gesell focused on normal children in an average expectable environment and emphasized four areas of development: motor, adaptive, language, and personal social (Table 14–1). He found that development is controlled by biologically predetermined pat-

TABLE 14–1.   Four Developmental Models

	Developmental Landmarks (Gesell and Other Authors)	Psychosexual Stages: Psychosocial Stages, Tasks, and Values (Erikson)	Attachment Theory (Bowlby): Psychological Characteristics	Intellectual Development (Piaget)
Infancy				
Birth	Reflex smile/grimace Develops eye/head control	Incorporative mode Trust vs. mistrust Outcome: **Hope**	**Preattachment (0 to 8-10 wk)** Orientation and signals without discrimination of a figure	**Sensorimotor stage** Reflex (0-1 mo) Primary circular reaction (2-6 mo)
2 mo	Social smile 180-degree visual pursuit		**Attachment in the making (4-10 wk to 6 mo)** Orientation and signals directed toward one (or more) discriminated figures	Secondary circular reaction (2-8 mo) Secondary schemata (8-12 mo)
3 mo	Reaches for objects Rolls over			Tertiary circular reaction (12-16 mo)
6 mo	Transfers objects Raking grasp		**Clear-cut attachment (6 mo to end of life)** Maintenance of proximity to a discriminated figure by means of local motion as signals	Invention of new means through mental combinations (16 mo on)
9 mo	Sits up well Purposeful release Prehension deft Cruises at rail			
1 yr	Walks unassisted 3-4 words Builds towers of 2 cubes	Retentive-eliminative mode Autonomy vs. shame and doubt Outcome: **Will**	Exuberant exploration Realizes omnipotence is limited, becomes more conservative	**Stage of preoperational thought (prelogical)** Development of symbolic functions
18 mo	Scribbles with crayon 10-20 words Builds towers of 5-6 cubes Names a few pictures		Oppositional behavior Messiness Parallel play Pleasure in looking and being looked at	Differentiation between signs and symbols
2 yr	Runs (and falls) Uses 3-word sentences Names several body parts Uses appropriate personal pronouns			
Preschool			**Goal-corrected partnership**	
3 yr	Rides tricycle Copies a circle Can stand on one foot Talks of self and others	Intrusive-inclusive mode Initiative vs. guilt Outcome: **Purpose**	Disgust Orderliness possible Fantasy play Masturbation begins	Use of language Observational learning; representation vs. direct action
4 yr	Buttons clothes Throws ball overhand Copies square Draws a person Says ABCs		Curiosity heightened Cooperative play Imaginary companion Task perseverance Rivalry with parent of opposite sex	Egocentrism Thinking by intuition
5 yr	Copies triangle and diamond Ties knots in string Complete toilet self-help		Problem solving Games with rules begin	

Adapted from Metcalf, A., in Review of General Psychiatry, ed. 2, H. Goldman (ed.). Norwalk, Conn., Appleton & Lange, 1988.

TABLE 14–1.   Four Developmental Models—cont'd

	Developmental Landmarks (Gesell and Other Authors)	Psychosexual Stages: Psychosocial Stages, Tasks, and Values (Erikson)	Attachment Theory (Bowlby): Psychological Characteristics	Intellectual Development (Piaget)
School Age				
6 yr	Can roller-skate Prints name Ties shoelaces	Industry vs. inferiority Outcome: **Skillfulness**	Hobbies Ritualistic play Rational attitudes about foods	**Stage of concrete operations** Child begins to be rational and more stable in thought. An orderly conceptual framework is applied in understanding the world. Physical quantities such as weight and volume are now viewed as constants despite changes in shape and size.
7 yr	Knows seasons of the year Rides two-wheeled bicycle		Enjoys friends and "best friends" Invests self in teachers and older leaders	
8 yr	Ideas shared Names days of the week Repeats 5 digits forward			
9 yr	Can define sympathy and foolishness			
10 yr	Able to rhyme Repeats 4 digits in reverse			
11 yr	Understands pity, grief, surprise Knows where the sun sets			
Adolescence				
12 yr	Can define complex scientific concepts such as entropy			
13 yr		Identity vs. identity diffusion Outcome: **Fidelity**	Rebelliousness Loosens family ties Runs in cliques	**Stage of formal operations** Child can now deal deductively not only with the reality he can see but also with abstractions and propositional statements. The adolescent uses deductive reasoning and can evaluate the logic and quality of his own thinking. Increased powers of abstraction enable him to deal with laws and principles. Although egocentrism is still evident, balanced idealistic attitudes emerge in late adolescence. Some "normal" people do not advance this far in intellectual development. Many do not lose their essential egocentrism at all; it returns at senescence.
14 yr	Can divide small number in head		Responsible independence emerges in fragments	
15 yr	Can repeat 6 digits forward and 5 digits backward		Work habits solidify Obvious heterosexual interests (girls usually before boys)	
16 yr				
17 yr				
18 yr				
Youth Early adulthood		Intimacy vs. isolation Outcome: **Love**	Preparation for occupational choice Occupational choice (or advanced schooling) Elaborate recreational activity Marriage and parenting readiness	
Middle Adulthood		Generativity vs. self-absorption or stagnation Outcome: **Care**		
Late Adulthood		Integrity vs. despair and disgust Outcome: **Wisdom**		

terns of maturation that follow a relatively in-flexible pattern, although the rate may vary from one child to another. His investigations on motor development, on individual differences in rate of growth, and on personality patterns have been often replicated. One implication of Gesell's model is that pushing children to early task mastery is futile. This has resulted in the concept that the child should show "readiness" for new experiences before premature interventions during the developmental period. Gesell emphasized internal regulation, used age as a marker, provided guidelines for developmental levels, noted a sensitivity to responses at certain times in development, observed discontinuity in development, appreciated individual differences, and understood the impact of the environment on amplifying or reducing behavioral effects. His methods and the data-based approach that he pioneered continue to be models in approaching behavioral study. However, it must be kept in mind that his studies are based on children in a normal environment.

The *ethological model* addresses the roots and mechanisms of behavior in both humans and animals. It focuses on classes of behavior that are biologically based: reflexes, taxes, and fixed action patterns. Behaviors that are innate occur without learning and are species typical, for example, imprinting in birds. Primitive reflexes such as the tonic neck reflex and the walking reflex in infants are examples. At least 25 such reflexes have been identified in the human neonate. The taxes are locomotor or orienting responses and include responses that require more than one reflex, such as cuddling. The fixed action pattern is a sequence of coordinated motor actions. It is made up of innate releasing mechanisms associated with a signed stimulus; for example, a mother leaves the room and that departure is associated with the infant crying. The departure is a signed stimulus leading to an innate releasing mechanism followed by a fixed action pattern. Another example is the infant's facial appearance, with large head, bulging cheeks, and large eyes, which acts as a signed stimulus for care-eliciting behavior toward the infant. Many parenting behaviors may have an ethological origin.

Genetically based behaviors take place in a natural social context and are studied by preparing an ethogram that categorizes behaviors that are observed in a natural environmental context, allowing links to be established. J. Bowlby has utilized this approach in infant study; using the example of mother-infant attachment, he found four separate phases. The first is preattachment, which is demonstrated by

orienting behavior toward caregivers, for example, early following with the eyes, smiling, and vocalization. This is followed by "attachment in the making" and then clear-cut attachment as the toddler walks away and then returns to the caregiver. The last phase of attachment occurs in the second year of life and is known as the "goal-corrected partnership." Here, the young child begins to understand the adult's behavior and adapts his behavior accordingly. The goal of attachment is to increase physical proximity between parent and child and to facilitate nurturance. The ethological view takes into account both genetic and environmental factors.

An extension of ethology is sociobiology. The sociobiologists, unlike the ethologists, describe all aspects of development as related to and controlled by specific genes, therefore attributing less importance to environmental factors. Rather than individual potential, the focus is on biological and psychological determinism. Sociobiology has been defined as the systematic study of the biological basis of all social behavior. An emphasis is placed on successful reproduction of the species. The sociobiologists have found that altruism is regularly demonstrated by parents in all mammalian species in providing care for the next generation of their species.

Psychodynamic Approaches

Psychoanalysis was one of the first attempts to offer a systemic theory of personality development. Psychoanalysts establish a therapeutic alliance with an individual and through the study of adult recollection of childhood experiences identify factors that are out of awareness or "unconscious" but which influence development. Using the energy models prevalent at the time, Sigmund Freud, the founder of psychoanalysis, described a hypothetical psychic energy that was conserved in a closed system. This component of his model, known as the dynamic or psychodynamic approach, was based on his studies of conversion symptoms, which occurred without a demonstrable organic disorder. The distribution of psychic energy depended on the organism's stage of development, experiential history, and current life setting. The primary source of psychic energy was instinctual, that is, unlearned psychological drives. The most powerful of these is the sexual instinct, which is important in the preservation of the species rather than of the individual alone.

Freud's investigations resulted in the description of psychic energy, the libido, which was conserved and distributed dynamically to various psychological functions. Libido is applied to biological processes, and thereby they are given psychological representation and referred to as instinctive drives. The reduction of tension generated by that instinctual drive is referred to as instinctual gratification. With development, instinctual energy that could not be discharged is converted into other energies related to more complex behavior. The bulk of psychic energy derived from biological impulses or instincts is referred to as "id" energy and is expressed in infants through their behavior in seeking pleasure and avoiding pain. Crying and increased motor activity, however, bring the infant into contact with the external world. As the infant adapts his responses, psychological structures are differentiated that mediate future behavior. With this energy transformation, the infant develops a sense of self-awareness or ego development that is made up of his complex of conscious associations. Finally, as societal mores are established, the young person develops a sense of morality or consciousness, which is referred to as the superego. This internalized awareness of social reality or parental expectations leads to inhibition of inappropriate behavior. Inhibition also takes place through a transformation of psychic energy. The hypothetical constructs of id, ego, and superego are referred to as Freud's structural system. The goal is the reduction of tension and the achievement of goals through the interaction of biological impulses, adaptive mediation of behavior, and the emergence of a sense of self-control and a sense of morality.

The dynamic and structural components interact by a set of defense mechanisms to minimize experienced anxiety. These mechanisms distort reality in the face of potential danger that might threaten ego functioning. They are designed to alleviate the conflicts or stressors that give rise to the anxiety signal. They may be adaptive or maladaptive, depending on the context in which they occur. The most common defense mechanisms are denial, displacement, dissociation, idealization, intellectualization, isolation, passive aggression, rejection, rationalization, reaction formation, repression, somatization, autistic fantasy, acting out, suppression, splitting, and undoing. Defense mechanisms aid in restructuring the personality as the child experiments with new experiences. They enable psychic energy to remain directed toward a goal rather than to be expressed as excessive anxiety. With development, the ego acts as a more effective mediator in modulating anxiety, thereby reducing the need for defense mechanisms in dealing with reality.

Finally, Freud offered a series of sequences or stages of development (psychosexual stages) to designate the child's progression through early development. He suggested that psychic energy is progressively focused on different areas of the body—erogenous zones; for example, the oral stage focuses on stimulation of the oral area and involves psychic energy related to hunger and eating behavior, and the anal and phallic stages refer to the subsequent awareness and focus on these body regions. Freud suggested that the sequence of the stages was the result of maturational or genetic factors but that the psychological mastery of each stage depended on child-rearing practices and early interpersonal experiences. Fixation at a stage is seen as a defense against anxiety and may influence later personality development. This approach is another example of the interaction of genetic endowment and environmental experiences. It was the first attempt to describe developmental change as an orderly and predictable process. Freud's work, by emphasizing reorganization and sequential restructuring at each stage rather than a continuous developmental process, has become the prototype for other stage theories. His emphasis is on the importance of early experience on later adult development; however, his emphasis on infantile sexuality as a universal phenomenon remains controversial. The current emphasis is on interactional factors, including parental attitudes, family circumstances, and life experiences as the essential elements in psychosocial development, with less emphasis on innate predisposition.

Psychosocial Model

The psychosocial model originated with Erik Erikson, who suggested that psychological development is the result of an interaction between maturational and social forces, but placed more emphasis on socialization than did Freud. Erikson's approach emphasizes socialization throughout the life span, making him the first life span psychologist. Erikson suggested a series of eight stages of development that deal with the task of identity formation. In each stage, a developmental crisis requires resolution, and therefore the importance of the ego is highlighted. Whereas Freud focused on the libido and its importance in psychological functioning, Erikson emphasized the importance of the ego and suggested that an immature ego is present at birth. He is referred to as an ego psychologist. Erikson also introduced the principle of epigenesis, based on an embryologic model, with each psychosocial stage emerging out of the previous one.

At each stage of development, a different conflict has particular significance for the individual. These conflicts are expressed as polarities that represent opposite tendencies that lead to a particular virtue when resolved. The first five stages deal with developmental tasks of children and adolescents, and the final stages address tasks for parents and grandparents. In the first stage, during the first year of life, the polarity between trust and mistrust is experienced. If it is resolved with a predominance of trust, the infant develops the virtue of hope. In the second stage, experienced in the second and third years of life, the polarity is between autonomy and shame or doubt. Resolution leads to confidence and a sense of self-control. For the third stage, at 4 to 5 years of age, the polarity is between initiative and guilt at a time when the child is internalizing adult roles and standards. The resolution of this conflict leads to a sense of purposefulness.

Erikson's adult stages can profitably be applied to parents and grandparents. The resolution of the earlier stages helps to prepare adults for marriage and effective parenting. With the resolution of role confusion in adolescence and the establishment of fidelity, the young adult is prepared to consider entering into marriage and establishing a family. For the young adult, the polarity is between intimacy and isolation, and its resolution is the experience of love in interpersonal relationships. Following the establishment of intimacy, the next stage presents the polarity between generativity and self-absorption. Its resolution is in the ability to provide care to one's children. The final stage in the life cycle addresses the polarity of integrity and despair. It is the task of old age to reflect on the degree to which one has established contentment and satisfaction in life. The satisfactory resolution of this phase is wisdom. Erikson's major contribution has been to stress the importance of the development of a strong ego identity. His formulations are widely used in medicine, psychology, and education.

Cognitive-Developmental Approach

The cognitive-developmental approach emphasizes that the infant and child are active in initiating behavior rather than reactive; development is a spontaneous process, and the child and infant play an active role. Jean Piaget is the most important theorist in this area, and his work addressing the growth of knowledge in infancy and childhood is referred to as genetic epistemology. He envisioned development as a spontaneous process with constant addition, modification, and reorganization. The child strives for order and seeks to find a self-regulatory equilibrium between internal motivation and environmental demands. Beginning with the study of his own children and then through developing an institute for child study, Piaget outlined a series of stages of increasing complexity. He described four stages of intellectual development: (1) the sensorimotor stage, (2) the preoperational stage, (3) the concrete operational stage, and (4) the stage of formal operations. The sensorimotor stage lasts from birth to 2 years of age, and the preoperational stage lasts from 2 through 7 years of age.

Piaget emphasized the structural transitions that take place in each stage rather than simply describing behavior. The child assimilates experiences and accommodates them to prior psychological schema. For example, in the sensorimotor stage, the child begins with simple reflexive behavior that gradually becomes intentional and comes under conscious control. The infant begins to coordinate motor experience into habits of behavior. Through intentional repetition of these behavioral patterns, the child learns cause and effect. Older behavioral schemes are then applied in new situations, and gradually novel approaches are applied to new problems. The child begins to internalize actions and experiment in the world. This sensorimotor learning through action is supplanted by preoperational thought as the child becomes older. Now, the toddler develops symbolic abilities and can intentionally manipulate symbols that represent objects in the real world. Imagination enters as a developmental phenomenon to be used by the child in task mastery. The onset and expression of language are the most important events during the preoperational stage. The child at this stage is bound by immediate perception and may make inappropriate generalizations. Subsequent cognitive development leads to further skill acquisition. In Piaget's model, the child's active participation in the world leads to changes in both psychological structure and content, adding a further dimension to the developmental process.

SUMMARY

To summarize, each of the following views is utilized in addressing behavior in children and adolescents. As the child matures and interacts with the environment, the development of the person, the personality, is the focus of the following developmental theorists. The earliest focus was that of Freud on psychosexual development, followed by Erikson on identity formation, and Piaget on cognitive development. Psychotherapies have been suggested based on these approaches. The term *psychological birth* has been introduced to indicate the emergence of a new individual; the phases of early development have been further refined into phases of separation and individuation. More recently, an emphasis has been placed on an ethological model of development that addresses behavior in a biological context. Patterns of behavior across species that serve the same purpose, natural selection of behavioral traits, and behavior that is biologically based, such as infant attachment, are included. Each of these frameworks of development makes assumptions about the capabilities of the infant and young child in regard to recognition and remembering of past experience, temperamental characteristics, and response to environmental uncertainty. These perspectives suggest an emphasis on socially important features, for example, self-control, moral development, intellectual stages in development, interpersonal behavior, and self-awareness as ideal goals. They indicate that there are developmental tasks that each child must accomplish. We must ask, "What are the capabilities of infants and young children and how do they relate to these developmental theories?"

BIBLIOGRAPHY

Ainsworth, M.D.: The development of mother-infant attachment, in Review of Child Development Research, vol. 3, B. Caldwell and N. Riccuiti (eds.). Chicago, University of Chicago Press, 1973.

Bowlby, J.: Attachment and Loss: III. Loss, Sadness and Depression. New York, Basic Books, 1980.

Bowlby, J.: Developmental psychiatry comes of age. Am. J. Psychiatry 145:1-10, 1988.

Carlson, M., Earls, F., Todd, R.D.: The importance of regressive changes in the nervous system: Towards a neurobiological theory of child development. Psychiatr. Dev. 1:1-22, 1988.

Coyle, J.T., Harris, J.C.: The development of neurotransmitters and neuropeptides, in Basic Handbook of Child Psychiatry, vol. 5, pp. 14-26. New York, Basic Books, 1987.

Davis, M.D., Wallbridge, D.: Boundary and Space: An Introduction to the Work of D.W. Winnicott. New York, Brunner/Mazel, 1981.

Erikson, E.H.: Childhood and Society. New York, Norton, 1950.

Gesell, A., Amatuda, C.S.: Developmental Diagnosis. New York, Holber, 1947.

Greenough, W.T., Black, J.E., Wallace, C.S.: Experience and brain development. Child Dev. 54:53-59, 1987.

Harris, J.: The biopsychosocial approach, in Principles and Practice of Pediatrics, F.A. Oski, C.D. DeAngelis, R.D. Feigin, and J.B. Warshaw (eds.). Philadelphia, Lippincott, 1990.

Marshall, W.A.: Development of the Brain. London, Oliver and Boyd, 1968.

Piaget, J.: Piaget's Theory. Handbook of Child Psychology. I. (P. Mussen [ed.]). New York, Wiley, 1983.

Salkind, N.J.: Theories of Human Development, ed. 2. New York, Wiley, 1985.

Chapter 15
The First Years of Life

James C. Harris, M.D.

This chapter discusses the prenatal period, infancy, and early childhood until the age of 5 years. Both theoretical formulations and prospective studies in child development are addressed. Progress in this area has been complicated by the complexity of studying thought, emotion, and intention in infants and young children, the ethical issues inherent in utilizing scientific approaches that are carried out more classically in animal studies, and the preferred societal interpretations of what is appropriate behavior.

PRENATAL PERIOD

Pregnancy

There are multiple and often complex motivations for becoming pregnant. Knowledge of the parental attitude toward pregnancy is essential to the developmental assessment. Although the usual attitude is a positive one, in some in-

stances pregnancy may have occurred to please others, such as grandparents, or with the wish to be nurtured oneself. In other instances, conception may occur in an attempt to save a marriage that is dysfunctional or to deal with anxiety about sterility. As the pregnancy itself ensues, there may be an initial period of enhanced preoccupation by the mother with herself until the infant's movement brings about a clearer awareness of the developing new person. At this time psychological responses to pregnancy or ambivalence about becoming pregnant may manifest itself. If delivery is complicated and painful, potentially negative attitudes toward the newborn infant may evolve. After birth, endocrine changes associated with delivery may be associated with psychiatric problems. In some instances, clinical depressive symptoms, often referred to as the "postpartum blues," may lead to withdrawal and partial rejection of the infant. This response may be associated with difficulties in feeding, and patterns of mother-child interaction may develop that require intervention. Psychological, genetic, and physiological predispositions play a role in the development of postpartum psychiatric symptoms.

Prenatal Development

Prenatal life is composed of both embryonic and fetal stages. In general, the embryonic period is designated as the first 8 weeks of growth, leading to gross anatomical features of the human form. Since organs continue to develop, the embryonic period is sometimes considered to last through the first trimester, or the first 12 weeks, of pregnancy. Subsequently, during the fetal period, growth is rapid; and at 24 to 26 weeks, the fetus is considered viable. Concurrent with the growth of the fetus is the psychological experience of the parent during each of the trimesters of pregnancy as the fetus is identified by the parent as a growing person. The parents develop a conception of an expected child from a psychological perspective and behave accordingly.

Neurological activity is manifested at about 8 weeks of gestation. By 9 weeks, the palms and soles are reflexogenic. By 13 to 14 weeks, movement may be produced by stimulation. It is around this time that fetal movements may first be felt by the mother. By 25 weeks, the earliest response can be demonstrated. In later pregnancy, the fetus is capable of habituation to sensory input, as demonstrated by fetal movement and acceleration of the fetal pulse to sound. There is considerable variation in the activity of the fetus, including evidence that fetal activity may be responsive to changes in maternal emotional state, possibly through the intrauterine transfer of epinephrine and other substances. A reciprocal psychosocial interaction has already begun in the prenatal period between mother and infant. The parent begins to plan for an imagined and expected child as she responds to movements of the fetus in utero.

Influences on Prenatal Development

Perhaps the most important influence on prenatal development is the presence of a supportive emotional environment during the pregnancy. This will be strongly influenced by losses, illness, or separations that occur during the pregnancy. If there have been multiple previous pregnancies, the attitude toward the current pregnancy will be affected; and the new child may be burdened with unrealistic expectations. If the child is unwanted, if an abortion has been attempted, or if there are hereditary disorders in the family, the parents' attitude toward the child may be affected. The attitude toward the fetus is influenced by the phase of pregnancy; attitudes may gradually change, becoming more positive as the pregnancy ensues and signs of life are experienced.

Involvement of Other Family Members

Both parents and extended family undergo psychological adaptation to pregnancy. The father's role has been emphasized recently. On the one hand, there is the issue of paternal providing, emphasized in the psychological literature; on the other hand, the possibility exists of paternal ambivalence about the pregnancy. Maturity and motivation for parenting evolve with both parents as the pregnancy progresses. The relationship of the father with his own father, through identification, deserves consideration. Anxieties about providing for the mother and infant, as well as agreement on the respective roles of the parents, need clarification.

Prematurity

The fetus born prematurely has the best chance of survival after 26 to 28 weeks of gestation. Those infants whose birth weights are 1000 to 1500 g show little muscle tone and maintain the tonic neck posture with little movement of their extremities. Sucking, vocalization, grasp, and general responsiveness are diminished. It may be difficult to clarify their degree of alertness. The infant who weighs 1500 to 2000 g has better muscle tone, is more alert, and has a sleep pattern that is more easily determined. These infants can fixate on the environment and may be able to breast-feed. Premature infants who weigh 2000 to 2500 g look like small full-term infants and, on developmental examination, have similar responsiveness with good muscle tone and cry. Despite this appearance, the actual developmental level requires time to attain that of a normal full-term newborn. However, developmental differences between them will generally not be apparent by 2 years of age. The premature infant is at risk because of the immaturity of enzymatic, metabolic, and physiological systems. Developmental defects more commonly occur in premature infants, who are vulnerable to sensory and social deprivation.

The mother's involvement with even the

smallest baby in providing care as early as possible is extremely important to facilitate mutual emotional bonding and the attachment relationship. Infants born prematurely are at greater risk for problems in parenting, since they show less social responsiveness than the full-term infant; they may be more prone to neglect and abuse. Observations of the mother interacting with the premature infant in the nursery should be recorded and often are a good indicator of adjustment to the infant. Because the premature infant is less active in responding to the parent, the period of early adaptation and bonding may be delayed. There are associated anxieties about complications associated with prematurity, as well as the risks of behavioral difficulties and learning problems in later life in premature infants who have complicated courses in the nursery.

It is essential that both the physical and psychological environment, including the attitudes of the primary family members involved with the infant, be taken into account. Most infants are born into conventional, stable, and supportive environments. It is important to look carefully at the environment, which should be "good enough," neither one where everything must be perfect, nor one that is lacking in resources. The infant makes a substantial contribution to optimizing the environment through active interaction with the parent. Complications in the early beginnings with the infant can best be dealt with by means of anticipatory guidance. Anticipatory guidance addresses normally expected difficulties and provides basic information on physical growth and development. Psychosocial expectations and particular anxieties are discussed with both parents and involved members of the extended family.

INFANCY AND FIRST YEAR OF LIFE

The newborn infant increasingly begins to shape the environment through his preattachment behavior, which ordinarily elicits pleasurable parental responses. Active infants who cry more and those who show early temperamental traits of responsiveness may elicit different maternal behavior from quiet and apparently contented infants. As early as 2 to 6 weeks of age, infants seem more comfortable with familiar people than with strangers.

Initially, there is a lack of discrimination between people and objects, and smiling is nonspecific. Newborns and some premature infants may show fragmentary smiles in response to internal stimuli. These may occur during REM sleep or during moments of drowsiness. Smiling may be elicited by dots on a card located to represent the eyes of the parent. With time, normally at about 5 to 6 months, the smile becomes social and is elicited only by the human face. At first, this social smiling is in response to familiar persons but then extends to others. It is one ingredient in the gradual emergence of infant attachment.

As awareness through the specific senses is developed, the senses become linked as different skills are utilized. For example, the infant sees objects and has the ability to move his arm, but it is only at about 5 months that these skills are combined to reach for an object and touch it. The infant can distinguish sounds, but it takes several months to understand specifically what is heard. From the beginning, there is a responsiveness to others' interest and attention, but discriminating among different people is a developmental task. Social landmarks, such as following with the eyes and smiling, initially appear without specific social qualities. However, this orientation toward others gradually leads to attachment by the seventh to eighth month of life. Then the smile is elicited only by the human face, and the child responds only to familiar people. Subsequently, discriminating familiar people, the child becomes aware of strangers and begins to show "stranger anxiety" when confronted with a new person. Concomitant with the development of attachment is vocalization, following with the eyes, and anticipatory reaching up, leading to the separation response. It is this response to separation that is the landmark demonstrating that an individual bond to another person has occurred.

There are individual differences in temperament that affect attachment. Attachments, as they develop, are not specific to one person; the child becomes attached to other people in the environment as well. Later relationships build on what has happened earlier in life. There is no specific and limited critical period for the development of attachment between the child and family members. However, if through neglect or physical circumstance, the child does not develop bonds of attachment by 2 to 3 years of age, it is more difficult later on. Extreme situations, such as an institutional setting in which the child is cared for by a large number of adults without special responsibility for a particular child, have alerted investigators to the importance of an average expectable environment for every child. However, providing simple physical care and stimulation is not enough. The quality of the relationship is important, and the security of the child's attachment is demonstrated by the ability to maintain bonds during a period of separation.

Individual differences among infants are initially seen in heart rate, blood pressure, and other physiological responses, such as muscle movements, response to stimulation, the routine of wake/sleep cycles, emotional responses of particular types and intensities, and sensory threshold. Three temperament patterns in infants that seem to persist throughout maturation have been identified: the easy child, the difficult child, and the slow-to-warm-up child. The origin of individual differences may be genetic (as noted in twin studies), a consequence of the differences in the two sexes, or related to the degree of physical maturation. However, complications at birth, poor nutrition, illness, injuries, and life experiences lead to individual differences as well. The premature child is especially vulnerable because of metabolic needs for warmth and a constant nutritional source of support. Individual differences are the result of the interaction between the child's temperament and life experiences that are unique to a particular family. Individual differences affect how other people respond to the child, what stimuli are presented to the child, and how others relate in an interpersonal way.

Landmarks in First Year of Life

The emergence of an attachment relationship through social and language interactions is the primary and perhaps the most important feature of the first year in personality development. Concurrent with these advances is the development of skills that allow coordination and reaching for things, sitting without support, crawling, and standing. There is a progression from mouthing objects to the use of the hands and then to reliance on vision and hearing in response to the environment. Language develops as more complex sounds are made and their meaning is understood. Language development leads to understanding the pragmatic, or practical, use of language, in reciprocal communication with others.

Fears are first noted in the first year of life in relation to unexpected sights and sounds. These fears are followed by anxiety with regard to strangers, as the child begins to differentiate adults. Mastery of these fears leads to increased self-control and enhanced motivation to explore the environment, utilizing new cognitive abilities and applying past experiences to new situations. In the first year, the infant is developing the skills that would allow him to become more independent during the second year of life. From a cognitive point of view, by 10 months of age the child is able to search for a lost object and also is aware of a lost person. By retaining in memory an image of another person, the child is on the way to seeing himself as an individual distinct from others.

SECOND YEAR OF LIFE

During the second year of life, there is a slowing in the rate of growth. The average child gains 5 to 6 pounds and about 5 inches during this year. Appetite decreases, and, as a result, the plump infant changes into a more lean and muscular child. Brain growth progresses at a less rapid rate during the second year. The head circumference increases about 12 cm during the first year but increases only 2 cm during the second. At the end of the first year, the brain has reached about two thirds of its adult size; at the end of the second year, it reaches four fifths of its adult size. The eruption of teeth continues, and eight more teeth appear during this year. The child's motor skills progress in the second year, moving from an awkward posture to a high degree of locomotor control. By 18 months, the child can go upstairs with assistance and, by 20 months, can walk downstairs with assistance. At 24 months, the child is able to run and move quickly, requiring protection and regular observation. Finger grasp is refined during this year, as the child develops a more effective pincer grasp. With the new ability to use the hands, the child begins to build towers and can scribble with a pencil and imitate vertical strokes by 18 months. Jargon speech, which shows the intonations and rhythm or prosody of speech, is followed by the meaningful use of words. As the second year proceeds, two words are put together, and then three are used together.

In the second year, the child's attachment to people becomes stronger; there is a second phase of attachment as the child moves and explores the environment and then returns to the parent for security. It is during this year that the child begins to imitate others, to show the first evidence of symbolic play activity, and to recognize himself in a mirror. At this age, children are most often disturbed by change and new situations. The presence of a familiar person is essential to help with these adjustments. With the development of an intense attachment response, the child is able to demonstrate new attachments to others. Shaking the head "no" meaningfully first occurs; this "no" response becomes characteristic of the second year. Toward the end of the year, nodding "yes" is noted, as are other nonverbal gestures, such as the shyness response when strangers approach.

With newly formed abilities to explore the environment, there is a sense of apparent confidence and an environmental mastery that is enhanced by new skill development. Fears of unexpected noises decrease, as do those of strangers. However, new fears with uncertainty about the unfamiliar may emerge, such as a fear of dogs and other animals or situations where pain has been experienced. Ethological studies are consistent with Erik Erikson's emphasis on self-reliance and autonomy as important developmental tasks. In the first year of life, Erikson suggested that the development of trust is the most important milestone; in the second year, it is independence of action. During the second year, children often want to do things on their own but may not be able to do them safely and may take unnecessary risks. As a consequence of this independent exploring, accidents are common at this age. The adult facilitates the child's social competence by providing limits to prevent excessive failure. This approach of filling in the gaps and trying to guarantee success is referred to as scaffolding. Self-mastery also includes toilet training, an important task during the second year of life. The issue of control over toileting often leads to oppositional behavior on the child's part. The conflict that occurs involving the child's autonomy and self-control leads to difficulty with noncompliance.

Emotional Development in Second Year

Beginning in the second year, anger is often expressed through tantrums, kicking, screaming, and breath holding. Most often, tantrums occur in situations where parents place demands or restrict the child or the child is frustrated in not being able to accomplish something. This often extends to speech, when children are unable to make themselves understood because of lack of speech skills. Tantrums may occur at bedtime, around toileting, or around dressing or other activities that require parental assistance. Change in the routine may also result in tantrums. A natural opposition and noncompliance emerge during this time, as the child seeks autonomy. Fluctuations in mood are common, particularly those related to changes in physiological state around mealtimes or when the child is hungry, tired, or ill.

In dealing with emotional difficulties in the second year, it is important to focus on helping the child master the situation and not attend specifically to tantrums per se. Through an awareness of what the child's needs are when he is not having a tantrum, and clarifying known precipitants of anger, as well as redirecting the child's attention and providing alternative activities, tantrums can generally be alleviated. In working with tantrums in children, the reason for the tantrum should be established before specifically ignoring the behavior. The focus is on helping the child reestablish self-control. Emotional problems shift in the second year of life. In the first year, sleeping and eating difficulties are the most common problems; in the second year, separation anxiety and oppositional behavior are more common occurrences. With the rapid developments that occur during the second year of life, parents often become concerned about delays in development or in bowel or bladder control.

Language Development in Second Year

At about 18 months, the vocabulary increases substantially; by 2 years, the child has a vocabulary of several hundred words that he understands, about 200 of which are used regularly. There is considerable variation, however, and a few children may have only a dozen or so words at their second birthday. Initially, language in the first year of life is essentially signal language, where words are associated with events; in the latter half of the second year, words become clearly associated with meaning. Now, flexibility in word use begins and intonation patterns may be applied to words, so that one word or phrase, such as "mommy" or "want this," may be expressed in different ways. With these new understandings, sentences are used for the first time. Increased receptive and expressive vocabulary allows the child to follow simple instructions and begin to listen carefully to speech. Language skill is enhanced through hearing the same story over again and attending to the rhythms of nursery rhymes.

The beginnings of symbolic play emerge during the second year of life. First, the child demonstrates functional play, using objects for their intended purposes. Subsequently, the child begins to pretend to eat a meal or answer the telephone in imaginary play. By around 20 months of age, in symbolic play, the child uses miniature toy people in an imaginative fashion and starts to participate in games that involve gestures, such as bye-bye. At this age, the child plays alongside other children, but interactions with them have not yet become important.

In the last half of the second year, the most striking changes are noted, particularly in regard to an awareness of adult standards and the emergence of awareness of the child's own actions, intentions, states, and competencies. Self-awareness is indicated by mastery smiles, making directives toward adults, and self-descriptive talk. Between 18 and 22 months, there is an increase in foresight. The child begins to make inferences. For example, a crack in a toy is now caused by someone's action. At this age, children are able to evaluate actions and events as good or bad; this awareness of adult standards suggests the beginning of moral development. An appreciation of what is appropriate and inappropriate behavior may result in the inhibition of aggression and substitution of other more appropriate behavior.

This stage is often called "the terrible twos" because of the child's awareness of the standards set by adults and how he tests their validity to reduce uncertainty over enforcement. These tests are not always motivated by hostility but may be motivated by attempts to gain knowledge. Unlike the first year of life, where learning develops primarily through active trial-and-error experiment, by the end of the second year, imagery and symbols are beginning to play a part in problem solving as a child learns to use language more effectively. This new ability in problem solving is applied with the beginnings of self-awareness. As objects and actions have names and functions, events can then have meaning. It is this seeking after meaning and trying to understand the names and purposes of things that distinguish the child's language development from that of higher apes, who do not inquire, although they may be able to associate names. The ability to impose meaning develops beyond the second year into the preschool years.

PRESCHOOL YEARS

During the third, fourth, and fifth years, there are steady gains in height and weight, about 4.5 pounds and 2.5 to 3.5 inches per year, respectively. The lordosis and protuberant abdomen of infancy have disappeared by the fourth year;

by 3 years of age 20 deciduous teeth have erupted. The configuration of the face begins to change, and the jaw is widened in preparation for the eruption of the new and permanent teeth. Developmentally, motor skills have progressed; by 3 years the child can stand on one foot, and by 5 years the children can hop on one foot. Perceptually, at 3 years of age he is able to draw a cross, and by 4 to 5 years, copy figures with slanting lines, such as triangles. Toward the end of this period, by 6 years, the ability to construct figures, such as letters of the alphabet, and to use symbols for numbers has emerged. This is a period of rapid development in personality and includes language development, play, activity, identification with others, and an awareness of one's own gender identity. It is a period when moral development progresses and guilt is expressed about behavior.

Perceptual developments aid in the recognition of symbols. By 4 years of age, a child can differentiate closures in letters (for example, the letters O and C) but continues to have problems when line-to-curve transformation must occur (as in U and V). It is not until school age that rotational transformations (such as the B and D, or M and W) can be accurately carried out. These skills are important in the development of reading and writing. The child learns that the way a letter faces and the combination of elements, such as circles and straight lines, determine its use.

Language Development in Preschool Years

In the preschool years vocabulary increases from approximately 200 to 7000 words; the child speaks in sentences and begins to use appropriate syntax. This learning involves meaning and understanding rather than simple association. Concurrently, children learn rules in speech and begin to ask more specific questions about what things are, where they are, and who people are. By the fourth and fifth years, children are asking more questions; now, they ask why as they seek new information. During this time, the same question may be asked repeatedly, although the child knows the answer, as adult phrasing of words teaches more and more about language. Children talk to themselves during this time, trying out different word combinations. Pronunciation is improving; the majority of children can speak intelligibly by school age, although approximately 4 percent are still difficult to understand.

Development of Imaginative Play

In the preschool years, particularly between 3 and 4 years of age, there is a rapid increase in the use of imaginary and pretend play. The child practices skills to master or plays out fantasy games about experiences, such as cops and robbers, games about school, and stories about the family. Developmentally, make-believe is expressed most strikingly between 18 months and 7 years of life. The child invents items in the imagination and may have imaginary playmates. Initially, the imagination does not show coherence, but gradually it comes in ordered sequences, so that, by 5 years, children are producing meaningful stories.

The development of play is particularly important in the mastery of experience in the preschool years. Play may serve several functions. (1) Play may lessen fears through reenactment of frightening events. The repetition of the event in safety may help the child to come to terms with the experience. (2) Play may serve the function of exploring emotions, as a child pretends to be frightened about unlikely situations. (3) Play may completely reenact events the way the child would have liked them to have happened and, in this way, be compensatory or wishful. (4) Play may be presented in the form of a question, as the child plays out events by asking the parent to observe and see if this is actually what is anticipated. (5) Play may be a response to an unstimulating environment as a way of overcoming boredom.

Play allows the child to explore feelings, lessen fears, increase excitement, understand puzzling events, seek confirmation, or alter events in fantasy. Besides playing alone, in the preschool years children begin to move from solitary play to parallel play and to associative play with other children. By 3 years of age, play has become cooperative, as small groups of children join together, first in groups of two and then in groups of four or five later in the preschool years. Interpersonal responses become important in development, as rivalry and competition emerge through shared play activities; the ability to share is a developmental task that is mastered during this time.

Commonly, a specific object becomes the first possession and is utilized in play. It might be a toy, for example, a soft bear or a blanket. Its texture is important, and so is the time of ownership. The object is used for comfort when the child is anxious or tired, most frequently at bedtime. These objects have been characterized as "transitional objects" and are linked with the parent as a source of comfort. Both the object and the parent may be necessary at stressful times. The objects are transitional in allowing the child to move from a dependent to a more independent posture. As children mature, transitional objects assume a symbolic nature, for example, the songs and memories they use to comfort themselves.

In addition to independent play and play with other children, objects are also investigated and time is spent trying to find out how things work. In doing this, children may accidentally be destructive as they take objects apart. Putting objects together is important in the use of bricks and construction toys, as well as in the exploration of tools around the house. There are individual variations in children, as well as in their parents, in terms of this exploratory play activity. Exploration takes place when children are most at ease. Each form of play involves repetition of items that are familiar, so that preschool children like to play games in exactly the same way each time. There is comfort in the familiar and anxiety on separating from it; for this reason, bedtime rituals become important, since separation occurs at bedtime. Separations from home during hospitalization or in beginning a nursery school, where routines are unfamiliar, are distressing and require the presence of a reassuring adult.

Self-awareness continues to develop as the child begins to identify with other children and particularly with parents or older siblings. Children often act out the personal characteristics of another person as they participate in role playing. There may be a sharing of emotions as well as an imitation of habits. As this process of identification progresses, the child may gradually absorb the moral standards and behaviors of adults as well as their prohibitions. The types of identification with parents in the form of moral behavior must be considered in terms of both degree and type, rather than whether identification with one parent is present or absent.

Development of Sexual Identity in Preschool Years

The child's initial identifications with adults are best seen in reference to gender role, which is ordinarily established by 3 or 4 years. At this age, the child becomes aware of the differences in the sexes. It takes longer to recognize sexual differences in adults, however. Both endocrine factors and psychological experience influence gender role identity. Children often show by 3 years of age a same-sex preference. This happens earlier in boys than in girls, and some girls continue to play out the roles of the other sex over a prolonged period. The differences in children's behavior between the sexes are to some extent biologically determined, but they definitely involve learning sexual standards. Sex differences in attitudes, game choice, and other activities are clearly noted by 4 or 5 years of age and continue up to 8 or 9 years.

Since preferences are partially defined by society, the variation of behavior between the sexes is considerable. Both boys and girls may enjoy activities traditionally ascribed to the other sex. There are a few children who identify strongly with the opposite sex and, in a rare instance, develop a gender identity disorder. Sexual curiosity is a contant feature by age 4 to 6 years, when particular interest is shown in genital sex differences. This curiosity may be reflected in children's games. Both masturbation and sexual exploration are common curiosities in the preschool years. The themes of sexual rivalry and fears about sexual mutilation (castration) have been noted, particularly in children who are emotionally disturbed. In the normal school-age child, such concerns ordinarily do not lead to adjustment difficulties.

As children sacrifice the perogatives of the earlier years and move to increasing responsibilities, they may identify more with the parent who is outside the home and may develop antipathy toward the mother if she remains protective and is a reminder of an earlier phase in their development. Family circumstances and attitudes toward children at this age are important in psychological development; a focus on age-appropriate limit setting by the parent is essential in behavioral management.

Emotional Development in Preschool Years

In the preschool years, emotions are often intense and fluctuating. The child may quickly go from anger and impatience to excitement. Socially acceptable means of expressing emotion and displeasure require new learning. Anger in young children is generally explosive and not adaptive but is often short lived. Conflicts between young children frequently occur over a possession; however, it is only later that children use planning to seek revenge. Interpersonal problems involving competition or rivalry for an adult's attention, particularly in reference to brothers and sisters, are regularly seen. Be-

tween 2 and 4 years of age sibling rivalry is most commonly noted. A younger child, from 12 to 18 months, tends to be less concerned about the arrival of a sibling than an older child. The emergence of rivalry is affected by the parents' response and how they deal with the situation.

Negativism, resistance, and opposition toward a sibling gradually diminish during the preschool period, as children become more aware of their capabilities and of appropriate societal standards. Temper tantrums also become less common as the child reaches school age. Tantrums, however, may continue to occur in a family setting when the child regresses at times of stress. Fears of animals seen in the early preschool years are replaced as the child becomes older by fears of imaginary dangers, such as ghosts and nightmares; these are common in preschoolers. Some fears are learned from family members, but others result from unpleasant experiences, such as a dog jumping on a child and also the child's own imagination.

The psychiatric problems seen in the preschool years may be extensions of earlier developmental patterns that are not resolved, such as separation anxiety, oppositional behavior, and avoidance behavior. Anxiety symptoms are expected when preschool children are separated from a parent; however, when symptoms are severe, preschool children who have not mastered separation experiences may manifest a separation anxiety disorder. With this condition, the child demonstrates excessive anxiety to the point of panic when separated from those to whom he is attached. The child may show unrealistic and persistent worry that the parent will abandon him or will be harmed, may be reluctant to go out alone or sleep without the parent nearby, have physical symptoms when separation is anticipated, experience nightmares, or demonstrate excessive distress when separated from home. A related disorder that may be seen in this age group is avoidant disorder. Younger children may be normally fearful of strangers; however, when avoidance of contact with unfamiliar people is sufficiently severe to interfere with social functioning, this disorder should be considered. The child is actively involved with family members but socially withdrawn and timid with strangers and may become anxious when they make minor requests. The degree of anxiety may result in difficulty speaking or muteness.

With oppositional disorder, the child continues to have difficulty with autonomy after 3 years of age. If the parent interprets the normal phase of oppositional behavior as a need for control, power struggles may ensue that, by excessively focusing on the oppositional behavior, reinforce it. A normal effort to become independent may become an attempt to be free of external control and perceived overprotection. The child shows frequent loss of temper, defiance of adult requests, argumentativeness, and apparently deliberate acts to annoy others.

Developmental disorders, such as delays in language and speech and particular temperamental patterns, make the child more vulnerable to psychiatric disorders at these ages. The most common concerns are fears and worries associated with difficulty in sleep and eating. However, specific developmental disorders, such as infantile autism, are also recognized in the preschool period. Infantile autism, a severe pervasive developmental disorder, is most commonly recognized in the second and third years of life. Children with this condition have qualitative impairments in reciprocal social interaction and in interpersonal communication, along with delayed and deviant language development and stereotyped patterns of interests and activities. The child has difficulty interpreting the meaning of voice tone, posture, and facial expression and demonstrates a severe deficit in initiating social communication. These problems are associated with abnormal motor behavior and frequent hand stereotypies. The majority of children with this condition are mentally subnormal and therefore doubly handicapped.

Attention deficit disorder is another condition that is recognized in the preschool years, although it may not require specific treatment until school age. It is marked by overactivity, inattention, and impulsivity. It is described in detail in Chapter 18: Childhood Psychopathology: Diagnosis and Treatment.

Psychiatric Assessment

Preschool children are brought for assessment by their parents who are concerned about their behavior. The reason for referral at this particular time is elicited, and a statement of the current difficulties involving the child and parent is recorded. This includes questions in regard to behavior, emotions, and interpersonal relationships. Developmental considerations are taken into account in regard to the child's level of development and the appropriateness of the parent's response. A family history addresses the parent's rearing as well as a history of psychiatric problems in the family.

The use of play in psychiatric assessment of the child's behavioral, emotional, and interpersonal problems is particularly important in the preschool years. Play can be helpful in evaluating normally developing children and those who are delayed in development. Assessment focuses on how toys are used, patterns of play, the extent that the child can deal with situations introduced, and whether objects are utilized meaningfully. Fantasy play is observed for the expression of anxieties and concerns. A view of the child's wishes, fears, and attitudes in specific situations may be presented through play. The child overtly expresses feelings by putting thoughts into characters that are in a game. Since younger children do not ordinarily talk about their feelings directly, these indirect means are essential in child assessment. However, since the means are indirect, caution must be used in interpretation. In observing play with other children, the style and manner of interactions, in addition to the quality of the interactions, are essential elements in assessment.

BIBLIOGRAPHY

Behrman, R.E., Vaughn, V.C.: Textbook of Pediatrics. Philadelphia, Saunders, 1987.
Fraiberg, S.H.: The Magic Years. New York, Scribner's, 1959.
Frith, U.: Autism: Explaining the Enigma. Cambridge, England, Basil Blackwell, 1989.
Graham, P.: Child Psychiatry: A Developmental Approach. Oxford, Oxford University Press, 1986, p. 1023.
Harris, P.L.: Children and Emotion: The Development of Psychological Understanding. New York, Basil Blackwell, 1989.
Lewis, M.: Clinical Aspects of Child Development. Philadelphia, Lea & Febiger, 1982.
Osofsky, J. (ed.): Handbook of Infant Development. New York, Wiley, 1987.
Rubin, K.H., Fein, G.G., Vandenberg, B.: Play, in Handbook of Child Psychology, IV, E.M. Hetherington (ed.). New York, Wiley, 1983, pp. 693-774.
Rutter, M.: Helping Troubled Children. New York, Penguin Books, 1975.
Rutter, M., Schopler, E.: Autism and pervasive developmental disorders: Concepts and diagnostic issues. J. Autism Dev. Dis. 17:159-185, 1987.

Chapter 16

Elementary-School-Age Child

Gail A. Edelsohn, M.D., M.S.P.H.

Trainees in child psychiatry often ask how they can tell if their patients are entering latency, the developmental stage of middle childhood. One could reply, "Check to see if they have sprouted latency legs, if they have started telling stupid knock, knock jokes, and if they like games that have rules and numbers." There are many changes during the period referred to as latency. Growth and developmental changes occur along physical lines, in the cognitive sphere, and in the social or emotional sphere. At this stage, children learn new motor skills, such as balancing on a bicycle, they develop better language skills, and they become more capable of abstract thought. This is a period marked by the consolidation of all earlier stages of development. It is generally characterized by the behavior of a child who is calm, pliable, and educable.

It is not merely by chance that by 6 years old or so children are expected to start their formal education and to handle greater responsibility. This major transition is not unique to Western society but is accompanied by a similar shift for children in other cultures with regard to the expectations for them in their roles and responsibilities.

The important developmental tasks of the latency stage cross domains; understanding of those tasks allows one to anticipate where the conflict and problems will arise for these children. The main developmental tasks are (1) to be capable of learning in school, (2) to develop peer relations outside the family, and (3) to be less in conflict with parents through identifying with same-sex parent while continuing to value and learn from the other parent.

Maturation of certain defense mechanisms and reality testing is more clearly seen at this stage. Certain concepts of inevitability, such as death, birth, and sex differences, become established. Logical thinking is clearly dominant, and the child becomes much more able to delay impulses. Children in this stage can take care of their bodies fairly well and usually consider food as nourishment rather than as a symbol. The psychological defenses are stronger and are reinforced by awareness of shame, disgust, and guilt.

These feelings can counteract wishes to be exhibitionistic, messy, or aggressive.

There is a lessening of observable sexuality; the conflicts of triangular issues with the parents are less intense. The child is more responsive to the environment. Because the child no longer has to expend so much energy to control impulses, the child is more free to move on to other activities such as learning, exploring, and deepening relationships with others. In this context, one can appreciate how a sexually abused child has to expend so much energy in dealing with the sexual conflict at home or wherever it occurred that he is likely to suffer academic problems in school.

The major areas of developmental change during latency are reviewed in this chapter, with a particular focus on the key tasks, skills, and challenges of each area.

COGNITIVE DEVELOPMENT

Concrete Operations

Jean Piaget studied the age of 7 to 11 years in detail and called this period the stage of concrete operations. Although many cognitive changes occur, only a few of the most critical ones are covered here. The word *operations* refers to the child's ability to manipulate information. The word *concrete* is used in the sense that the child's capacity to perform these operations is limited to concrete objects or signs representing these objects (that is, words or numbers). The main components of concrete operational thought can be summarized as the following abilities: conservation, classification, and combinatorial skills (ability to manipulate numbers). Children in this stage are capable of performing mental operations; that is, they can manipulate oral and visual information according to logical rules. Reversibility refers to the ability to return to the starting point of a mental operation and turn it around; a common example is a child who can say "6 + 4 = 10" but also can say "10 − 4 = 6." During the period of formal operations, the next developmental cognitive stage, which coincides with adolescence, the child develops the ability to manipulate abstract ideas.

The capacity to classify relies on class inclusion, that is, understanding hierarchical relationships, and seriation, which means the ability to place objects in an orderly series, such as in ascending order. Also coming into play during this period, is transitive reasoning, or the ability to deduce the relationship between two objects, given their relationship to a third object. Attaining these reasoning powers allows a child to engage in logical and systematic thinking.

It is useful to briefly expand on a few key concepts of the stage of concrete operations and to recall one of Piaget's classic experiments. The concept of reversibility extends beyond mathematical manipulation, and includes the ability to reverse a sequence of actions. The term *decenter* refers to the ability to concentrate on more than one aspect of an object at the same time. The child who is preoperational can only focus on the height of a glass, whereas the concrete operational child can take in other aspects, such as width. In Piaget's famous demonstration of the conservation of liquids, the child is presented with two identical glasses of liquid. Then the content of one container is poured into a taller, thinner glass and the child is asked which glass contains more liquid. The child who has not yet reached operational thinking will answer that the taller glass does. The operational child can recognize that the volume of liquid remains constant despite being transferred to another container. There are various types of conservation, including that of numbers, matter, length, volume, and area, which all have analogous experiments.

Another concept is that of reciprocity, which is the ability to see that one characteristic can compensate for another; for example, the height of the glass can compensate for the width.

Piaget and more recent researchers have noted that there is unevenness in development, as can be seen in a child's acquiring conservation of some properties and not of others, usually in a specific order. A number of theories have been proposed to explain this unevenness. Transitional changes take place even within stages that occur at different times, and this diminishes the utility of using stages. However, in general, using stages to describe cognitive development is viewed as useful and has wide acceptance. Findings from recent research support that the onset of a particular stage of emotional or social growth may be earlier than was once thought, may exhibit more variability than is considered normal, or may have certain features that transcend stages, as is also true of other developmental stages.

An alternative view of cognitive development considers information processing as the initial variable. This viewpoint focuses on attention and aspects of memory, particularly the different memory storage systems (sensory, short-term, long-term). Information processing is often described by using the analogy of the computer, with the processes of encoding, or receiving information, organizing and storing information, and being capable of retrieving information. Theorists point out that, as the child becomes older, these processes are changing in a quantitative sense, and thus it is the greater ability to process information that allows the child's problem-solving abilities to advance. In the school environment, children are expected to be able to focus their attention. The ability to pay attention is critical for information processing. The capacity to screen out irrelevant aspects and hone in on the relevant aspects of the environment is called *selective attention*.

Attention and memory go hand in hand in the learning process. As just mentioned, there are three different kinds of storage systems: sensory memory (retention of less than a second), short-term memory (about 30 seconds), and long-term memory. During the elementary school years, children develop the ability to remember much larger blocks of information and retain the information for a longer time. The capacity for greater memory requires the use of different strategies, such as rehearsal (repeating the information over and over again) and organization (grouping the items to be remembered). During latency, children gain an appreciation of how memory works and are able to use memory-enhancing techniques in a deliberate fashion, whereas preschool children cannot.

Language Development

Grade-school-age children are able to understand intuitively how language works; their communicative skills are enhanced by their capacity to think about language. During this stage of development, children understand syntax and no longer confuse words, having learned the precise meaning of them. For example, a pre-school child may confuse "heavy" and "strong" and use the words interchangeably.

Between the ages of 6 and 7 years children gain appreciation of narrative grammar. The elements of narrative grammar are those of a traditional story: (1) the setting (characters and description), (2) the initiating events (conflict), (3) the internal response including goals and plans, (4) the attempt to address the problem, (5) the direct consequences, and (6) the reaction. Children of this age are able to relate a true plot or narrative with the essential features of an episode (elements 2 or 3, 4, and 5). This differs from the stories of 2- to 3-year-old children,

which contain only a central topic or theme, and the primitive narrative of 3- and 4-year-olds, which includes emotions and relations between events but does not have sequence or resolution of the true plot or true narrative. Narrative discourse allows the child to interpret experiences, appreciate causal relationships, share information, and employ story grammar. Narrative discourse is the form employed when a child reports on a book or a film or tells a story. The ability to use the narrative is a necessity in social and educational settings.

In addition to being able to think about language and becoming more competent in communicating, latency-age children are able to appreciate metaphors. Although some aspects of metaphors are understood at 7 or 8 years of age, children cannot fully explain metaphors and comprehend their psychological meanings until 10 or 11 years of age.

As language and the processes involved in concrete operations develop, the child begins to appreciate humor, particularly jokes, riddles, and puns. Latency-age children like to play on words and enjoy situations in which both meanings of a word have to be kept in mind at the same time in order to appreciate the joke or riddle.

Capacity to Learn in School and Acquisition of Skills

As noted, one of the main developmental tasks of this period is the capacity to learn in school. This ability depends on the successful mastery of the skills acquired in the cognitive, emotional, and social spheres. These skills could be described in a number of domains; however, it seems sensible to group them here, because they are so important to the educational experience. One skill that is uniquely significant in giving the child the opportunity to acquire information is that of reading. A child's success or failure at reading can have a major impact on the entire tone of the early educational experience. Reading well offers the child more independence with respect to learning new information and is linked to achieving other skills. Poor reading achievement in early school years has been viewed as a risk factor and has been associated with psychiatric symptoms, particularly adolescent depression. A major reason for clinical referral in this age group is related to academic achievement and behavioral problems in the school setting.

Since learning disabilities are so prevalent

during this developmental period, a brief summary of the scope of the problem merits mention. Learning disabilities affect at least 1.8 million schoolchildren and are a major concern of teachers. The *Diagnostic and Statistical Manual of Mental Disorders, Third Edition, Revised* (DSM-III-R), definition of a learning disability is that it is a basic difficulty in learning to read, write, or do arithmetic that is *not* due to mental retardation, impairment of vision or hearing, psychological problems, or lack of cultural and educational opportunity. The consequences of a learning disorder are widespread and can seriously affect a child's otherwise normal development. They include the failure to acquire basic academic skills and may result in lifelong handicaps. Many aspects of adaptation may be affected, and social and behavioral problems may arise. These social and behavioral problems include rejection by peers, low self-esteem, poor attitude toward learning, and being seen as less cooperative, less attentive, and less able to cope with new situations. It is critical that learning problems be detected early, their etiology determined, and appropriate intervention instituted.

Other skills that bear on the school experience are athletic skills, creativity (such as the ability to create stories), and skills in music and graphic arts.

SOCIAL DEVELOPMENT

Psychosocial Crisis: Industry vs. Inferiority

The latency child is a more social being, aware of time for play and work. This stage, referred to as "industry vs. inferiority," is, according to Erikson, the period when attitudes toward work are established. Industry refers to eagerness for building skills and performing meaningful work. The child must achieve the ability to enjoy work, a sense of growing possibilities, and a feeling of capability. Besides adults, peers are a source of encouragement. The danger at this stage is the development of a sense of inadequacy and inferiority. Worthlessness and inadequacy come from two sources. Self organ inferiority has been described by Alfred Adler as any physical or mental limitation that prevents an individual from gaining certain skills. If a skill cannot be mastered, the child experiences some degree of inferiority. Since the social environment reinforces certain skills more than others, it cannot be assumed that success in one area will compensate for another. Second, the process of social comparison can foster feelings of inferiority. The school setting offers opportunities for social comparison such as grouping by ability, grading, and public criticism. Although there is a developmental push that encourages a child to take on new challenges, feelings of self-consciousness, competitivism, and doubt are also aroused. One can see how the fear of failure or doing poorly as compared to one's peers could inhibit a child from trying a new task.

There are psychodynamic as well as psychosocial reasons that contribute to feelings of inferiority and inadequacy. Erikson described the scenario of earlier conflicts remaining unresolved, such as the child who may still want his mother more than knowledge; he may still rather be the baby at home than the big child in school; he still compares himself with his father, and the comparison arouses a sense of guilt as well as a sense of anatomical inferiority. Family life may not have prepared him for school life, or school life may fail to sustain the promises of earlier stages in that nothing that he has learned to do well already seems to count with the teacher. This stage differs from the others, because there is no violent upheaval. Sigmund Freud called this stage "latency" because the strong aggressive and sexual drives associated with the previous oedipal period or subsequent adolescence, remain fairly quiet during this period. This is a socially important stage, since industry involves doing things beside and with others; a sense of division of labor and of equal opportunity develops at this time.

Play Development

During latency, play is typically cooperative, with team games and board games being prominent. By being a member of a team, the child has the opportunity to learn about the division of labor, to learn about group goals, which are secondary to personal goals, and to learn about competition. Through team play, children learn more about rules, strategies, and evaluating their peers. There are certain social consequences of team play that further the child's concept that one plays to win and that there should be antagonism between teams. Although children learn that team members rely on each other, the child who is viewed as poor in athletic ability is likely to be singled out and criticized, especially if the team loses. Team sports do provide an opportunity for cognitive and social learning. Problem-solving capacities are challenged as players consider a range of strategies. Team sports require the mastery of rules that are often more complex than those of other games. Engaging in a team sport can prompt a child to evaluate his own assets and weaknesses as well as those of peers.

The latency child also enjoys memberships in special clubs and organizations, such as scouts, or extracurricular activities focused on a particular shared interest or skill, such as gymnastics or cooking. During this stage, groups and clubs are typically made up of same-sex peers, with emphasis on the exclusion of the opposite sex. The latency child delights in the rules and rituals associated with group membership. However, it is not uncommon for secret clubs and groups to be relatively short lived.

Peer Group and Friendship

The peer group offers the youngster in middle childhood an opportunity to learn that there are many points of view, to experience rules of society and peer pressure, and to experience the intimacy offered by a same-sex friendship. Working and playing in a peer group permit a child to grow away from the egocentric view predominating in early childhood. There is a reciprocity between the ability to be sensitive to the views of others and having peers view one favorably. The peer group develops norms for acceptance and rejection. Conforming to the peer group takes on greater importance, whereas earlier the teacher in the class setting was the most significant in terms of approval and acceptance. This is the time when the role of class clown or hero comes of age.

Being rejected by peers can lead to feelings of loneliness. Rejected children have been noted to be inclined toward aggressive and disruptive behavior toward peers. Rejected children are at risk for continuing to have psychosocial adjustment problems through adolescence and into adulthood.

The peer group has been found to provide a very perceptive source of information concerning fellow classmates. One technique for tapping into peer assessment is referred to as peer nominations, in which each child in a class is asked to nominate fellow classmates who best fit the description given. An example of one such instrument is the Pupil Evaluation Inventory, which includes items such as "those who always get into trouble" and "those whom everybody likes." Peer ratings have been used along with self-ratings and teacher ratings to provide dif-

ferent perspectives to behaviors or feelings of interest, such as aggression and depression. Studies have found significant correlations between self- and peer-reported depression. Higher rates of depression have been found in unpopular peers.

The development of close friendships is unique during this stage. This is the time children have "best friends," tell each other secrets, and come to each other's aid. Children also learn how to resolve conflicts with each other. Children now have significant relationships outside the context of the family, and these relationships are with peers rather than other adults. These same-sex friendships have been viewed as laying the foundation for later adult heterosexual relationships. When children begin school, they do not generally have the capacity to be close friends but have relationships more like companions or playmates. However, by 10 years old, children have a more complex understanding of the elements of close friendship, placing great value on the exchange of personal information and trust.

SOCIAL AND EMOTIONAL DEVELOPMENT

Moral Development

There have been two main theoretical approaches to moral development, the psychoanalytic and the cognitive-developmental approach.

The psychoanalytic framework has focused on the development of guilt and the successful identification with the same-sex parent, culminating in the resolution of the oedipal conflict. The formation of a conscience is promoted by the identification with the same-sex parent. The oedipal child fears the loss of parental love and feels guilty over yearnings for the parent of the opposite sex. Fear, anxiety, and guilt are seen as necessary for the formation of internalized moral rules.

The cognitive-developmental approach is exemplified by Piaget and Lawrence Kohlberg, who attribute moral development to cognitive growth. How children approach rules held great interest for Piaget. Children begin to play by rules during the period of concrete operations and are generally fairly rigid about them. It is not until 11 or 12 years of age that children can be more flexible about rules and view the more general objectives of rules. Piaget also studied moral development by presenting children with moral stories. The classic stories present one boy who accidentally breaks 15 cups and one boy who breaks one cup while doing something wrong. Children are asked which boy is naughtier; Piaget found that children between 5 and 10 years old based their judgment on consequences, that is, the more broken cups is worse, whereas children aged 11 years and older based their judgment on intentions.

Kohlberg expanded on Piaget's work and proposed three levels of moral thought that contain six stages. The three levels parallel the cognitive periods and are outlined as follows. The most primitive level of moral judgment is the preconventional level. This level approximates preoperational thought, between 2 and 7 years. Moral judgment at this level is guided by the child's concern with obtaining rewards and avoiding punishment. The next level, referred to as conventional, parallels the cognitive period of concrete operations, between 7 and 12 years. This stage is characterized by a focus on approval, social rules, and social expectations (law and order). The highest level is called postconventional or autonomous and corresponds most closely to the cognitive period of formal operations, from 12 years to adulthood. This level focuses on the individual's own attempts to clarify moral values and a sense of duty to society. At this stage, there is more critical thinking about individual rights and rules of society.

Like Piaget, Kohlberg used stories with moral dilemmas in his interviews with children and adults to build his theory of moral development. One of the classic moral dilemma stories is about a man who steals medication from a druggist for his sick wife. Kohlberg and others found support for the universality of the developmental sequence of stages of moral development by studying children in other cultures. However, some have questioned this finding. Although Kohlberg's work has played a major role in this area, it has been criticized with respect to its close tie to cognitive development. Others believe that children build their moral code more socially out of their interactions with others. The link between moral judgment and moral behavior has been questioned; some of Kohlberg's assumptions have been criticized through questioning the reliability of the moral judgment scale, the validity of Kohlberg's stages, the relevance of Kohlberg's moral development dilemmas to real life, and the lack of affective factors that may contribute to motivation. The validity for women of the levels of development has also been questioned, with some studies suggesting that women use different types of reasoning than men in making decisions.

Moral knowledge does not always go hand in hand with moral behavior. Behavior of others, one's own personality, and society's standards, as well as moral knowledge, influence one's moral behavior.

Social Cognition and Perspective Taking

Perspective taking, also referred to as role taking, is the ability to think about how others think and feel in a situation. This is another ability children gain during the latency period. Perspective taking, along with reinforcements, punishments, and observational learning, also influences moral behavior. It has been observed that in his earlier theoretical writings, Piaget held to a unity of social and intellectual development in fostering the capacity for perspective taking; in fact, social interaction with the peer group and the social push to accommodate to the views of others were seen as critical to advancing from egocentrism to perspective taking. Although Piaget later retracted this position, placing greater emphasis on the cognitive structures and downplaying the role of social experience, recent research has found support for the enhancement of cognitive development through social interaction.

Four levels of role taking that children progress through between 4 and 12 years of age have been proposed: level 0, egocentric role taking; level 1, subjective role taking; level 2, self-reflective role taking; and level 3, mutual role taking. Generally, children below 7 years old are egocentric and do not yet comprehend that other people may have inner thoughts and feelings that differ from their own. As has been the case with other developmental stages, and as more recent research employing different tests has revealed, gradation and variability in role-taking abilities exist, accounting for the sensitivity found among children under 7 years of age. At level 1, children understand that others may view the situation differently from themselves; however, they are not able to "step into the shoes" of the other person, nor can they think about their own perspective at the same time as thinking about others' perspectives. At level 2, children can attribute different perspectives to differences in interests and values, not only to others being in different situations or having access to different pieces of information (as children at level 1 would). Children at this level begin to develop an awareness of how others perceive them and begin to think about the reactions they will elicit. Also at this level, children can "step into the shoes" of others. At level 3 (mutual role taking), children are capable of thinking about their perspective and that of others at the same time.

The opportunity for social interaction with peers is critical to gaining ability in perspective taking. Researchers have found that children who perform at the same cognitive level and are of the same socioeconomic status demonstrate different levels of role taking, based on the extent of their time spent in peer interactions. In addition to strides being made in role taking during the period of middle childhood, advances are also made in the capacity for empathy.

PROBLEMS AND DISORDERS TYPICALLY APPEARING IN LATENCY

Three developmental tasks of latency have received emphasis in this chapter, namely, learning in school, developing peer relations outside the family, and having less conflicted relationships with parents. This section reviews some selected problems and disorders that may be seen as either posing obstacles to mastery of these particular developmental tasks or representing failure in the tasks. This framework is not intended as a statement about etiology of disorder, since research continues to address questions of causality, risk factors, and protective factors. Rather, the main point is to allow the student of normal child development to have a sense of the continuum from adaptive to maladaptive behaviors and to begin to appreciate the relatively new field of developmental psychopathology. Developmental psychopathology offers the perspective of trying to view maladaptive behavior against the milestones, tasks, and challenges that occur throughout the life span. Developmental psychopathology draws on a number of perspectives, including cognitive, biological, social-emotional, genetic, educational, and neurobiological. Two of the disorders used to illustrate the interrelationship between adaptive development and psychopathology—attention-deficit disorder and separation anxiety—are covered more extensively in Chapter 18, Childhood Psychopathology: Diagnosis and Treatment, and are discussed here with a developmental and contextual focus.

Attention-Deficit Hyperactivity Disorder

As mentioned earlier, one of the main developmental tasks of the latency-age child is to learn in school. The most referrals of hyperactive children to clinical settings occur during the elementary school years. This particular pattern of referral does not answer the question of prior hyperactivity in the preschool period or continuation or cessation of hyperactivity during adolescence. It is likely that a child with preexisting hyperactivity will soon be noticed in the school environment where there are clear standards of acceptable behavior. The expectations are to pay attention, to sit still, to refrain from impulsive activity, and to finish one's work. One has merely to preface these expectations with the phrase "failure to" and one has a number of the key criteria, according to DSM-III-R, for the diagnosis of attention-deficit hyperactivity disorder (ADHD), which is characterized by impulsivity, inattention, and overactivity.

As reviewed in Chapter 18, one must carefully consider the differential diagnosis for attention-deficit hyperactivity disorder, which includes anxiety, mental retardation, age-appropriate overactivity, affective disorders, and pervasive developmental disorders. Learning disabilities require careful evaluation and the provision of specialized educational services. Learning disabilities can occur independently of other disorders or may occur in association with attention-deficit hyperactivity disorder.

A number of changes and stresses may occur in the child's environment and may affect the latency child's capacity to learn in school. These stresses may have both fairly time-limited and longer-term consequences with regard to school success. Children living in a chaotic environment may be seen in a similar manner to children with attention-deficit disorder. The clinical literature of abuse (physical and sexual) and neglect reports a variety of signs and symptoms, including the clinical picture of hyperactivity, decline in academic performance, and behavioral problems that can manifest themselves in the school environment as well as at home. The research on children of divorce has found latency-age children exhibiting behavioral problems in school, such as inattention, decreased work effort, and a decline in academic performance.

In summary, because the latency period is a time when there is a tremendous emphasis on learning and a time when future attitudes about academic success are formed, the development of difficulties in the capacity to learn deserves comprehensive study to clearly identify the etiology and institute an appropriate intervention.

Anxiety Disorders

Anxiety disorders such as separation anxiety, avoidant disorder of childhood, and overanxious disorder can each interfere with the development of peer relations, and separation anxiety and overanxious disorder have serious implications for school learning. Both separation anxiety and overanxious disorder may have school refusal as a complication. In separation anxiety the main feature is the anxiety surrounding separation from a primary attachment figure. The development of peer relations is compromised, because children with separation anxiety are so apprehensive about being apart from the attachment figure that they may refuse to go on outings with friends or stay overnight at a friend's home. Since organized interest groups (such as scouts) and team sports require an ability to enter new and unfamiliar situations away from home, the child with separation anxiety often is unable to take advantage of the usual opportunities provided for enhancing peer contact.

In overanxious disorder the anxiety is more global and manifested by self-consciousness, worries about competence, and anxiety about future events. Overanxious disorder may be accompanied by a social or a simple phobia. Children with overanxious disorder may worry so much about their performance that they may avoid peer group activities. A high level of anxiety can interfere with performance on school examinations and the ability to meet deadlines. The extent of impairment in social and school functioning depends on the severity of the disorder.

Avoidant disorder of childhood or adolescence is characterized by an excessive withdrawal from contact with unfamiliar people in the face of a clear desire for social contact and good relationships with familiar people, such as family members and peers the child knows very well. Although the disorder is not thought to be common, the degree of impairment in socialization is often severe.

Conduct Disorder

A number of developmental tasks of latency are affected by the presence of aggressive, hostile, and defiant behavior. The three main tasks involving learning, peers, and family are clearly compromised by the disorders currently classified as conduct disorder and oppositional defiant disorder. According to DSM-III-R, the conduct disorders have been delineated into three types: group type, solitary aggressive type, and undifferentiated type. In the previous system of DSM-III, there were four types: socialized aggressive, undersocialized aggressive (similar to solitary aggressive), socialized nonaggressive (similar to group type), and undersocialized nonaggressive. These types require further investigation in support of their validity and utility. For ease of understanding and for emphasis on the relationship of disorders and failures in developmental tasks, conduct disorders are discussed here as a single entity. The DSM-III-R diagnostic criteria for conduct disorder include a duration of conduct disturbance of at least 6 months, during which three of the following have been present:

(1) has stolen without confrontation of a victim on more than one occasion (including forgery)

(2) has run away from home overnight at least twice while living in parental or parental surrogate home (or once without returning)

(3) often lies (other than to avoid physical or sexual abuse)

(4) has deliberately engaged in fire setting

(5) is often truant from school (for older person, absent from work)

(6) has broken into someone else's house, building, or car

(7) has deliberately destroyed others' property (other than by fire setting)

(8) has been physically cruel to animals

(9) has forced someone into sexual activity

(10) has used a weapon in more than one fight

(11) often initiates physical fights

(12) has stolen with confrontation of a victim (e.g., mugging, purse-snatching, extortion, armed robbery)

(13) has been physically cruel to people

If 18 years or older, the individual does not meet criteria for antisocial personality disorder. Usually the onset is before puberty; however, postpubertal onset is more common among females than males.

It is clear that a child with conduct disorder has already experienced failure in adapting to rules at home, at school, and in the community. In studies comparing sociopathic children to subcultural delinquents, neurotic delinquents, and normal children, sociopathic children were found to have lower levels of moral judgment (using Kohlberg's moral dilemmas) than any of the other groups. Although moral judgment was significantly correlated with cognitive development, the finding of lower moral judgment in sociopathic children persisted when the effects of cognitive level were controlled.

It is beyond the scope of this chapter to review the various theoretical frameworks of the development of aggression and delinquency; however, the cognitive-behavioral approach is useful in illustrating the difficulties aggressive boys have in the area of social cognition. Kenneth Dodge studied grade school boys' responses to hostile, benign, and ambiguous social cues. In comparing aggressive to nonaggressive boys, he found that aggressive boys had no difficulty in interpreting clear-cut cues, but when cues were ambiguous, they attributed hostile intentions to others. In addition, Dodge found that other boys attributed more hostile intentions to aggressive boys than to nonaggressive boys when the cues were ambiguous, thus exaggerating the hostility of aggressive peers.

The problems of aggressive and delinquent children with respect to school and the peer group have been reviewed; the difficulties such children have in establishing less conflicted satisfying relationships with parents are extensive, particularly in the area of identification with parents' prosocial behavior and values. Although there are many explanations for the aggression, it is known that parents can exert a tremendous influence on social-emotional development during latency. A number of factors have been found to increase and reinforce children's aggression, including parental deviance, quarrelsomeness, rejection, permissiveness, and encouragement of aggression.

Oppositional Defiant Disorder

The essential element for the diagnosis of oppositional defiant disorder is a pattern of negative, hostile, and defiant behavior, without more serious violations of the basic rights of others. The DSM-III-R criteria require a disturbance of at least 6 months, during which at least five of the following are present:

(1) often loses temper
(2) often argues with adults
(3) often actively defies or refuses adult requests or rules, e.g., refuses to do chores at home

(4) often deliberately does things to annoy other people, e.g., grabs other children's hats
(5) often blames others for his own mistakes
(6) is often touchy or easily annoyed by others
(7) is often angry and resentful
(8) is often spiteful and vindictive
(9) often swears or uses obscene language

The child does not meet the criteria for conduct disorder, and the behavior does not occur exclusively during the course of a psychotic disorder, dysthymia, or a major depressive, hypomanic, or manic episode. The behavior must be more frequent than that of other children the same mental age.

These children may also exhibit low self-esteem, low frustration tolerance, labile mood, and temper outbursts. They may become users of illegal substances and alcohol before legal age. In reviewing the diagnostic criteria, it becomes apparent that these children will be engaged in conflict at home, in school, and with peers. The argumentative quality of their interactions, usually accompanied by a failure to take on age-appropriate responsibilities and a marked tendency to blame others, prevent these children from responding in an appropriate fashion to the increasing demands at school and home for compliance and from assuming greater responsibility for their behavior. It is not uncommon for a child with oppositional defiant disorder to be viewed as the class clown or to find his way to the principal's office with regularity. Children with oppositional defiant disorder may have a rather poor self-concept beneath their defiant immature image. Although the course is not known, this disorder may evolve into a conduct disorder or mood disorder.

BIBLIOGRAPHY

Achenbach, T.M.: Developmental Psychopathology, ed. 2. New York, Wiley, 1982.
Erikson, E.: Childhood and Society. New York, Norton, 1963.
Guidubaldi, J., Perry, J.D.: Divorce and mental health sequelae for children: A two-year follow-up of a nationwide sample. J. Am. Acad. Child Psychiatry 24:531-537, 1985.
Guidubaldi, J., et al.: The impact of parental divorce on children: Report of the nationwide NASP study. School Psychol. Rev. 12:300-323, 1983.
Kellam, S.G., et al.: Mental Health and Going to School. Chicago, The University of Chicago Press, 1975.
Lefkowitz, M., Tesiny, E.: Depression in children: Prevalence and correlates. J. Consulting Child Psychol. 53:647-656, 1985.

Lewis, M.: Clinical Aspects of Child Development, ed. 2. Philadelphia, Lea & Febiger, 1982.

Light, P.: Piaget and egocentrism: A perspective on recent developmental research. Early Child Dev. Care 12:7-18, 1983.

Morrison, D., Siegal, M., Francis, R.: Control, autonomy, and the development of moral behavior: A social cognitive perspective. Imagination, Cognition Personality 3:337-351, 1983-84.

Schneider, M.J., Leitenberg, H.: A comparison of aggressive and withdrawn children's self-esteem, optimism and pessimism and causal attributions for success and failure. J. Abnorm. Child Psychol. 17(2):133-144, 1989.

Selman, R., Selman, A.: Children's ideas about friendship: A new theory. Psychol. Today 13:70-80, 114, 1979.

Tesch, S.A.: Review of friendship development across the lifespan. Hum. Dev. 26:266-276, 1983.

Vosk, B., et al.: A multi-method comparison of popular and unpopular children. Dev. Psychol. 18:571-575, 1982.

Zigler, E.F., Finn-Stevenson, M.: Children Development and Social Issues. Lexington, Heath, 1987.

Chapter 17
Adolescence

Charles S. Grob, M.D.

Adolescence is a period of life marked by rapid change. The individual during these years transitions from the psychological and social world of the child to the mature experience of the young adult. Adolescence can be both frightening and exhilarating, not only to the individual adolescent, but also to the family, community, and society. It is a period often marked by intense emotions in individual experience as well as in the reactions of those in close proximity. The adolescent period is a phase of life that has been idealized and glamorized by American culture, while at the same time evoking anger and resentment. The surging and intense emotional states of young people, coupled with the particular newness of the process of discovery, inevitably provoke strong reactions. Whether favorable or hostile, one can always be assured that the adolescent period will elicit a marked response from the surrounding world.

ADOLESCENT DEVELOPMENT

Adolescence is defined as the state or process of growing up from puberty to maturity. It in-

cludes physiological, cognitive, psychological, social, and family changes. The initiation of adolescence is marked by the onset of the physiological process of puberty. The termination of adolescence, however, is ill defined and depends on a variety of psychosocial variables.

Puberty

Puberty is defined as the period of first becoming capable of reproducing sexually, as manifested by the maturing of genital organs, development of secondary sex characteristics, first occurrence of menstruation in the female, and first occurrence of seminal emissions in the male. The age of onset of puberty varies, with a range of several years marking the initiation of this physiological process. Puberty may begin as early as 10 years in girls and 11 years in boys, although the average age of onset is 2 to 3 years later. The psychosocial process of adolescence evolves with puberty but often at a different rate. The psychological responses to the physical changes of puberty are influenced by prevailing socioeconomic conditions and cultural values. One intriguing phenomenon of modern society has been the increasingly early average age of onset of puberty in girls. Over the course of 120 years, from 1860 to 1980, the average age of onset of menses has dropped from 16.5 years to 12.5 years. The earlier appearance of these physiological changes has been attributed to improvements in health, nutrition, hygiene, and sanitation that have occurred during this span. The age at menarche is a sensitive indicator of the physical well-being of the population. Unfortunately, the psychological concomitants of puberty have generally not undergone a similarly early maturation. This psychological lag in development, compared to the more rapid expression of physiological development, has created a heightened risk for the emergence of emotional problems during this critical period.

The growth spurt of puberty proceeds according to different physiological patterns in the two sexes and progresses in a manner that takes into account individual variation in tempo, or rhythm, of growth. A widely accepted classification for sexual maturity has been established. For females, this classification system stages the development of pubic hair, breast development, and menarche from immature prepubescent patterns progressively through the various stages of puberty to mature adult female expression. Likewise, a system has been developed for males undergoing puberty that classifies the progressive stages of pubic hair and penile and testes development from prepubescent status to mature adult male expression. Pubertal initiation and evolution depend on significant alterations in the relative levels of the sex hormones. In adolescents of both sexes, the surge in production of androgens and estrogens is due to increasing gonadal stimulation by gonadotropins secreted by the anterior pituitary.

In addition to the physiological changes associated with the development of secondary sex characteristics, puberty also entails a rapid increase in the rate of growth. A peculiar circumstance commonly observed at the beginning of puberty is the sudden surge in height in girls relative to boys. Between approximately 11 and 15 years of age, girls are taller than boys of the same age. Both before and after this period of several years, males are commonly of greater stature than females. Whereas the average maximal growth spurt in girls is around 12 or 13 years old, the maximal growth spurt for boys is around 14 or 15 years old. Pubertal males and females also differ in the relative degree of acquisition of muscle bulk and the relative distribution of body fat.

As a general rule, early versus late onset of maturation has different behavioral and emotional implications in boys and girls. Studies have revealed that early maturing girls are faced with more psychological and social difficulties than girls who mature at a later age. Early maturing girls often experience considerable self-consciousness and anxiety and often attempt to conceal breast development through alterations in posture. On the other hand, among boys it is the late maturers who have been observed to have significantly more adjustment difficulties, including poor self-confidence, low assertiveness, and social anxiety. They are often late in initiating heterosexual activity and are frequently plagued with introspective self-doubt. Interestingly, early maturers of both sexes tend to have a higher IQ and greater academic accomplishment at all ages.

Cognitive Changes

The stage of adolescence is marked by a transition from the concrete thinking processes of the latency and preadolescent child to the more evolved and intricate cognitive capacity observed in mature adults. Jean Piaget defined this mature process, first observed in the developing adolescent, as the stage of formal operational thinking. This period is marked by a growth of intellectual activity, increased awareness, and capacity for insight. The successfully maturing individual during adolescence, as part of the acquisition of formal thought operations, develops the capacity to understand and utilize abstract concepts, becomes more introspective, and cultivates the ability for self-critical reflection. Further, as psychological growth progresses, the adolescent develops the capacity to think beyond the concrete here and now of the present and to ponder and reflect on the future. Adolescence is also the phase of development in which one becomes acutely aware of the passage of time, the finiteness of life, and the inevitability of death.

Psychosocial Tasks of Adolescent Development

Adolescence is a time of upheaval and challenge, the successful resolution of which leads to the rewards of healthy and adaptive adult functioning. It is also a time of potential danger. In the process of surmounting the inevitable hurdles of adolescent development, stresses arise, taxing the young person's coping skills and psychological strength and resilience. The degree to which an individual is able to resolve the inevitable conflicts of adolescent development determines the degree to which mature functioning is eventually attained.

A primary task of adolescent development is the acceptance of a changing body image. The profound physiological alterations associated with the pubertal process drastically and irrevocably alter the self-concept of the developing individual. Within a relatively short period of time, the body has grown considerably, developed secondary sexual characteristics, and experienced an overall redefinition of intrinsic body image. It is often a confusing and frightening experience to undergo such rapid progression from the relatively quiescent physical and hormonal state of a child to the rapid state of flux experienced in puberty. Adolescents commonly feel awkward and ill at ease with their changing bodies. Sexual drive also heightens and intensifies during this period, in both boys and girls, thus necessitating further accommodation to the profound change in body image and self-concept.

A critical challenge of the adolescent period is the acquisition of a mature personal identity. Whereas during childhood the family and peer associations are often integral to identity formation, with the onset of adolescence the individual begins to develop the capacity to conceptualize as a more autonomous being, apart from those in close proximity. As cognitive processes mature, the adolescent begins to be able to project into the future and anticipate and plan for an eventual career identity. This is a critical process in the development of a work identity, a vital element of healthy adult functioning. Another phenomenon that often evokes a struggle during adolescence is that of establishing gender identity. Particularly during early adolescence, the individual struggles with the definition of male and female heterosexual identity.

Adolescence is also the time during which the individual begins to separate from his family of origin and seeks to function independently. Particularly in early adolescence, the individual often feels not only the need to separate and become somewhat autonomous from family, but also the regressive pull to hold on to and remain intimately bonded to family. This period has been described by the psychoanalyst Peter Blos as the second phase of separation-individuation.

The first phase of separation-individuation occurs earlier in development, during the toddler period, with the young child first venturing out and exploring the world on his own and then hastening back into the reassuring and secure presence of the mother. The second phase of separation-individuation implies a synonymous process for the adolescent, with a maturational push into separation followed by a regressive pull back to the parent or parents. The ultimate goal for the adolescent is to function as an independent and autonomous individual while establishing and consolidating more mature and healthier adult ties to one's family of origin.

During the adolescent period, it is critical that a process of healthy reality testing be attained, particularly with regard to the establishment of personal goals for both the near and the distant future. Through trial and error, and aided by a maturing sense of identity, the psychologically healthy adolescent begins to develop a realistic perspective on what the future may hold. As development evolves, the maturing adolescent's self-concept begins to incorporate and elaborate on themes and goals of healthy adult identity and function.

Another task critical to the process of maturing adolescent development is that of obtaining the capacity to defer gratification. By experience, one gradually realizes the inevitability of life's stresses and learns the process of reestablishing a state of equilibrium after a discordant (disruptive) event. In the process of healthy development, the growing adolescent needs to accept that there are times when it is in one's own best interest to pursue short- and long-term goals by resisting the temptation to escape into transient but maladaptive stress-free states. The adolescent who develops the habit of coping with stress by fleeing from the stressor and, instead, seeking out means of instant gratification (such as drug-induced euphoria) has failed to develop a capacity essential for healthy and optimal maturation, that of deferred gratification.

A final psychosocial task necessary for the eventual acquisition of healthy adult functioning is the development of the capacity for empathic and intimate relationships. During adolescence, the need to explore relationships, particularly with a member of the opposite sex, achieves great strength. This is often a stressful and discordant process. However, the capacity to relate to another individual in a caring and unselfish manner is in many respects one of the most positive attributes of the mature personality.

Family Development during Adolescence

As the identified adolescent engages in the struggle for autonomy, so the family of origin often experiences its own regressive push-pull of separation-individuation. The entry of the child into adolescence may precipitate a crisis within the family as parents and siblings struggle to accommodate to this new and often frightening developmental transition. Many parents of adolescents undergo personal as well as marital crises during this period. Further, volatile and destructive altercations between adolescent and parents are not uncommon and, if not resolved, can cause prolonged rupture within the family system. There must ultimately be an accommodation to this new phase of individual and family development, as well as a redefinition of family identity. As with the individual, the family of the adolescent must adapt to change and successfully master its own psychosocial tasks of development to facilitate growth and fulfillment.

Adolescence—Historical Perspective

Contrary to popular mythology, adolescence is not a simple creation of modern civilization. The adolescent period, previously known as youth, was both recognized and held in high esteem by the ancient civilizations of Greece, Rome, and Egypt. Among the Greeks, in particular, youth was considered to be the epitome of both physical and mental development. Greek philosophers stressed that privileged youth be provided with optimal philosophical discourse and education.

In Western Europe, following the fall of the Roman Empire, the conceptualization of adolescence as a discrete period was discarded. Throughout the Middle Ages of Europe, life was barely separated between childhood and adulthood, with social and economic conditions necessitating extraordinarily early entry of children into adult work and procreative roles. Only with the emergence of the Renaissance was there rediscovery (albeit limited to the privileged classes) of the idealized concept of youth.

Many primitive cultures studied by anthropologists have also revealed the presence of an equivalent of adolescence. The transition between childhood and adulthood has been almost universally recognized as a critical period of development. Many of these so-called "primitive" cultures symbolically demonstrate the importance of the adolescent period by pubertal initiation rituals. These puberty rites are ceremonial occasions that generally last from several days to several weeks. They range from the simple changing of garments and recitation of sacred verse to the tatooing of skin, prolonged isolation and fasting, and the experience of painful body mutilation. All successful pubertal initiation rites culminate with the entry of the young individual into mature adult society.

The modern concept of adolescence as a period of prolonged preparation for mature adult roles originated with the industrialization of Western society in the mid to late nineteenth century. Since then, the length of adolescence has gradually increased, reflecting the growing affluence of society. The first modern theorist who defined adolescence as a discrete and identifiable stage of development was the educator G. Stanley Hall. Hall, writing in the early twentieth century, was strongly influenced by Darwinian theory and emphasized the biogenetic determinants of personality development. He stated that normal adolescence was an "era of storm and stress analogous to mankind's tumultuous progression from primitiveness to higher civilization." Hall conceptualized that, amid the turmoil and upheaval of adolescence, there occurred the Darwinian phenomenon of "survival of the fittest" enacted on a contemporary human field.

The early twentieth century also saw the inception of the psychoanalytical movement. Although Sigmund Freud did not focus his writings extensively on the discrete period of adolescence, his emphasis on libidinal (sexual) drives was certainly pertinent to the psychosexual experience of adolescence. Freud defined the psychophysiological "transformation of puberty" as a bridge from infantile and childhood sexuality to adult sexuality. Freud, however, left the detailed exploration of this particular period of development to his successors.

Turmoil versus Normality

Many of the preeminent psychoanalysts of the last 50 years have written extensively on the varieties of psychopathological experience observed in adolescence. Impressed with the extreme degrees of disturbance they observed, many psychoanalysts began to attribute a psychopathological core to all of adolescence. The propensity to generalize to an entire developmental stage from the case examples of a few select patients exerted a profound influence on the understanding of "normal" adolescent development. Unfortunately, such a perspective has also contributed to a pervasive bias in conceptualizing adolescent phenomena, as well as in intervening in apparent disturbance.

Anna Freud

Anna Freud, the disciple and youngest child of Sigmund Freud, described adolescence as being marked by a sudden increase in instinctual drives and a "libidinization" of infantile ties. She described the utilization of "pathological defenses" to ward off such drives, as well as for protection from threatening parental attachments. She defined the period of adolescence as being, in essence, a "developmental disturbance," and emphasized that adolescent turmoil is not only normal but desirable. According to Anna Freud, if an adolescent does not show a pronounced degree of "turmoil," it is a virtual certainty that he will be developmentally immature, emotionally constricted, and poorly differentiated. To Anna Freud, therefore, it was essential that all individuals undergoing adolescence must wrestle with and overcome the universal and inevitable conflicts associated with that phase of development.

Erik Erikson

Erik Erikson espoused a similar perspective. Erikson wrote that periodic crises during adolescence are developmentally normal. Such episodes of emotional and behavioral turmoil are ultimately directed toward the consolidation of identity. For Erikson the resolution of each crisis reinforces a strong sense of identity. The failure of crisis resolution would inexorably culminate in role diffusion, a state of identity weakening and fragmentation. Erikson further theorized that before each sequential consolidation of identity, intermittent states of identity diffusion are experienced. Such states of crisis precipitate "acting out" behaviors, social alienation, marked fluctuations of mood, pervasive anxiety, feelings of "inner emptiness," distorted concepts of time, difficulty making decisions, marked inability to work, impaired concentration, and a desperate sense of hopelessness about the future. Such states of crisis, according to Erikson, are *always* active during adolescent development. The degree to which one resolves these inevitable crises will determine future health and development.

Peter Blos

The contemporary psychoanalyst Peter Blos theorized that it is essential during adolescence to experience a series of phase-specific regressions to achieve developmental progression. These "phase-specific regressions" are defined as being manifested by maladaptive behavioral patterns and heightened emotional turbulence. During periods of individuation, in which the stage of adolescence figures prominently, a state of intensified vulnerability of personality organization is experienced. As mentioned previously, Blos contrasts this phenomenon of reemergent separation-individuation during adolescence with the first individuation process, which is completed by the end of the third year of life. According to the early childhood theorist Margaret Mahler, this process is marked by a "hatching from the symbiotic membrane" on the path to becoming an individuated toddler. The second individuation process of adolescence, of which Blos wrote at length, is defined as the shedding of family dependencies and loosening of its symbiotic ties as one successfully matures and progresses from adolescence to adulthood. As the adolescent experiences an intensification of drives and rejects parental support, further intensification of psychological distress and turmoil is anticipated. Blos viewed virtually all disturbances in adolescence as reflecting the existence of developmental impasses sustained at earlier stages, the resolutions of which are essential for emotional health and normal functioning.

Daniel Offer

Anna Freud, Erikson, and Blos, as representative of psychoanalytical theory over the past 50 years, reflect the contention that adolescence is a potential period of turmoil and conflict, frequently to pronounced degrees. It is pertinent to note that the primary field from which such conclusions were drawn was the domain of the seriously disturbed adolescent patient. To these psychoanalysts, access to a more normative population of adolescents seems to have been limited. Although many valuable insights on disturbed adolescent function were achieved, a regrettable overgeneralization of an entire stage of development occurred.

A contrasting perspective, however, has been offered over the past decade by the psychiatric researcher and epidemiologist Daniel Offer. Offer, who performed extensive surveys of mainstream adolescent populations, concluded that emotional health and well-being in adolescence are quite the norm, rather than the exception. On the basis of his extensive studies, Offer concluded that the majority of adolescents are hopeful about the future, are free from severe behavioral dysfunction, have warm feelings toward their parents, have positive peer relationships, have a positive work ethic, have positive self-esteem, and have adapted without severe conflict or stress to their changing body image and emerging sexuality. Offer's concept of adolescence is that of individuals predominantly "enjoying life" and being "happy most of the time." Offer stated that although approximately one half of these "normal" adolescents do admit to sporadic situational anxiety, they are otherwise free of psychiatric symptoms.

In his definitive study, Offer identified four developmental groups into which all adolescents can be divided. The first group, which he assessed as comprising approximately 25 percent of the adolescent population surveyed, is described as having excellent biogenetic and environmental backgrounds, having good impulse control, being comfortable with and accepting of general cultural and societal norms, and having emotional mastery of previous developmental stages. This high-functioning group has been defined as the "continuous growth group." The second group, the "surgent growth group," comprising 35 percent of the population studied, is defined as possessing mild degrees of biogenetic vulnerability and environmental disturbance. An additional 20 percent of Offer's study population comprised a mixed continuous and surgent group. The final group, the "tumultuous growth group," also comprising 20 percent of adolescents, are described as having family psychiatric histories, parental marital discord, and family financial difficulties and being comprised of individuals prone to intermittent depressed moods. Offer concluded that this tumultuous growth group, the final and most unhealthy group defined, is quite similar to the patient population studied by psychoanalytical theorists over the past half century.

One of the most compelling points that Offer made was that the other groups, comprising approximately 80% of the population he extensively surveyed, are free or relatively free of serious psychopathological disorder. This does not mean, however, that such individuals are without significant problems. Conflict and stressors are inevitable in development. Nevertheless, most adolescents appear to have sufficient emotional resources and resilience to be able to weather the periodic storms of adolescence and attain healthy functioning and progressive development.

It is critical to realize that psychopathology during adolescence is not a normative experience and that the approximately 20 percent of adolescents with severe emotional turmoil do not simply "grow out of" the extreme difficulties they experience during this period. Such individuals are often in desperate need of intensive treatment, without which they will likely not be able to weather the raging storms of their intrinsic condition. When extreme turmoil and maladaptation are observed in an adolescent, one should be alerted that severe emotional disturbance exists, necessitating the rapid application of appropriate intervention. An adolescent, burdened with a serious psychopathological condition, must be provided with necessary treatment. It is a great disservice to the disturbed adolescent, as well as to the family, to regard the adolescent as just "going through a stage" from which "normality" will spontaneously evolve. The physician has the responsibility to identify the adolescent and family in need of treatment and to initiate appropriate intervention as rapidly and effectively as possible.

ADOLESCENT PSYCHOPATHOLOGY

According to Offer's extensive survey, approximately 20 percent of adolescents experience sufficient disruptions in states of internal mood, thought regulation, and external behaviors that some form of competent treatment is essential for healthy functioning. Although some authorities criticize this assessment as conservative, nevertheless, Offer's 20 percent figure poses staggering implications for the delivery of primary mental health services.

Currently, there are approximately 17 million adolescents in the United States, of which 20 percent, or 3.4 million, are identified as in need of treatment. Of these 3.4 million, only 1 million have been seen by a mental health professional. And of these 1 million, only 250,000 have received psychiatric assessment and treatment. In other words, of the substantial and ever-increasing number of adolescents in serious need of expert mental health intervention, only a fraction will be provided with effective treatment. For the individuals in question, their families, their communities, and the greater society, the impact of failure to provide adequate treatment at a critical time will be tremendous. Great costs will be felt in terms of human life and happiness, family and community stability, and economic depletion. This is the ultimate price for failing to identify and provide treatment for the serious emotional and behavioral disorders of adolescents.

With many psychiatric disorders, the risk of occurrence is related to both the degree of individual biological-genetic vulnerability and the degree of chronic and unrelenting environmental stress. Modern psychiatry has established that a family history of mental illness is a strong predictor for its occurrence. The greater the biogenetic endowment, the greater the eventual risks. A relative protective factor, however, is the maintenance of a nurturing, caring, and health-enhancing home environment. Such an environment may minimize the ultimate severity of illness and dysfunction even in individuals with strong biological-genetic predispositions. On the other hand, a profoundly pathological environment can magnify the risks of illness in individuals with only mild degrees of biological and genetic vulnerability.

Adolescent Depression

Traditionally, depression in adolescence has been an underdiagnosed disorder. Before the past two decades, the prevailing psychoanalytical viewpoint had been that psychopathological signs and symptoms, which would have predicted a deteriorating clinical course in adults, were not particularly alarming in adolescents. From this perspective, adolescents were perceived to be experiencing only the inevitable and necessary turmoil of their age. Unfortunately, many ill adolescents of earlier generations were deprived of appropriate intervention. More recently, however, significant advances have been made. Depressive psychopathology in adolescence is now seen on a direct continuum with adult illness. In fact, formal diagnostic criteria utilized to diagnose depression in adults are now accepted as being equally valid for adolescents. Risk factors, manifestations, and prognosis of depression in adolescents and adults are perceived as relatively synonymous, although the state of adolescent development does provide a unique coloration to the phenomenon. The experience of depressive illness in adolescence will have a major impact on the developmental tasks of identity formation, establishment of goals, autonomy from the family, and the experience of intimate and empathic relationships outside the family. The more pro-

nounced the psychopathological state, the greater the likelihood a severe developmental fixation, and even regression, will occur.

Standardized DSM-III-R criteria have been successfully applied to depressed patients of all age groups, with only mild age-specific variation. Yet, diagnoses with adolescents can be a more difficult task than with adults. One reason is that adolescents have greater difficulty articulating internal feelings and emotional states. It may also be difficult for young individuals to sufficiently trust an adult in a position of authority with such intimate personal material. Since this is often the first episode of a major depression for the adolescent, the relative "newness" of the experience can create a heightened state of severe anxiety and demoralization. Depression is frequently cyclical. As an individual ages and experiences a number of episodes, some understanding of the process, including the phase of recovery, will be incorporated. For the young patient, often in the throes of a first episode, fear mounts that there will be "no way out." A sense of pervasive hopelessness ensues. In such a state the capacity for reflection and insight is limited. Instead, the depressed adolescent often begins to "act out" the internal state of turbulence, despair, and fear. This acting out often takes the form of alcohol and substance abuse, sexual promiscuity, school truancy, juvenile delinquency, violence, and dangerous risk-taking behavior (which are often disguised forms of suicide). It is critical for those called on to evaluate such "out of control" adolescents to recognize that the core precipitant for these maladaptive and dangerous behaviors is often depressive illness.

Adolescent Bipolar Disorder

Bipolar illness (or manic-depressive illness) is intrinsically related to depression as one of the primary affective disorders. As with major depression, bipolar disorder in adolescents has also had an extensive history of misdiagnosis and mistreatment. Similarly, it has been only relatively recently that bipolar conditions have been identified and accurately diagnosed with some consistency in adolescents. Not only have established criteria for bipolar disorder been applied to younger patients, but also various patterns specific for early age of onset have been described. These include the identification that a particular subset of individuals with an early onset of depressive illness is at risk for escalation into a bipolar state. Such progression, frequently at early adolescence, from major depression to bipolar illness is often predictive of a particularly severe course, poor prognosis, and resistance to conventional psychopharmacological treatment. A major risk factor for the development of bipolar illness is not only a biological family history of bipolar disorder, but also a high genetic "loading" for all the affective disorders. Another predictor for future evolution of bipolar disorder from major depression in an adolescent is the association of the depression with active hallucinations and delusions (psychotic symptoms). Two additional features of bipolar illness in adolescence that are often present are irritability and anger (which can be explosive).

As with adolescents who have major depression, it is often very difficult when assessing these young patients who have underlying bipolar illness to perceive the core disorder beyond what is often an idiosyncratic adolescent behavioral expression (that is, aggressive behaviors, drug abuse). Developmental considerations must be accounted for when identifying the specific expression of bipolar disorder and when exploring the developmental impact of the condition. It is imperative that an accurate diagnosis be established as early as possible, so as to avoid the potentially dangerous treatments of an incorrect diagnosis, as well as to optimize the therapeutic effects of interventions derived from an accurate assessment. As in adolescents with major depression who are not diagnosed or treated correctly, the ultimate developmental impact on an untreated or mistreated adolescent with bipolar illness may be devastating. Not only does healthy developmental progression depend on a relatively consistent and normative mood, but also the attribution of an errant condition to an affectively ill adolescent can be severely injurious. Such a situation will take an enormous toll on the individual's self-esteem, self-confidence, and capacity to avoid the abyss of absolute hopelessness and despair. Relevant to this is the fact that the period of greatest risk for suicide in an individual with bipolar illness is within the first year from initial onset of the disorder.

Consequences of Adolescent Sexuality

Adolescence is a period when the individual, having entered puberty, with its associated surges of endogenous hormones and development of external genitalia, begins to experience stronger sexual feelings and preoccupations. This experience may be initially one of anxiety or fear, because the transition into puberty is often quite abrupt and dramatic. Yet, it is the prelude to one of the most critical experiences of the mature individual—the establishment of intimate relationships.

Adolescence is a time of exploration and experimentation. The sexual self-stimulation of masturbation, particularly in early adolescent males, is quite common and frequently a source of conflict for the individual. Today, masturbation is no longer condemned, as it once was. An important psychosocial task of adolescent development is the establishment of gender identity. Early in adolescence, experimentation with sexual activity is common. Specifically, participation in homosexual play (generally among same-age peers) during this period does not necessarily indicate permanent gender identification.

With the earlier onset of puberty, intermixed with changes over the years in cultural values and standards, there has been an escalation in overall sexual activity in adolescents. Initiation into sexual activity is occurring at earlier ages, often with frequent rotation of partners. Unfortunately, the judgment utilized in such activity is often limited. Furthermore, in spite of periodic attention to sex education in the schools, adolescents' knowledge of critical information overall is usually quite limited. As a result, the rates of teenage venereal disease and pregnancy are increasing. Although the adolescent age group has not as yet been identified with known cases of the current epidemic of acquired immune deficiency syndrome (AIDS), the extent of sexual activity, combined with poor judgment, probably places many adolescents in the high-risk category. One can only speculate whether the endemic fear of AIDS will mobilize greater efforts at education and preventive intervention and thereby reduce the serious multiple risks associated with sexual activity in today's adolescents.

Pregnancy in adolescence is a problem of major societal significance. Twenty percent of all live births in the United States are to adolescent mothers. The adolescent pregnancy rate in the United States is greater than in any other Western country. The offspring of adolescent mothers are at significantly higher risk for "failure to thrive" syndromes, physical abuse, school failure, behavioral disturbances, and delinquency. Most adolescent mothers are not married and will have great difficulties in the future achieving success with their education, employment, and stable relationships. Most adolescent fathers will neither provide assistance nor maintain contact.

Many adolescent girls who become pregnant may have been preoccupied with the fantasy of becoming autonomous and independent from their families and surroundings. However, close examination has revealed that many of these girls are burdened both before and after the pregnancy with persistent low mood and poor self-esteem. The reality for these adolescent girls is often one of dependence, passivity, and sadness. The developmental tasks of adolescence—including separation and disengagement from the family of origin, movement toward extrafamilial relationships, pursuit of academic and career goals, and growing experience of individuation—may all be short-circuited as the adolescent girl is forced to increasingly rely on her family throughout the pregnancy and frequently beyond. With many pregnant adolescents, the fantasies of freedom, happiness, and mature identity rapidly erode, to be replaced by the painful, numbing reality of reinforced dependence, helplessness, and hopelessness.

Adolescent Delinquency

Juvenile delinquency, or conduct disorder, as it is referred to in modern nomenclature, comprises the largest single group of psychiatric disorders in adolescence. Officially, the rate of delinquency is approximately 20 percent in adolescent boys and 2 percent in adolescent girls. Since this figure pertains only to individuals apprehended and identified by legal authorities, the actual rate may be considerably higher. Adolescents are also responsible for a substantial proportion of violent crimes, accounting for over 18 percent of all arrests for violence. Although increasing criminal and violent behavior is a general societal phenomenon, the escalation of such deviant behavior in adolescents is twice that of the adult rate.

From a developmental perspective, severe delinquent behavior often implies a failure to successfully consolidate many of the psychosocial tasks of healthy adolescent functioning. The violence-prone adolescent, in particular, often has low self-esteem, poor empathic capacity, a low threshold for frustration, ineffective impulse control, and repressed rage. Juvenile detention facilities have become rapidly overwhelmed with the burden of an increasingly violent and severely psychopathological population. The recidivism rate for adolescent offenders is growing,

with many eventually reincarcerated in adult prisons. The prognosis for delinquency in adolescence is poor, with approximately 50 percent progressing to serious antisocial behavior as adults. Adolescent delinquency also predicts a high rate of alcohol abuse in adulthood. Intervention efforts with adolescent delinquents have primarily failed, necessitating greater efforts in reassessment and treatment.

Both social and biological factors play a role in the development of conduct disorders. Major factors predictive of later aggressive and delinquent behavior include poverty, overcrowding, parental unemployment, broken homes, and parental rejection. Poor parenting technique is common, with erratic utilization of harsh and punitive discipline alternating with deficiencies in consistent parental supervision and limit setting. For many individuals who progress from adolescent delinquency to antisocial behaviors of adulthood, the home environment becomes a learned model for negative behaviors.

A genetic etiology has also been identified as playing a role in conduct disorders. Most boys with conduct disorders have fathers not only who engaged in delinquent behavior as adolescents, but also who later developed antisocial disorders and alcohol abuse as adults. This appears to go beyond direct environmental influence that is learned, because such patterns exist even when the father left the home before the child was born.

Adolescent delinquents, particularly those with aggressive characteristics, often have a history of serious medical and neurological illness. They are far more accident prone than their peers and have often been the victims of significant perinatal problems (birth injury), head and face injuries, and physical abuse. A surprisingly high percentage of adolescent boys with histories of aggressive behaviors have also been found to have sustained major neurological injury, including seizure disorders (especially psychomotor epilepsy). Such neurological vulnerability appears to have predisposed these individuals to violence, impulsivity, school failure, and overall maladaptive behavior. Cognitive deficits have also been associated with delinquency in adolescence. Whether or not linked to identifiable neurological injury, aggression and antisocial behaviors have been associated with low IQ, specific reading disability, articulation disturbances, and delayed language development.

Another potent factor in the development of delinquency in adolescence is the presence of a preexisting depressive disorder. Aggressive and antisocial behaviors may be the externalized expressions of an underlying depression. Evidence is increasing that depression may predispose vulnerable individuals to a variety of delinquent behaviors. Studies are also beginning to establish that definitive treatment of an underlying depression may induce a remission of the aggressive and antisocial behaviors associated with the conduct disorder.

Although adolescent delinquency is often perceived as an intractable condition, recent advances in understanding the psychosocial, genetic, environmental, and biological roots do offer etiological insight as well as more specific avenues of treatment. While those with conduct disorders frequently suffer from the feelings of hopelessness, helplessness, and despair endemic to the impoverished socioeconomic underclasses, hope at this time does exist at least for those individuals who are afflicted with identifiable and treatable neurological and psychiatric disorders.

Adolescent Substance Abuse

A significant alteration in attitudes of adolescents toward experimenting with illicit substances has occurred over the past two decades. Experimentation with unsanctioned intoxicants has become so widespread that it is now statistically normative for adolescents to engage in some degree of illegal drug taking. This phenomenon can be observed by examining the precipitous rise of marijuana use, the most commonly utilized illicit substance, among successive cohorts of graduating high school seniors. For the cohort born in 1945 and graduating from high school in 1963, there was a 2 percent lifetime prevalence of marijuana use by 18 years of age. This figure increases to 19 percent for the class of 1968 (born in 1950), 48 percent for the class of 1973 (born in 1955), and 60 percent for the class of 1978 (born in 1960). Although recent statistics indicate a modest decline during the 1980s (lifetime prevalence dropping to 54 percent for the class of 1985), the United States continues to have a more severe and pervasive substance abuse problem than any other industrialized nation. The 1987 statistics reveal that 61 percent of high school seniors have used an illicit substance at some time in their lives.

Another very disturbing trend has been the progressive reduction of the mean age of first use of an illegal substance. In the late 1960s, the mean age was 19 to 20 years old; by the late 1970s, it was 15 years old. One serious consequence of this trend is the increasing tendency for rapid progression to multiple drug abuse.

To date, most educational and media attention has been directed at the illegal substances of abuse and not toward the legal (and presumably socially acceptable) substances of alcohol and tobacco. Except for cocaine, which has shown an alarming increase in frequent usage over the past decade, most of the illegal substances have sustained a modest decline in prevalence among adolescents. Alcohol and cigarettes, however, have remained quite popular with the younger population. By the end of high school, the great majority of seniors have tried these two substances, with lifetime prevalence of 92 percent for alcohol use by 18 years of age and 69 percent for cigarette use by 18 years of age. Of greater concern is the substantial proportion who are active and heavy users of these two substances. With alcohol, the 30-day prevalence among high school seniors is 66 percent, with 5 percent daily drinkers and 37 percent admitting to binge drinking of five or more consecutive alcoholic drinks in the 2-week period before being surveyed—this figure is higher for males (45 percent) than for females (28 percent). With cigarettes, 30 percent of high school seniors admit to smoking on an intermittent basis, with 20 percent smoking daily. Taking into account that either alcohol or tobacco products alone will eventually cause far greater overall morbidity and mortality than all illicit substances combined, the degree to which their use is sanctioned and even encouraged by prevailing societal attitudes is alarming.

The greatest predictor of all levels of substance abuse is having friends whose lives are centered around the acquisition and self-administration of sanctioned and unsanctioned substances. Many factors known to be associated with substance abuse—poor academic performance, delinquency, rebelliousness, and, most importantly, low self-esteem and depression—precede rather than follow the initiation of the abuse. It is critical that efforts at preventive intervention not only recognize the profound effects of adolescent peer influence, but also clarify the profile of those young individuals who are most vulnerable for later substance abuse. Early intervention into a developing life-style of habitual substance abuse is necessary to prevent serious consequences to long-term health and development.

The period of adolescent development is often a time of considerable stress and insecurity. "Mind-altering" substances can be tempting as an escape from the painful and discordant processes of adolescence. Yet, this attraction is deceptive; the habitual escape into a drug-induced euphoria inevitably results in failure to acquire the developmental tasks necessary for future health and well-being. Further, the chronic and compulsive utilization of powerful mood-altering substances has a significant dulling effect on cortical tone, thus impeding the attainment of optimal cognitive functioning and obstructing the path of developmental growth. Developmental fixation and regression are among the serious risks of chronic substance abuse. Because of the rapidity and scope of physiological growth and change, the adolescent is particularly sensitive to these effects. The adverse developmental consequences of substance abuse in adolescence include persistent identity diffusion, lack of clarity about goals, creation of a false sense of autonomy, impaired capacity for deferred gratification, and a fixation of the negative identity characteristics of early adolescence.

The "amotivational syndrome" has also been described in long-term substance-abusing adolescents. It is defined as the apathetic withdrawal of interest and energy from activity requiring effort and is manifested by withdrawing from demanding social stimuli, diminishing expression of creativity, and increasing mental and physical lethargy. The passive process of chronic substance abuse also creates the illusion of power, control, and achievement without the actual effort necessary for true accomplishment. Although mood-altering drugs may not necessarily create de novo an amotivational state, they ultimately consolidate and intensify a preexisting condition when repeatedly abused by a vulnerable adolescent. The need to perseveratively alter and dull the emotional and drive states eventually results in a pronounced state of mental and physical depletion. This process jeopardizes the adolescent's adaptation to the stresses and challenges of development.

The long-term substance-abusing adolescent inevitably experiences deterioration in psychosocial functioning. The capacity to develop empathic and intimate relationships is attenuated as the dysfunctional adolescent seeks to escape the anxiety-provoking demands of social interaction through repeated drug abuse. The need to avoid new and challenging human contact heightens. The development of mature social and interactive skills is obstructed as experiences that could lead to a consolidation of personal identity are avoided in favor of the regressive experience of chronic substance intoxication. In addition, the long-term drug-using adolescent experiences the evolution of a rigidified external locus of control, along with avoidance of personal responsibility. In the process of desperately modifying their internal states of stress and painful emotions, long-term drug-abusing adolescents flee from the potential of a mature and responsible social role.

As the extent and duration of substance abuse and dependence increase, the dysfunctional adolescent experiences greater alienation and estrangement from the mainstream of cultural life. Intensified degrees of loneliness and isolation, along with pronounced feelings of hopelessness and helplessness, perpetuate the need for further drug-induced refuge and escape. As the process intensifies and loses any semblance of responding to efforts of internal control, self-esteem progressively deteriorates. The concurrent and cumulative effects of impaired developmental maturation, declining psychosocial functioning, and deteriorating self-esteem place the adolescent at greater risk for dangerous and potentially lethal behaviors, including suicide.

Intervention efforts must focus not only on preventive education at the preadolescent level, but also on identification of those at risk for progression from casual use to chronic dependence. Preexisting depression has been identified as a critical predictive factor in the transition from being drug free to experimentation and later dependence on marijuana. Furthermore, persistent depression in habitual marijuana users predicts the develpment of polysubstance abuse. Early identification and treatment of these depressed adolescents who are at risk for the initiation and evolution of serious drug-abuse behaviors are essential. To avoid profound and often irreversible degrees of developmental fixation and regression, with their drastic impact on future health and functioning, it is imperative that sufficient attention and treatment resources be provided for these vulnerable adolescents.

Adolescent Suicide

Certainly the most tragic outcome of the admixture of disturbed adolescent development and severe psychopathology is the premature termination of life. Since the end of World War II, all age groups in the United States have experienced an overall decline in relative mortality, except for adolescents and young adults. The frightening rise in adolescent mortality is entirely attributable to violent death. Rates of suicide, homicide, and motor vehicle fatalities have all risen dramatically. Overall violent death rates for young Americans are now 50 percent higher than for the same age groups of other industrialized nations.

Suicide rates specifically have climbed for adolescents. Over the past two decades, the adolescent suicide rate in the United States has risen twofold, and over the past three decades, it has risen threefold. Experts speculate that even these alarming statistics are in all likelihood underestimates, owing to the frequent failure of identifying the suicide-prone victim of a homicide or a motor vehicle accident. Psychiatric epidemiologists ominously predict that, as recent generations of adolescents and young adults age, the relative suicide rates of the later developmental stages of life will increase with the entry of these vulnerable generations. This phenomenon has been termed the "cohort effect."

A critical question is, "Why has violent death in adolescents risen to such alarming, epidemic proportions?" Clearly, the changing nature of American society over the last several decades plays a substantial role. Since the 1950s, there have been dramatic alterations of basic societal structures. With the massive geographical migrations in search of economic and "life-style" opportunity, traditional social ties have fragmented, extended family networks have weakened, and the nuclear family has experienced widespread disintegration. The "modern" adolescent no longer grows and matures within the relatively protective, supportive, and traditional family and community of prior generations. Dissolution of the strong family network, in particular, has led to increased divorce rates, illegitimate pregnancy, and child abuse, all of which are strong risk factors for self-destructive behaviors. A societal deemphasis on religious and moral values, which have traditionally been protective against individual suicide, has also occurred.

Recent economic and political trends play a role in the youth suicide epidemic. Not since the great economic depression of the 1930s has there been such a dearth of opportunity for young people entering the job market. (Interestingly, the last historical period in the United States with an identifiable upsurge of suicide was the 1930s.) Employment opportunities that offer the safe, traditional road to prosperity and family security have eroded, being replaced by the desperate, competitive struggle for survival. Another ecopolitical development over the last two decades that contributes to the problem of escalating violence (both inwardly and outwardly directed) is the deteriorating government support to community health and mental health programs, which are intended as primary resources for preventive health and mental health. Their dissolution has led to the denial of intervention to families of children and adolescents desperately in need of help. When critical professional attention is not received at early stages of development, the eventual risks for severe psychopathological and maladaptive behavior escalate exponentially. It is a tragedy of our time that such vulnerable and victimized young people are often provided psychiatric assessment and treatment only when their aberrant development and psychopathological status have reached severe, intractable proportions.

A further disturbing sociocultural trend is the increasing exposure to violence. The continual passive viewing of violence on television news and shows renders an audience desensitized to violent death. Children and adolescents in American society have become culturally conditioned to and dependent on television and movie representations of reality. By the time the average, contemporary child reaches adolescence, he has witnessed on television literally thousands of wantonly violent deaths. Both in fantasy and in daily reality, violence is assuming a more visible and omnipresent role. On the streets and in homes, deadly violence is increasing. Handguns have proliferated and are now present in at least half of all American households. The increasing availability of handguns has contributed heavily to the rising rates of suicide and homicide among the young. During the time period spanning the early 1950s to the late 1970s, alternative methods of suicide did not increase, but the rate of gunshot-inflicted suicide rose by 45 percent. More recent research data substantiate this strong association between increased availability of firearms and the high rate of lethal suicide in youth. Currently, handguns account for 83 percent of all completed suicides in the United States. A recent phenomenon has been the increasing lethality of female suicide attempts. Traditionally, suicidal females were far less likely to kill themselves than their male counterparts; over the past several years, there has been an upsurge of suicide in females. This has been attributed to the increasing availability of guns and the increasing likelihood that women and adolescent girls will use such irreparably destructive tools of self-destruction.

From a psychiatric perspective, the two groups at greatest risk for suicide are patients with affective disorders (both depression and bipolar illness) and patients with alcohol and substance abuse. Of individuals with affective illness, 15 percent will eventually die of suicide.

This represents a thirty-fold risk compared to the general population. The adolescent with affective illness is at particular risk for self-destructive behavior. Professional mental health attention is often denied to these vulnerable young people. Even when it is provided, however, such patients have traditionally been difficult to diagnose accurately. Careful psychological autopsies have been conducted of adolescents who have committed suicide. One recent study determined that most of the adolescents who had died by suicide had not been recognized as having severe emotional disorders and had not received competent professional intervention. Of the group retrospectively studied, over 75 percent had suffered from a significant affective disorder (predominately depression), and 70 percent had had active alcohol and substance abuse disorders. Many of these adolescents had histories of aggressive and violent behaviors directed at others as well. Further, 85 percent of the victims had spoken of suicidal intention before their deaths, and 40 percent had a history of past attempt. Suicidal ideation and self-destructive behavior in an adolescent, especially in the presence of an active affective disorder and impairment in healthy development, must be taken seriously as indicative of serious risk for future suicide.

BIBLIOGRAPHY

Bailey, G.W.: Current perspectives on substance abuse in youth. J. Am. Acad. Child Adol. Psychiatry 28:151, 1989.

Barglow, P., Bornstein, M., Exum, D.: Psychiatric aspects of illegitimate pregnancy in early adolescents. Am. J. Orthopsychiatry 38:672, 1968.

Baumrind, D., Moselle, K.A.: A developmental perspective on adolescent drug abuse. Adv. Alcohol Substance Abuse 4:41, 1985.

Blos, P.: The second individuation process of adolescence. Psychoanal. Study Child 22:162, 1967.

Boyd, J.H.: The increasing rate of suicide by firearms. N. Engl. J. Med. 308:872-874, 1983.

Boyd, J.H., Moscicki, E.K.: Firearms and youth suicide. Am. J. Public Health 76:1240-1242, 1986.

Brent, D.A., et al.: Alcohol, firearms and suicide among youth. J.A.M.A. 257:3369-3372, 1987.

Brent, D.A., et al.: Risk factors for adolescent suicide. Arch. Gen. Psychiatry 45:581-588, 1988.

Clayton, R.R., Ritter, C.: The epidemiology of alcohol and drug abuse among adolescents. Adv. Alcohol Substance Abuse 4:69, 1985.

Colletta, N.D.: At risk for depression: A study of young mothers. J. Genet. Psychol. 142:301, 1983.

Eisenberg, L.: The epidemiology of suicide in adolescents. Psychiatr. Ann. 13:47, 1984.

Erikson, E.H.: Childhood and Society, ed. 2. New York, Norton, 1963.

Freud, A.: Adolescence. Psychoanal. Study Child 13:255, 1958.

Grob, C.S.: Substance abuse: What turns casual use into chronic dependence. Contemp. Pediatrics 3:26, 1986.

Johnston, L.D., O'Malley, P.M., Bachman, J.G.: Psychotherapeutic, licit, and illicit use of drugs among adolescents: An epidemiologic perspective. J. Adolescent Health Care 8:36, 1987.

Kandel, D.B.: Epidemiological and psychosocial perspective on adolescent drug use. J. Am. Acad. Child Psychiatry 21:328, 1982.

Kay, R.L., Kay, J.: Adolescent conduct disorders. Annual Rev. Psychiatry 5:480, 1986.

Lewis, D.O., et al.: Violent juvenile delinquents: Psychiatric, neurological, psychological and abuse factors, J. Am. Acad. Child Psychiatry 18:307, 1979.

Offer, D.: Adolescent development: A normative perspective. Annual Rev. Psychiatry 5:404, 1986.

Paton, S., Kessler, R., Kandel, D.: Depressive mood and adolescent illicit drug use. J. Genet. Psychol. 131:267, 1977.

Piaget, J.: Six Psychological Studies. New York, Vintage Books, 1968.

Rutter, M.: Normal psychosexual development. J. Child Psychol. Psychiatry 11:259, 1971.

Ryan, N.D., Puig-Antich, J.: Affective illness in adolescence. Annual Rev. Psychiatry 5:420, 1986.

Shaffer, D., et al.: Preventing teenage suicide: A critical review. J. Am. Acad. Child Adol. Psychiatry 27:675, 1988.

Shaffi, M., et al.: Psychological autopsy of completed suicide in children and adolescents. Am. J. Psychiatry 142:1061, 1985.

Stewart, M.A., deBlois, C.S.: Diagnostic criteria for aggressive conduct disorder. Psychopathology 18:11, 1985.

Strober, M., Carlson, G.: Bipolar illness in adolescents with major depression. Arch. Gen. Psychiatry 39:549, 1982.

Tanner, J.M.: Issues and advances in adolescent growth and development. J. Adolescent Health Care 8:470, 1987.

Chapter 18

Childhood Psychopathology: Diagnosis and Treatment

Barbara H. Sohmer, M.D., and Joseph T. Coyle, M.D.

Childhood psychopathology is not rare. A recent study of the prevalence of *Diagnostic and Statistical Manual of Mental Disorders, ed. 3* (DSM-III), disorders in an unselected sample of nearly 800 eleven-year-olds in the general population revealed an overall prevalence of 17.6 percent, with a male/female ratio of 1.7:1, a prevalence rate consistent with other reports. Disorders reported by more than one source and therefore deemed to be clinically significant had an overall prevalence of 7.3 percent. Fifty-five percent of the disorders occurred in combination with other disorders, whereas the remainder occurred as single disorders. The most common disorders were attention deficit, oppositional, and separation anxiety disorders; intermediate in prevalence were conduct disorder, overanxious disorder, and simple phobia. The least prevalent were depression and social phobia. Notably, treatment was sought by parents in only 25 percent of the identified cases.

This chapter reviews five of the more serious childhood psychiatric disorders and approaches to their treatment: attention-deficit hyperactiv-

ity disorder, major depression, pervasive developmental disorders, schizophrenia, and separation anxiety disorder. The nomenclature and diagnostic criteria used are based on the 1987 revision of the DSM-III, the DSM-III-R.

ATTENTION-DEFICIT HYPERACTIVITY DISORDER

Clinical Description

Children with attention-deficit hyperactivity disorder (ADHD) have *developmentally* excessive degrees of impulsivity, inattention, and overactivity. Thus, in considering this diagnosis, the mental age [(IQ × Chronological age) / 100] of the child must be taken into account. The extent of disturbance in each of these three areas (impulsivity, inattention, and overactivity) generally is not uniform in any given child. However, ADHD is usually, but not always, manifest in all environments: home, school, and other social situations. In addition, the character of each environment impinges on the disorder, often causing it to seem more or less severe. For example, very structured or novel settings can facilitate control of symptoms by the child, while unstructured or chaotic settings exacerbate symptoms. In situations requiring sustained attention, symptoms typically become more evident.

Some of the manifestations of ADHD are age specific. Preschoolers have prominent gross motor overactivity with inattention and impulsivity characterized largely by endless flitting from one activity to another. Such children often appear to be driven and difficult to contain. The older child or adolescent tends to be excessively fidgety or restless with inattention and impulsivity evident in failure to complete assignments and careless, sloppy, quick performance. In addition, adolescents with ADHD display exaggerated impulsivity in social activities.

Children and adolescents with ADHD generally have a great deal of academic or cognitive difficulties, only in part due to specific concomitant developmental learning disorders. Time lost from studies because of inattention, impulsivity, and overactivity can be crucial. Resultant poor self-image, frustration, and decreased motivation can potentiate these difficulties. Emotional lability is common. In addition, the very symptoms listed in the diagnostic criteria below predispose these children to have less than satisfactory peer relationships. This often persists into adulthood.

Diagnostic Criteria

Diagnostic criteria (DSM-III-R) include onset before 7 years of age and duration of at least 6 months. (See Chapter 19 for complete DSM-III-R diagnostic criteria.) The disturbance must include 8 of the following 14 symptoms:

1.   often fidgets with hands or feet or squirms in seat (in adolescents, may be limited to subjective feelings of restlessness)
2.   has difficulty remaining seated when required to do so
3.   is easily distracted by extraneous stimuli
4.   has difficulty awaiting turn in games or group situations
5.   often blurts out answers to questions before they have been completed
6.   has difficulty following through on instructions from others (not due to oppositional behavior or failure of comprehension), e.g., fails to finish chores

7.   has difficulty sustaining attention in tasks or play activities
8.   often shifts from one uncompleted activity to another
9.   has difficulty playing quietly
10.   often talks excessively
11.   often interrupts or intrudes on others, e.g., butts into other children's games
12.   often does not seem to listen to what is being said to him
13.   often loses things necessary for tasks or activities at school or at home (e.g., toys, pencils, books, assignments)
14.   often engages in physically dangerous activities without considering possible consequences (not for the purpose of thrill-seeking), e.g., runs into street without looking

Differential Diagnosis

The differential diagnosis of patients with symptoms of ADHD must include mental age–appropriate "overactivity," that is, some particularly active children may appear so because of their relatively younger chronological age (in a given situation) or relatively lower IQ. These children do not exhibit haphazard, disorganized activity, as do children with ADHD. Inadequate, disorganized, or chaotic home environments can cause a clinical picture that is practically indistinguishable from ADHD. In such a case, every effort must be made to determine wherein the cause lies—the child or the family—since treatment considerations depend on this assessment. Further, it is important to differentiate an apparently hyperactive child from an anxious child; with the anxious child, the overactivity and impulsivity are generally restricted to situations prompting anxiety.

In mentally retarded children, the diagnosis of ADHD is made only when the presenting symptoms are abnormal given the developmental level of the child, that is, mental age. For example, a 12-year-old with an IQ of 50 would be expected to exhibit the activity, attention, and impulsivity of a 6-year-old. If a child is diagnosed as having pervasive developmental disorder, the diagnosis of ADHD is preempted. Mood disorders must also be differentiated from ADHD, since they often are seen in children with psychomotor agitation, overactivity, impulsivity, and poor attention and concentration. A thoroughly ascertained family history of psychiatric disorder can be very helpful in distinguishing these cases.

Epidemiology

Attention-deficit hyperactivity disorder is common; estimates of its prevalence range from 3 to 5 percent of elementary schoolchildren. Reliable estimates of ADHD's prevalence in adolescents do not exist, since, until recently, diagnosis and treatment of ADHD in adolescents occurred only reluctantly. Although the onset of ADHD occurs before 4 years of age in approximately half of the cases, the syndrome is often not recognized until the child enters school, because these behaviors become most evident in the classroom setting, which requires sustained attention, impulse control, and prolonged inactivity. In children seen for treatment, the male/female ratio is between 6:1 and 9:1, whereas in community samples, the male/female ratio is only 3:1.

In clinic populations, many children who fulfill diagnostic criteria for ADHD also have some or all of the features of oppositional defiant disorder, conduct disorder, and specific developmental disorders. These diagnoses should be made in addition to the diagnosis of ADHD whenever appropriate. Functional enuresis and encopresis are sometimes present as well. Neurological "soft signs," which involve subtle but reproducible problems with eye-hand coordination, rapid alternation, or hemispheric dominance and motor-perceptual dysfunctions, are also common in children with ADHD.

A number of risk factors for ADHD have been identified. Central nervous system abnormalities as manifest by neurological soft signs have led to the suggestion that intrauterine or perinatal difficulties are a significant factor. In this regard, minor physical congenital abnormalities are more prevalent in children with ADHD than in the general population. Increasing evidence for a genetic predisposition is also being considered, because the disorder is more common in first-degree relatives. The interplay between these two factors and environmental circumstances remains an open question, since alcohol abuse, drug abuse, and antisocial personality are overrepresented in the families of children with ADHD.

Course

In the majority of children with ADHD, the disorder persists throughout childhood and into or through adolescence, although its presentation may vary in time because of developmental changes and maturation of the child. Recent studies suggest that one third of the children with ADHD continue to be symptomatic in adulthood. However, studies indicate a marked reduction of symptomatology in adolescence in many cases. The childhood disorder does not predispose to schizophrenia or alcoholism. It is associated with antisocial personality disorder in a minority of cases, primarily in children who also fulfill criteria for conduct disorder. When conduct disorder, low IQ, or severe parental mental disorder coexists with ADHD, the prognosis can be poor.

Treatment

Treatment of ADHD is best accomplished when attention is given to *all of the factors* that impinge on the manifestations of the disorder. Thus school placement commensurate with the degree of disability caused by the ADHD and concomitant disorders (in particular, developmental learning disorders) can be crucial with regard to academic achievement. Behavioral management, which may include structuring of heretofore chaotic environments, is often helpful. Family and/or individual psychotherapy, when indicated, can decrease the degree of the symptomatology displayed. The child who can benefit from psychopharmacological treatment *alone* is rare. However, it is the latter treatment modality that often has the most dramatic effects and has the best scientifically documented efficacy. Indeed, although stimulant treatment may not eliminate later educational, work, or life difficulties, it may result in decreased social ostracism and improved self-esteem and social skills. It should be noted that stimulant therapy is now known to be efficacious in adolescents with this disorder. If appropriate pharmacotherapy were continued routinely in adolescence in those children who remain symptomatic, perhaps the emotional benefits (improved self-image and peer relations) accrued would be even greater.

The psychostimulants methylphenidate and dextroamphetamine are the most common psychopharmacological agents appropriately employed in the treatment of ADHD. Dosage titration must be accomplished in conjunction with school reports. Preferably the baseline ratings of the patient's behavior on the Connors' Abbreviated Teacher Questionnaire should be compared to ratings obtained while the child is receiving varying doses of chosen medication until the desired balance between therapeutic and adverse drug effects is achieved. This can take considerable effort and time on the part of the treating physician. There has been great controversy over whether stimulant treatment results in academic gain. A recent double-blind placebo controlled trial across a reasonable dosage range of methylphenidate found improved behavioral, cognitive, and academic performance in children given 0.7 mg/kg/d.

Both methylphenidate and dextroamphetamine are short-acting drugs. Thus their often dramatic behavioral effects are rarely evident outside the school environment if the last dose is administered at noon. It is necessary to advise parents of this fact before beginning therapy to minimize discouragement and noncompliance as a result of unrealistic expectations. Because of controversy over the adverse effects of stimulants on physical growth, it is customary to discontinue treatment on weekends, holidays, and summer vacations whenever feasible. Height, weight, blood pressure, and pulse rate should be monitored every 4 to 6 weeks. It is especially important to be sure that the child is not being prescribed imipramine for bedwetting. Concomitant treatment with methylphenidate and tricyclic antidepressants can lead to dangerously high blood levels, at least of the latter, and can cause delirium as well as life-threatening side effects.

Tricyclic antidepressants have also been noted to ameliorate symptoms of ADHD. However, the bulk of the literature to date suggests that stimulants are superior to imipramine, a tricyclic antidepressant, in the treatment of ADHD. It may be that children with features of anxiety or depression, as well as ADHD, comprise a subgroup that responds better to treatment with tricyclic antidepressants. Neuroleptic drugs can ameliorate some of the symptoms of ADHD. However, because of their deleterious effects on cognitive functioning and the potential of development of tardive dyskinesia, a frequently disabling and rarely reversible movement disorder, these agents are not recommended except in the most dire of circumstances.

MAJOR DEPRESSION

Historical Development

Until the recent advent of standardized diagnostic criteria and interviews, the consensus was that depression either did not occur in children and adolescents or was not diagnosable by the same criteria applied to adults. Over the past 15 years, multiple studies of clinical populations of both children and adolescents have documented the occurrence of major depressive disorder (MDD) fulfilling the same diagnostic criteria used for adults. However, associated syndromes in young children are common and at times affect the symptomatic manifestations of depression. Children with identified anxiety disorders—for example, separation anxiety disorder and school phobia—if thoroughly evaluated, have high rates of concurrent depressive symptoms. This is true of children and adolescents with conduct disorder, as well. The reverse is also true: children initially referred for and diagnosed as meeting criteria for MDD have high rates of anxiety, oppositional-defiant, or conduct disorders. Indeed, it is sometimes difficult to determine which disorder, if any, is the primary one.

Clinical Description

Recent studies have compared the clinical phenomenology of depression in children and adolescents in primarily outpatient populations using the same diagnostic interview. Little or no differences in type, frequency, or severity of symptoms endorsed were observed when children and adolescents were compared; and the overall frequency of symptoms was high. Depressive mood was the most common symptom, followed by the inability to experience pleasure (anhedonia), loss of interest in usual activities, decreased concentration, irritability and anger, fatigue, negative self-image, insomnia, social withdrawal, psychomotor retardation, suicidal ideation, guilt, and loss of appetite. The percentages reported for the prevalence of these symptoms across studies have been remarkably consistent. Prepubertal children exhibited depressed appearance, somatic complaints, psychomotor agitation, and auditory hallucinations with depressive themes significantly more often and with greater severity. In contrast, adolescents exhibited hopelessness, hypersomnia, weight loss or gain, anhedonia, or lack of interest more often and with greater severity. Rates of suicidal thinking and suicide attempts were similar, but suicide attempts by adolescents were more serious and potentially lethal. These studies found high comorbidity rates (for example, a second diagnosable psychiatric disorder); but it is unclear whether these rates are different across age groups.

Diagnostic Criteria

The diagnostic criteria for MDD are essentially the same for children and adolescents as for adults, except that mood can be irritable instead of depressed and failure to make expected weight gain in children should be considered as weight loss.

Epidemiology

MDD clearly occurs in children and adolescents, but it is much less common in these age groups than in adulthood. Nevertheless, it is not rare, with two recent studies suggesting a prevalence of 1 to 2 percent in school-age children. Onset of MDD is much more likely to occur in adolescence than in childhood. Age of onset of depression is much earlier in children with one or both parents having a history of a primary mood disorder. In childhood, some studies suggest that MDD occurs more frequently in males than females, although there is disagreement on this issue. Nevertheless, during adolescence, there is a marked rise in rates among girls with only a gradual increase among boys, leading to the well-known preponderance of women with MDD.

The incidence of this disorder in children and adolescents is difficult to evaluate, as are risk factors, because generally accepted methods of assessment and diagnostic criteria have not existed until recently. It appears that although the incidence is relatively low in the general population, approximately 1.9 percent, it can be quite high in clinic populations. Prevalence, too, depends heavily on the populations sampled and the methods of assessment and varies from 0.14 to 59 percent.

Course

Early follow-up studies of prepubertal children with MDD reported a generally favorable outcome, whereas more recent studies, perhaps because of more sophisticated research methodologies, find a prognosis of continuing or recurrent episodes. Studies suggest that individual episodes of MDD are self-limited, lasting approximately 6 to 9 months. However, dysthymia, a less severe form of the disorder, may have a more chronic course, with episodes lasting 3 years or more. A recent follow-up study of adolescents 8 years after hospitalization for an episode of affective disorder found a high rate of subsequent MDD episodes as well as significant problems with social maladjustment.

Treatment

Owing to the relative lack of research until this decade, treatment research of any type in the area of MDD in children and adolescents is relatively sparse. However, the limited findings available suggest that the same strategies found efficacious in treating adults with MDD are applicable to children and adolescents. Thus pharmacotherapy with a tricyclic antidepressant or one of the newer antidepressants remains the main therapeutic approach. J. Puig-Antich and his colleagues have carried out placebo controlled double-blind studies of the tricyclic antidepressant imipramine on children with MDD. Although there was no statistical difference in success of treatment between placebo and imipramine-treated children, these investigators did demonstrate a correlation between the plasma level of the tricyclic and clinical response.

As with other drugs, children may exhibit high catabolic rates for antidepressants in comparison to adults. For this reason, monitoring plasma levels can be quite helpful in adjusting dosage to achieve therapeutic plasma levels, since the milligram per kilogram dose can be substantially higher in children than adults. Because of the cardiotoxic effects of antidepressants, baseline and follow-up ECGs should be obtained to monitor potential toxicity. In treating the suicidal child, it should be remembered that as little as a 1-week supply of tricyclic antidepressants, when taken at once, can result in a fatal overdose.

The value of cognitive therapy has not been scrutinized in children. However, supportive psychotherapy as well as family therapy should be undertaken in conjunction with pharmacotherapy. The patient's school may also need to be involved, because MDD can cause impairments in concentration and cognition that temporarily compromise school performance.

PERVASIVE DEVELOPMENTAL DISORDERS

Historical Development

Case reports of very young children with marked distortions of the processes of psychosocial development have occurred in the literature over the past hundred years. Until the 1970s, these severe mental disorders were referred to by a plethora of confusing diagnostic terms, most of which were defined as subgroups of the general term "childhood schizophrenia."

Some of those categories—each was not necessarily distinct from all of the others—included dementia precocissima, childhood schizophrenia, dementia infantilis, atypical development, childhood psychosis, symbiotic psychosis, and autism. With the exception of Leo Kanner's description of the syndrome of infantile autism in 1943, the other terms and assumptions underlying these disorders reflected the notion that they were simply early manifestations of adult psychoses. However, even the syndrome of infantile autism came to be considered by many as an unusual type of early-onset schizophrenia.

In 1980 in the DSM-III, the term *pervasive developmental disorders* (PDDs) was adopted to make clear the distinction between syndromes that arise in infancy and those that occur later in childhood or adolescence. The latter disorders, exemplified by schizophrenia, involve a loss of contact with reality and the development of hallucinations, delusions, and thought disorders in individuals who previously functioned in a normal manner. The PDDs, on the other hand, are considered to be serious deviations from the normal developmental process. It is unlikely that autism and schizophrenia are manifestations of one disorder. Evidence against this once widely held construct includes the markedly different ages of onset; lack of schizophrenia in families of individuals with autistic disorder and vice versa; phenomenological differences, since hallucinations and delusions are rare in autism; persistent course or lack of remissions in autism; and the strong association of seizures with autism and not with schizophrenia. Of all of the terms popular in earlier times, only autistic disorder has emerged as a generally recognized and valid psychiatric syndrome. Because of the difficulties and lack of accuracy inherent in establishing age of onset with the PDDs, the revised DSM-III-R, as opposed to DSM-III, does not require establishment of onset before 30 months for diagnosis of autistic disorder. The residual category of pervasive developmental disorder not otherwise specified (PDDNOS) includes those cases in whom the general description of a PDD, but not autistic disorder, is met. In fact, PDDNOS may be more prevalent than autistic disorder in the general population.

Clinical Description and Diagnostic Criteria

Diagnostic criteria for autistic disorder include evidence of qualitative impairment for developmental age in reciprocal social interactions, in verbal and nonverbal communication, and in imaginative activity, as well as a markedly restricted repertoire of activities and interests. Onset must occur during infancy or childhood (the latter should be specified if onset is after 36 months of age). The category of PDDNOS is used when there is a qualitative impairment in the development of reciprocal social interactions and of verbal and nonverbal communication skills but criteria are not met for autistic disorder, schizophrenia, or schizotypal or schizoid personality disorder. DSM-III-R lists 16 items, 8 of which must be present to diagnose autistic disorder (at least two from A, one from B, and one from C):

A. Qualitative impairment in reciprocal social interaction as manifested by the following:
   1. marked lack of awareness of the existence or feelings of others
   2. no or abnormal seeking of comfort at times of distress
   3. no or impaired imitation
   4. no or abnormal social play
   5. gross impairment in the ability to make peer friendships
B. Qualitative impairment in verbal or nonverbal communication, and in imaginative activity, as manifested by the following:
   1. no mode of communication, such as communicative babbling, facial expression, gesture, mime, or spoken language
   2. markedly abnormal nonverbal communication, as in the use of eye-to-eye gaze, facial expression, body posture, or gestures to initiate or modulate social interaction
   3. absence of imaginative activity, such as playacting of adult roles, fantasy characters, or animals; lack of interest in stories about imaginary events
   4. marked abnormalities in the production of speech, including volume, pitch, stress, rhythm, rate, and intonation
   5. marked abnormalities in the form or content of speech, including stereotyped and repetitive use of speech
   6. marked impairment in the ability to initiate or sustain a conversation with others, despite adequate speech
C. Markedly restricted repertoire of activities and interests as manifested by the following:
   1. stereotyped body movements, e.g., hand flicking or twisting, spinning, head banging, complex whole body movements
   2. persistent preoccupation with parts of objects or attachment to unusual objects
   3. marked distress over changes in trivial

aspects of environment, e.g., when a vase is moved from usual position

4. unreasonable insistence on following routines in precise detail, e.g., insisting that exactly the same route always be followed when shopping

5. markedly restricted range of interests and a preoccupation with one narrow interest, e.g., interested only in lining up objects, in amassing facts about meteorology, or in pretending to be a fantasy character

In general, the earlier the age of onset, the more severe is the impairment. Early onset is also associated with a number of additional features, including abnormal cognitive skill development; posture and motor abnormalities; odd responses to sensory stimulation; self-injurious behavior; eating, drinking, or sleep abnormalities; mood lability; and disturbed quality or quantity of affective response.

Differential Diagnosis

PDD often coexists with mental retardation; however, children who are mentally retarded, unless profoundly so, generally are sociable and communicate—if necessary by nonverbal methods. If interest in and pleasure from social approaches are evident, the diagnosis of PDD should not be made. When severe or profound mental retardation exists, differential diagnosis can be quite difficult.

If a diagnosis of schizophrenia can be made, it preempts a diagnosis of PDDNOS. However, if the criteria for autistic disorder are met, an additional diagnosis of schizophrenia should be made only when there are prominent hallucinations or delusions that meet the criteria for schizophrenia. This question occurs most commonly in adults with PDD, since they may exhibit many of the "negative symptoms" of adults with schizophrenia in the residual phase. The diagnosis of schizophrenia is extremely rare in childhood, whereas a diagnosis of PDD of any type is almost always made during infancy or childhood.

Epidemiology

The prevalence of autistic disorder is approximately 4 to 5 per 10,000 children; when autistic disorder and PDDNOS are considered together, combined prevalence is thought to be 10 to 15 per 10,000 children. A recent study of PDD in North Dakota found lower prevalence rates, which might be explained on the basis of the diffcrent age groups studied. Autistic disorder is three to four times more common in boys. This sex differential is maintained for all types of PDD, with the male/female ratio estimated to be between 2:1 and 5:1.

The list of risk factors associated with autistic disorder is long and includes many prenatal, perinatal, and postnatal conditions that can cause brain damage or dysfunction. Maternal rubella, untreated phenylketonuria, tuberous sclerosis, encephalitis, birth anoxia, infantile spasms, and fragile X syndrome are among the conditions that have been noted to be associated with autistic disorder. In addition, genetic factors have also been implicated, since autistic disorder is more common in siblings of children with the disorder, and there is greater concordance for the disorder among monozygotic than dizygotic twins.

Course

The PDDs are manifest throughout life, and severity of the disorders varies with chronological age. In some children, there is an improvement in some skills at age 5 to 6 years. The influence of puberty is unpredictable in any given child with regard to social skills and cognitive function. Aggressive and oppositional behaviors usually increase at adolescence and persist for years. Even in the small percentage who are able to lead independent lives, social awkwardness and behavioral oddities persist. Flat affect, generalized anxiety, concrete thinking, lack of normal prosody of speech, peculiar uses of speech, and stereotypies are present even in high-functioning adults with autistic disorder, with few being competitively employed.

Treatment

Thus far, it seems that behavioral and educational methods of treatment are the most effective for PDDs, with the marked interindividual variations in response seemingly accounted for by the degree of cognitive and language impairment. Many psychotropic medications have been tried, with some resultant reductions in tension, agitation, and overactivity. Fenfluramine, which lowers serum serotonin levels, was initially thought to be effective in treatment of children with autistic disorder but no longer seems as promising now that multicenter studies have occurred. Stimulants and occasionally neuroleptics can be helpful in reducing target symptoms such as hyperactivity, aggressiveness, stereotypies, and self-injurious behavior. Nevertheless, further treatment research is sorely needed.

SCHIZOPHRENIA

Since the epidemiology, clinical description, and DSM-III-R diagnostic criteria of schizophrenia (see Table 21–1) are the same for children, adolescents, and adults, they will not be listed here. Also, as reviewed in the previous section, PDD and schizophrenia in children tend to be intertwined in the psychiatric literature, a fact that has made reliable estimates of either the incidence or prevalence of schizophrenia in childhood difficult to determine based on existing reports. However, best estimates of the incidence of schizophrenia diagnosed by DSM-III criteria are 1 to 2 per 10,000 for prepubertal children. Schizophrenia, as defined in DSM-III-R, can be found in children as young as 5 years of age but is rare before 8 years of age. In fact, prepubertal onset of schizophrenia is thought to be much more rare than autistic disorder. When it does occur, schizophrenia is so disabling and disruptive that, despite the apparent rarity of this diagnosis in children, this disorder deserves continued investigation.

Historically, there has been debate as to whether autistic disorder and schizophrenia represent opposite ends of a clinical spectrum. However, only a few postpubertal-onset schizophrenics have an early history resembling autistic disorder in any way; and only rarely have any children with clearly diagnosed autistic disorder gone on to develop schizophrenia. Also, when a group of children with schizophrenia was compared to a group of autistic children of similar chronological age (5.2 to 12.1 years), the two groups were found to differ on most variables, including age of onset, intellectual functioning, complications of pregnancy and birth, and socioeconomic status; all schizophrenic children had thought disorders, most had hallucinations, and half had delusions. Thus it is unlikely that this notion can be correct, since although autistic children change with maturation, they do not develop symptoms indistinguishable from similarly aged children with schizophrenia. There is some evidence that children who are at high genetic risk for developing schizophrenia, because one or both parents are affected, may have an increased incidence of neurosensory and neuromotor deficits. It is not known, however, to what extent, if any, these signs, which are rather nonspecific, predict future development of schizophrenia or any other mental disorder.

Differential Diagnosis

The diagnosis of schizophrenia is made only when an organic factor does not seem to have initiated and perpetuated the syndrome. In addition, schizophrenia must be differentiated from psychotic forms of affective disorder and from schizoaffective disorder, a distinction that is not always easily made. If the duration of symptoms is less than 6 months, the diagnosis is schizophreniform disorder instead of schizophrenia. Delusional disorder lacks thought disorder and prominent hallucinations. Hallucinations and delusions do not occur in autistic disorder or PDDNOS. Children with mental retardation can develop a superimposed schizophrenia, but hallucinations, delusions, or thought disorder must be present, as well as a clear evidence of deterioration in functioning.

Course

Because the diagnosis of schizophrenia as defined by DSM-III or DSM-III-R has only recently been made in children, there is little known about the course of this syndrome in these children. One can suspect that it is chronic with a poor prognosis, but this has yet to be demonstrated unequivocally, since prospective studies have not been carried out.

Treatment

Few studies on the treatment of children with the diagnosis of schizophrenia based on DSM-III criteria have been published. Most studies on the utility of neuroleptics in childhood psychotic disorders relied on less rigorous diagnostic criteria lumping PDD children with schizophrenics. Nevertheless, current clinical experience suggests that childhood-onset schizophrenia responds to neuroleptic treatment in a fashion similar to adults. Hallucinations, delusions, thought disorganization, agitation, and withdrawal appear most sensitive to neuroleptics, whereas social incompetence, apathy, and oddities seem less responsive.

Consistent with the pharmacodynamics of other medications in children, the clearance rate for neuroleptics may be remarkably high in comparison to adults. This factor, which can be assessed by measuring plasma levels of the drug, may necessitate frequent administration of the neuroleptic (three or four times per day) to maintain constant blood levels. Also, therapeutic response may require doses for neuroleptics that, on a milligram per kilogram basis, are substantially higher than in adults. Nevertheless, care needs to be exercised to titrate drug dosage with clinical response and to maintain the lowest dose that affords optimal control of the symptoms.

Neuroleptics are associated with serious long- and short-term neurological side effects. Children are much more likely to experience acute dystonic reations as an extrapyramidal side effect than adults, whereas parkinsonian symptoms are less frequent in children. Akathisia can mimic the symptoms of ADHD in children because of the consequent overactivity, irritability, and distractability. An ethical concern is the risk of tardive dyskinesia with neuroleptic usage in children. Family members must be made aware of this risk; and tardive dyskinesia should be factored into the cost/benefit equation in the long-term management of childhood schizophrenia.

Although no treatment appears to be superior to neuroleptics in controlling the symptoms of schizophrenia, the pervasive and serious symptoms of schizophrenia in children require intense psychoeducational treatment. These children's effective education often requires intense, highly structured, personalized instruction; supportive and directive psychotherapy can be useful; and parents need to be informed of the nature of the disorder and involved in its treatment.

SEPARATION ANXIETY DISORDER

Clinical Description/Diagnostic Criteria

Separation anxiety disorder, according to DSM-III-R criteria, must have its onset before the age of 18 years; and the symptoms must persist a minimum of 2 weeks. In addition, the symptoms must occur at times other than in the middle of a pervasive developmental disorder, schizophrenia, or other psychotic disorder. For this diagnosis, there is essentially one criterion; there must be developmentally excessive anxiety concerning separation from those to whom

the child is attached. This is judged to exist if three of the following symptoms occur:

1.   unrealistic and persistent worry about possible harm befalling major attachment figures or fear that they will leave and not return

2.   unrealistic and persistent worry that an untoward calamitous event will separate the child from a major attachment figure, e.g., the child will be lost, kidnapped, killed, or be the victim of an accident

3.   persistent reluctance or refusal to go to school in order to stay with the major attachment figures or at home

4.   persistent reluctance or refusal to go to sleep without being near a major attachment figure or to go to sleep away from home

5.   persistent avoidance of being alone, including "clinging" to and "shadowing" major attachment figures

6.   repeated nightmares involving the theme of separation

7.   complaints of physical symptoms, e.g., headaches, stomachaches, nausea, or vomiting, on many school days or on other occasions when anticipating separation from major attachment figures

8.   recurrent signs or complaints of excessive distress in anticipation of separation from home or major attachment figures, e.g., temper tantrums or crying, pleading with parents not to leave

9.   recurrent signs or complaints of excessive distress when separated from home or major attachment figures, e.g., wants to return home, needs to call parents when they are absent or when child is away from home

Differential Diagnosis

One must determine whether the separation anxiety in a child is developmentally appropriate for the child's mental age. If so, the diagnosis of separation anxiety disorder is not made. For example, a 3-year-old often exhibits stranger anxiety and fear when placed in unfamiliar circumstances in the absence of the parent. Whereas this response is normal (that is, age appropriate) for the 3-year-old, it is deviant for a 10-year-old. The anxiety of the child with overanxious disorder does not focus on separation. If separation anxiety is one of the constellation of symptoms in a child with PDD or schizophrenia, a discrete diagnosis of separation anxiety disorder is not made. However, this diagnosis can be made in the presence of a diagnosis of MDD. In conduct disorder, truancy is common, but the child neither stays home when away from school nor is anxious about separation.

Epidemiology

Separation anxiety disorder is not uncommon; prevalence estimates range from 2 to 11 percent, depending on the population studied and the diagnostic interview used. The male/female ratio is thought to be 1:1, although some studies have found separation anxiety disorder to be 2.5 times more common in girls. Separation anxiety disorder also appears to be more common in first-degree relatives of affected individuals as compared to the general population and may occur more frequently in offspring of women with panic disorder with agoraphobia. A large percentage of children with separation anxiety disorder have parents with a history of major depression; the latter is often a concurrent diagnosis in these children, as well.

The syndrome is often precipitated by a life stress, usually involving a loss or threatened loss of a significant relationship, illness of the child, a move, or a change of schools. Anecdotally, it appears that two peaks of incidence occur, one at the beginning of the school year and the second after the long winter recess. The disorder appears to be more severe and much more difficult to treat in older children, whether recent in onset or chronic in duration.

Course

Typically, there are exacerbations and remissions over several years; this may persist into young adulthood. In fact, adult patients suffering panic disorder with agoraphobia often give a history of having had separation anxiety disorder in childhood. The course can be complicated by the simultaneous occurrence of a major depressive episode, with a concomitant increase in risk for suicide if the child is forced to return to school without appropriate support or pharmacotherapy. Recent studies indicate that nearly one third of a clinic population of children with separation anxiety disorder have a concomitant diagnosis of major depression, whereas in an early adolescent group of chronic school refusers, the rate approached 45 percent. Thus any child with separation anxiety disorder must be carefully evaluated for MDD before the treatment plan is devised.

Since many children with separation anxiety disorder have vague but disturbing somatic com-

plaints that keep them at home with their major attachment figures, these children are at risk for multiple hospitalizations and diagnostic procedures that are often invasive before the correct diagnosis of separation anxiety disorder has been made. Children with severe symptoms, if untreated, experience poor peer relationships because of social isolation, as well as great academic difficulties.

Treatment

Treatment of separation anxiety disorder is multifaceted. It should often involve individual psychotherapy with the child and intensive family work. A great deal of communication with the child's school is necessary if school refusal is a symptom. The pediatrician needs to be consulted and informed if the presentation is that of multiple somatic complaints. Although separation anxiety disorder alone can be an indication for treatment with imipramine, pharmacotherapy is especially important when MDD is a concurrent diagnosis. The results of pharmacotherapy are often dramatic; in uncomplicated separation anxiety disorder, marked symptom reduction can occur as soon as 1 week after initiation of imipramine treatment at an appropriate dose. Even when treatment with psychotropic agents produces great symptom amelioration and the child returns to school, much therapeutic work generally remains to be done with the patient and family.

BIBLIOGRAPHY

General

Anderson, J.C., et al.: DSM-III disorders in preadolescent children: Prevalence in a large sample from the general population. Arch. Gen. Psychiatry 44:69-76, 1987.

Attention Deficit Hyperactivity Disorder

Hechtman, L., Weiss, G., Perlman, T.: Young adult outcome of hyperactive children who received long-term stimulant treatment. J. Am. Acad. Child Psychiatry 23(3):591-594, 1984.
Klorman, R., Coons, H.W., Borgstedt, A.: Effects of methylphenidate on adolescents with a childhood history of attention deficit disorder. I. Clinical findings. J. Am. Acad. Child Adol. Psychiatry 26(3):363-367, 1987.
Kupietz, S.S., et al.: Effects of methylphenidate dosage in hyperactive reading-disabled children. I. Behavior and cognitive performance effects. J. Am. Acad. Child Adol. Psychiatry 27(1):70-77, 1988.
Mannuzza, S., et al.: Hyperactive boys almost grown up. II. Arch. Gen. Psychiatry 45:13-18, 1988.

Richardson, E., et al.: Effects of methylphenidate dosage in hyperactive reading-disabled children. II. Reading achievement. J. Am. Acad. Child Adol. Psychiatry 27(1):78-87, 1988.

Depression

Mitchell, J., et al.: Phenomenology of depression in children and adolescents. J. Am. Acad. Child Adol. Psychiatry 27(1):12-20, 1988.

Puig-Antich, J., et al.: Imipramine in prepubertal major depressive disorders. Arch. Gen. Psychiatry 44:81-89, 1987.

Ryan, N.D., et al.: The clinical picture of major depression in children and adolescents. Arch. Gen. Psychiatry 44:854-861, 1987.

Weissman, M.M., et al.: Children of depressed parents. Arch. Gen. Psychiatry 44:847-853, 1987.

Pervasive Developmental Disorders

Cohen, D.J., Volkmar, F., Paul, R.: Issues in the classification of pervasive developmental disorders: History and current status of nosology. J. Am. Acad. Child Adol. Psychiatry 25(2):158-161, 1986.

Folstein, S., Rutter, M.: Infantile autism: A genetic study of 21 twin pairs. J. Child Psychiatry Psychology 18:297-321, 1977.

Rumsey, J.M., Rapoport, J.L., Sceery, W.R.: Autistic children as adults: Psychiatric, social, and behavioral outcomes. J. Am. Acad. Child Psychiatry 24(4):465-473, 1985.

Rutter, M., Schopler, E.: Autism and pervasive developmental disorders: Concepts and diagnostic issues. J. Autism Develop. Disorders 17(2):159-186, 1987.

Schizophrenia

Green, W.H., et al.: A comparison of schizophrenic and autistic children. J. Am. Acad. Child Adol. Psychiatry 23(4):399-409, 1984.

Tanguay, P.E., Cantor, S.L.: Schizophrenia in children. J. Am. Acad. Child Adol. Psychiatry 25(5):591-594, 1986.

Separation Anxiety Disorder

Bernstein, G.A., Garfinkel, B.D.: School phobia: The overlap of affective and anxiety disorders. J. Am. Acad. Child Adol. Psychiatry 25(2):235-241, 1986.

Last, C.B., et al.: Separation anxiety and school phobia: A comparison using DSM-III criteria. Am. J. Psychiatry 144:653-657, 1987.

Chapter 19

Mental Retardation

Allan L. Reiss, M.D.

Mental retardation is a term well known to many but well understood by few. Even today, a review of the literature reveals considerable variation in how medical professionals define mental retardation. For the purposes of this chapter, the definition provided by the most recent edition of the *Diagnostic and Statistical Manual of Mental Disorders* (DSM-III-R) will be considered as most current (Table 19–1). As the DSM-III-R definition indicates, for a diagnosis of mental retardation, two criteria must be met. First, the individual must have significantly subaverage general intellectual functioning as measured by standardized testing instruments. Second, the individual showing subaverage intellectual functioning must also manifest impairment in adaptive behavior. The severity levels of mental retardation as defined by the DSM-III-R are also given in Table 19–1.

The first of the two DSM-III-R criteria, subaverage intellectual function, is generally not difficult to establish. As discussed later in this chapter, there are standardized and reliable test-

ing instruments for assessing intellectual functioning that utilize the general population as a reference group. Establishing the presence of deficits in adaptive behavior, however, may be more difficult. When mental health professionals utilize subjective clinical judgment in assessing level of adaptive behavior, this criterion becomes more difficult to standardize across professionals or settings. Thus reliance on standardized scales such as the AAMD Adaptive Behavior Scale or the Vineland Scales to supplement clinical assessment is usually recommended. The importance of the criterion of adaptive behavior deficits is twofold. First, there are many individuals with intelligence quotient (IQ) scores in the mild subaverage range who show little or no disability in day-to-day interpersonal or vocational functioning. It would not be useful or productive to label such individuals as mentally retarded. Second, factors such as cultural bias or environmental understimulation can potentially influence IQ scores and distort the true picture of an individual's intellectual

TABLE 19–1.   Diagnostic Criteria for Mental Retardation

A.   Significantly subaverage general intellectual functioning: an IQ of 70 or below on an individually administered IQ test (for infants, a clinical judgment of significantly subaverage intellectual functioning, since available intelligence tests do not yield numerical IQ values).

B.   Concurrent deficits or impairments in adaptive functioning, i.e., the person's effectiveness in meeting the standards expected for his or her age by his or her cultural group in areas such as social skills and responsibility, communication, daily living skills, personal independence, and self-sufficiency.

Degree of severity: There are four degrees of severity, reflecting the degree of intellectual impairment: Mild, Moderate, Severe, and Profound. IQ levels to be used as guides in distinguishing the four degrees of severity are:

Degree of Severity	IQ
Mild	50–55 to approx. 70
Moderate	35–40 to 50–55
Severe	20–25 to 35–40
Profound	Below 20 or 25

Reprinted with permission from the *Diagnostic and Statistical Manual of Mental Disorders, Third Edition, Revised.* Copyright 1987 American Psychiatric Association.

abilities. It would be expected that such individuals would not show prominent deficits in adaptive behavior.

STATIC VS. PROGRESSIVE MENTAL RETARDATION

This chapter primarily considers those conditions leading to mental retardation that do not significantly progress in severity. Conditions that arise in childhood that do lead to increasingly severe intellectual deterioration and developmental regression most often involve errors of metabolism or neurodegenerative disorders. These conditions usually arise after some period of normal development in the affected child. Examples of conditions that lead to progressive central nervous system deterioration are listed in Table 19–2.

Conditions which lead to mental retardation that will be reviewed in this chapter can be considered "static" in that the pathologic process has usually occurred in the prenatal or perinatal period and there is no expectation that the intellectual or adaptive behavior deficits will become significantly more severe over time. There are a few known causes of static mental retardation occurring in the postnatal period, such

as lead ingestion, trauma, and infection. These will be mentioned in a later section.

EPIDEMIOLOGICAL CONSIDERATIONS

When considering incidence and prevalence figures in mental retardation, one must take into account several potentially confounding factors. With respect to age of diagnosis, children with more severe delays in development will be identified earlier than those with more mild delays. There are several reasons for this phenomenon. First, children with severe developmental delay are likely to have accompanying physical and medical problems. An example is the characteristic facial appearance and cardiac malformations seen in the child with Down syndrome. Second, mildly retarded children will frequently not be identified until they reach an age when they are academically or socially compared to their peers. In addition to severity of retardation, other factors that are potential confounders to obtaining precise epidemiological data on mental retardation include (1) problems with standardization in definition of mental retardation, (2) increased mortality in children with severe mental retardation, and (3) changes in adaptive behavioral levels over time in mildly retarded individuals, leading to inconsistency in the applicability of the diagnosis within a single individual's lifetime.

It has been known for several decades that there is a male excess among diagnosed cases of mental retardation in the general population. The ratio of affected males to females is thought to be approximately 1.7:1. Conditions caused by genetic abnormalities occurring on the X chromosome (such as the fragile X syndrome) account for most of this male excess (see discussion below).

The current estimate of the prevalence of mental retardation in the United States is approximately 1 to 2 percent; that is, at any given time, 1 to 2 percent of the population would meet criteria for the diagnosis of mental retardation. The great majority of these individuals would fall into the mildly retarded range. The annual incidence of mental retardation is estimated to be approximately 50 per 100,000. This means that in a given community, approximately 50 individuals would be diagnosed as mentally retarded per 100,000 individuals each year. These 50 individuals would include children diagnosed in infancy with severe developmental

TABLE 19–2.   Examples of Conditions That Lead to Progressive Central Nervous System Damage

Condition	Etiology	Features
Phenylketonuria (PKU)	Autosomal recessive Deficiency of enzyme phenylalanine hydroxylase leading to accumulation of amino acid phenylalanine and its breakdown products	If untreated, normal development in early infancy (1-2 mo) followed by progressive and severe developmental delay; musky odor, light pigmentation, eczema, hyperactivity, seizures, autistic behavior; usually detected in routine infant screening; treated with dietary restriction of phenylalanine
Maple syrup urine disease (MSUD)	Autosomal recessive Defective oxidative decarboxylation of keto-acids of branch-chain amino acids, leading to accumulation of these substances	Normal development in early infancy (1-3 wk) followed by poor feeding, vomiting, lethargy, seizures, and severe developmental delay; usually detected in infant screening; some success in dietary restriction of branch-chain amino acids
Hurler syndrome	Autosomal recessive Deficiency of enzyme α-iduronidase leading to accumulation of incompletely degraded mucopolysaccharides in lysosomes	Coarse facies, corneal clouding, contractures of joints, enlargement of liver and spleen, severe and progressive developmental delay
Hunter syndrome	X-linked recessive Deficiency of enzyme iduronate sulfatase, leading to accumulation of incompletely degraded mucopolysaccharide in lysosomes	Similar to Hurler syndrome but less severe manifestations
Tay-Sachs disease	Autosomal recessive Deficiency of enzyme hexosaminidase A, leading to accumulation of GM_2 gangliosides in neurons	Normal development for 3-6 mo followed by severe neurological deterioration, blindness, deafness, seizures, cherry red spot on macula
Lesch-Nyhan syndrome	X-linked recessive Deficiency of enzyme hypoxanthine-guanine phosphoribosyltransferase (HPRT), resulting in purine metabolism abnormality	Normal development for 3-4 mo, followed by delayed growth and development, choreoathetosis, self-mutilation, gouty arthritis, spasticity
Metachromatic leukodystrophy	Autosomal recessive Deficiency of enzyme aryl sulfatase A, leading to accumulation of sulfatide and demyelination in CNS white matter	Normal development for 1 yr or more followed by neurological deterioration
Pelizaeus-Merzbacher disease	Predominately X-linked recessive	Normal development for several months or more followed by abnormal ocular movements, ataxia, gait abnormality, and mental deterioration
Adrenoleukodystrophy	X-linked recessive	Normal development for 5-10 yr, followed by mental deterioration; adrenal insufficiency, bronzing of skin, gait and speech abnormality, behavior disturbances; long-chain fatty acids accumulate in CNS
Menkes syndrome	X-linked recessive, causing deficient intestinal absorption and transport of copper into other cells	Normal development in early infancy, followed by decreased pigmentation; tangled, steely hair; pudgy face; osteoporosis; tortuous arteries; and progressive and severe developmental deterioration

delay, as well as milder cases diagnosed in later childhood.

IMPORTANCE TO PSYCHIATRY

Whether through direct (for example, central nervous system infection) or indirect (buildup of toxic metabolite) means, mental retardation results from abnormalities of, or insults to, the central nervous system. The prevalence figures given for mental retardation match or exceed the percentage of the general population that is thought to suffer from schizophrenia or bipolar disorder, both of which are also thought to result from central nervous system dysfunction. Despite this fact, there are few psychiatrists—and, in particular, child psychiatrists—who routinely work with mentally retarded individuals or who participate in research in mental retardation.

It is clear that mental retardation, like other mental health problems, is a heterogeneous condition with multiple etiologies. Mental retardation is a major cause of disability and potential stress to the affected individual, the family, and the economy. Mental retardation is usually diagnosed in childhood and is often associated with other psychiatric conditions that require highly specialized assessment and treatment. Thus mental retardation is very important to psychiatry in general and to the child psychiatrist in particular.

ASSESSMENT: IDENTIFICATION OF AFFECTED INDIVIDUALS

This section illustrates assessment of the mentally retarded child by giving specific examples of conditions that are identified at different developmental periods.

An example of early identification is the child with Down syndrome. This condition results from an extra copy of chromosome 21, resulting in the presence of 47 chromosomes, rather than the usual 46 making up the normal diploid chromosome complement. Children with Down syndrome are usually identified shortly after birth. Their facial appearance is quite characteristic, with a flat face, upwardly slanting palpepral fissure, epicanthal folds, small ears, and protruding tongue. Approximately one third of children with Down syndrome have congenital malformations of the heart, and a lesser proportion have numerous other medical problems reflecting developmental deviation of other organ systems. Children with Down syndrome generally have an IQ in the moderate to severely retarded range. Additional conditions commonly identified shortly after birth or in infancy include other chromosomal conditions, such as trisomy 18 or 13 or conditions leading to significant dysmorphic appearance or organ malformation such as Cornelia deLange syndrome. Most of the conditions identified in this early period have a known or suspected genetic or biological etiology.

Many children diagnosed as mentally retarded are first identified as being developmentally delayed from ages 1 through 3 years old. Such children are often first brought to their pediatrician by a parent because of failure to attain expected developmental milestones such as first words or steps. Referral is then made to a developmental specialist or community outreach program for further evaluation. An example of a condition that is now being identified in this early period is the fragile X syndrome. The presence of this condition is established by performing a specific chromosome test called a karyotype. If this condition is present, the karyotype reveals a specific and microscopically observable abnormality (fragile site) on the distal end of the long arm of the X chromosome. Parents of male children with fragile X syndrome frequently first note delays in language development when the child is 1 to 2 years of age. Other problems observed in early childhood include hyperactivity and autistic behavior. Adult men with fragile X syndrome have moderate to severe mental retardation. Although many other identifiable conditions also give rise to mental retardation detected in early childhood, there are also many children assessed in this age range in which a clear etiology for developmental delay cannot be established.

A proportion of children with mental retardation are identified during their first year or two of school. Most of these children have mild, and occasionally moderate, levels of mental retardation. Although the child is often noted by a parent as being mildly delayed in development as early as infancy, parents are frequently told their child will "catch up." When the child is placed in an environment in which he is academically compared to similar-aged peers, persistent scholastic failure brings these children to the attention of school personnel or the school psychologist. After preliminary testing, these children are frequently referred to developmental specialists or community outreach programs as described above. An example of an etiology for mental retardation commonly observed during early school years is that resulting from fetal alcohol exposure. Fetal alcohol syndrome is caused by exposure to alcohol in the prenatal period secondary to maternal alcohol ingestion. Children with fetal alcohol syndrome frequently have low birth weight, mild facial abnormalities, and organ malformations (particularly cardiac), in addition to mental retardation.

A group of individuals with mental retardation is not diagnosed until adolescence or early adulthood; the vast majority of these individuals have mild mental retardation. They are commonly brought to the attention of school personnel or a physician because of failure to meet normal societal expectations for adaptive behavior or self-sufficiency. An example is the individual who has been able to "get by" in school with special help or repetition of one or more grade levels until dropping out of high school. As this individual attempts to find employment or becomes involved in interpersonal relationships, his intellectual or emotional immaturity becomes more apparent to others. There are numerous biological, environmental, and multifactorial causes of this type of mild retardation, although in most cases a clear etiology cannot be established.

EVALUATION OF CHILD WITH SUSPECTED MENTAL RETARDATION

The most important component of the initial evaluation of a child with suspected developmental delay or mental retardation is the clinical history. In particular, a detailed pregnancy history must be obtained. Information about maternal illnesses during pregnancy, maternal diet, medications, illegal substances, alcohol use, and exposure to potential toxins or other factors potentially harmful to the developing embryo and fetus should be obtained. The child's developmental history must also be elucidated. Information about the four major developmental areas should be included: motor development, language development, development in social behavior, and sensory development. In addition to quantitative delays in these areas, the presence of qualitative abnormalities of behavior should be elicited, such as repetitive or stereotypic motor behavior, or language peculiarities such as echolalia (repetition of others' words) or perseveration. Particular attention must be given to the possibility of increasing severity in developmental delay or mental retardation, since this would indicate the presence of a metabolic or neurodegenerative disorder.

The medical history of the child is also important. Attention must be given to the occurrence of any congenital malformation, endocrinological problems, or coexistent neurological problems such as seizures. Often, such information can increase the developmental specialist's ability to identify the etiology of the child's mental retardation and potentially treat the condition.

The family history can often provide important information as well. Inquiry should be made about the occurrence of mental retardation, learning disability, speech and language disorders, hyperactivity, or other heritable conditions in biological family members from both sides of the family. Information should also be obtained about the presence of medical problems in the family, such as eye problems, abnormalities of stature, and dermatological conditions. For example, the presence of mental retardation in two maternal uncles of a mentally retarded boy would increase the likelihood of the fragile X syndrome or another X-linked mental retardation syndrome. The presence of multiple café au lait spots on either parent should raise the possibility of neurofibromatosis in a developmentally delayed child.

The clinical examination of the child is also important in the assessment of mental retardation. This examination should be thorough and include evaluation for ocular abnormalities, dysmorphic features, congenital anomalies, organ enlargement or malformation, skeletal features, sexual development, skin lesions, and general stature.

A multidisciplinary evaluation is often necessary in the evaluation of a child with mental retardation. This type of evaluation would commonly include developmental testing with standardized and reliable instruments, speech and language assessment, medical assessment, genetic evaluation, and psychiatric assessment. With such a multidisciplinary evaluation, a clear picture of the patient more readily emerges. Table 19–3 lists some of the common psychological and developmental testing instruments used in assessment of intellectual and adaptive function.

ETIOLOGY: GENETIC

Currently, genetic or other biological etiologies are identified for a larger percentage of cases of moderate to profound mental retardation than for cases of mild mental retardation. It is premature, however, to come to the conclusion that

TABLE 19–3.   Common Testing
Instruments Used for Intellectual and
Adaptive Behavior Assessment

Wechsler Intelligence Scale for Children–Revised (WISC-R)
Wechsler Adult Intelligence Scale–Revised (WAIS-R)
Stanford-Binet Intelligence Scale
Kaufman Assessment Battery for Children
Peabody Picture Vocabulary (PPVT)
Leiter International Performance Scale
Vineland Adaptive Behavior Scale
AAMD Adaptive Behavior Scales

children with mild mental retardation have non-genetic or multifactorial causes for their subaverage intellectual and adaptive function. It may be that there are many genetic causes of mild mental retardation that have not as yet been identified.

Chromosomal conditions leading to mental retardation result from abnormalities in the amount of chromosomal material present. Chromosomal etiologies can be divided into those affecting the nonsex chromosomes (autosomal conditions) and those affecting the sex chromosomes. As a general rule, excess chromosomal material is better tolerated than decreased material. This principle is shown by the presence of three well-known trisomic conditions (trisomy 21, 18, and 13) and the absence of known autosomal monosomic conditions that are compatible with life. Table 19–4 lists common autosomal chromosomal conditions that can lead to mental retardation, along with essential features of these conditions.

Nonautosomal conditions are those that involve the X or Y sex chromosomes. Although abnormalities in the number of sex chromosomes present, such as those found in Turner syndrome (XO), Klinefelter syndrome (XXY), or triple X (XXX) syndrome, appear to increase the likelihood of having subaverage intellectual functioning in the affected individual, the majority of such individuals are not mentally retarded.

Although not involving observable increases or decreases in the amount of material on the X chromosome, there are at least 16 mental retardation syndromes thought to result from a genetic abnormality on the X chromosome. X-linked mental retardation (XLMR) accounts for approximately 20 to 25 percent of all known mental retardation. XLMR is also thought to cause the male excess observed in the mentally retarded population. The most well-known XLMR is the fragile X syndrome. The syndrome is identified by the presence of a cytogenetic

abnormality seen on chromosome analysis (karyotype). As in the majority of X-linked conditions, males with this genetic abnormality have a greater degree of developmental disability than females. Males with this syndrome may exhibit some mild facial abnormalities, including long face, prominent jaw and forehead, and large and prominent ears. Other physical features include hypermobility of the joints, large testicles (macro-orchidism), and mitral valve prolapse. Male children with fragile X syndrome frequently demonstrate numerous behavioral problems, including hyperactivity, self-injury, and autistic behavior. Fragile X syndrome is the most common transmissible form of mental retardation currently known. Approximately one quarter to one third of females who carry the fragile X genetic abnormality are also mentally retarded, generally in the mild range of severity.

The next category of genetic etiology for mental retardation constitutes single-gene conditions. Under this category would be included both autosomal dominant and autosomal recessive conditions. Table 19–5 lists examples of more common single-gene conditions leading to mental retardation, with their essential features.

The last category of genetic etiology for mental retardation is made up of those syndromes or conditions that are thought to have a genetic etiology but for which there is no biological marker or confirmed mode of inheritance. Table 19–6 lists common syndromes thought to have a genetic basis with their essential features.

NONGENETIC ETIOLOGIES

Prenatal Etiologies

Although there are many nongenetic causes of mental retardation that occur during embryonic and fetal development, among the most important of these is maternal alcohol ingestion during pregnancy. Fetal alcohol syndrome (FAS) is now thought to be the leading known cause of mental retardation in the Western world. The incidence of FAS is approximately 2 per 1000 live births per year. The cardinal features of FAS are prenatal and postnatal growth retardation, a mild degree of dysmorphic facial features, and mental retardation. The facial features in the syndrome include short palpebral fissures, short nose, smooth philtrum and thin upper lip. Children with FAS frequently have a small head circumference and numerous organ malformations, particularly cardiac. Behavior problems are also present, including hyperactivity and problems

TABLE 19–4.   Examples of Autosomal Chromosomal Conditions That Cause Mental Retardation

Condition	Etiology	Features
Down syndrome (trisomy 21)	Extra copy of part or all of chromosome 21 (95% full trisomy, 5% mosaicism or translocation occurrence)	Low muscle tone and poor Moro reflex at birth, flat facial profile, slanted palpebral fissures, small ears, congenital heart defects, moderate to severe mental retardation
Trisomy 18	Extra copy of part or all of chromosome 18	Clenched hand with overlapping fingers, low-set and malformed ears, short sternum, frequent organ malformations, severe to profound mental retardation if child survives first year
Trisomy 13	Extra copy of part or all of chromosome 13	Multiple facial abnormalities, severe malformations of CNS, extra digits on hands and feet, severe to profound mental retardation if child survives first year
Cri du chat syndrome	Partial deletion of short arm of chromosome 5	Catlike cry in infancy, small head circumference, slow growth, severe to profound mental retardation
Prader-Willi syndrome	Partial deletion of long arm of chromosome 15 (50% of cases)	Low muscle tone in infancy, almond-shaped eyes, obesity, small hands and feet, behavioral problems, mild to moderate mental retardation

TABLE 19–5.   Examples of Single-Gene Conditions That Can Cause Mental Retardation

Condition	Etiology	Features
Tuberous sclerosis	Autosomal dominant mutation localized to chromosome 9	Fibrous-angiomatous skin lesions on face and body, retinal lesions, intracranial calcifications, bone lesions, seizures, propensity for autistic behavior, mental retardation in 50%–70%
Neurofibromatosis	Autosomal dominant mutation localized to chromosome 17	Multiple skin lesions including café au lait spots, neurofibromata and axillary freckling; bone lesions, pseudarthrosis, mental retardation in 5%–15%
Homocystinuria	Autosomal recessive (multiple forms)	Downward displacement of lens; myopia; slim build with long arms, legs, fingers, and toes; osteoporosis; skin abnormalities; mild to severe mental retardation with behavioral abnormalities; usually nonprogressive
Seckel syndrome	Autosomal recessive	Poor growth with short stature, microcephaly, unusual facies with prominent nose, moderate to severe mental retardation
Smith-Lemli-Opitz syndrome	Autosomal recessive	Microcephaly, poor muscle tone, genital abnormalities in males, short upturned nose, moderate to severe mental retardation
Sjögren-Larssen syndrome	Autosomal recessive	Skin abnormalities (icthyosis), spasticity, moderate to severe mental retardation with particular speech abnormalities
Bardet-Biedl syndrome	Autosomal recessive	Obesity, retinal abnormalities, small genitals, extra digits on hands and feet (polydactyly), moderate to severe mental retardation
Renpenning syndrome	X-linked recessive	Short stature, microcephaly, moderate to severe mental retardation

TABLE 19–6.   Examples of Conditions Causing Mental Retardation That Have a Probable Genetic Etiology

Condition	Features
Williams syndrome	Elfin facies including prominent lips, small nose, long philtrum, depressed nasal bridge; cardiac abnormalities, mild growth deficiency; behavioral problems; mild to severe mental retardation
Cornelia de Lange syndrome	Moderate to severe growth retardation; connected eyebrows (synophrys); small, up-turned nose; thin, down-turning upper lip; numerous limb abnormalities; severe to profound mental retardation
Beckwith-Wiedeman syndrome	Hypoglycemia in early infancy, large stature with large muscle mass and hemihypertrophy, large tongue (macroglossia), unusual ear creases, mild to moderate mental retardation in majority
Sotos syndrome	Large stature, large head with prominent forehead, large hands and feet, coarse-looking facies, most with mild mental retardation
Rubinstein-Taybi syndrome	Short stature, broad thumbs and toes, slanted palpebral fissures, hypoplastic maxilla, moderate mental retardation

with modulation of anxiety. Mental retardation caused by FAS may account for 10 percent or more of the annual cost of all institutionalized mentally retarded individuals in the United States. Although the figure of 2 per 1000 live births for FAS incidence is significant, it should be noted that this figure does not include those children who suffer milder or less readily identifiable developmental problems secondary to maternal alcohol use.

Numerous other medications and substances, such as sodium warfarin (Coumarin) and hydantoin derivatives, organic mercury, and antithyroid agents, if ingested during embryonic or fetal development, can lead to developmental deviation and, potentially, mental retardation. It is thus crucial to obtain an accurate and complete history of maternal medication, alcohol, and substance ingestion when assessing possible etiologies for mental retardation.

Prenatal infections are also a potential and important cause of mental retardation in children. Although the incidence is declining, congenital rubella still remains an important cause of mental retardation in the United States. Infection during the first or second trimester of pregnancy frequently leads to serious complications, such as sensorineural deafness, cataracts, cardiac defects, and mental retardation. Children with fetal rubella syndrome frequently have behavioral problems as well, including hyperactivity and autistic behavior. This syndrome can be identified at birth or, alternatively, may not be considered until later childhood. Other congenital infections potentially leading to mental retardation include toxoplasmosis (microcephaly, intracerebral calcification, and chorioretinitis), cytomegalovirus, and varicella. A history of maternal illness, infection, rash, or exposure to other individuals with infectious diseases can of-

ten lead the physician to suspect a congenital infection as the cause of mental retardation in a child.

Perinatal Etiologies

A large number of events occurring around the birth process can potentially damage the central nervous system of the newborn and cause mental retardation. These include anoxic events, anemia, hyperbilirubinemia, mechanical damage from the birth process itself, or toxic reactions to medication or anesthesia that the mother receives.

Among the most important potential causes of developmental abnormalities in children to be considered under the category of perinatal events is prematurity. With improving medical technology, the developmental age at which children are potentially viable has fallen progressively lower. Although many more children born from 24 to 30 weeks of gestation are surviving, many of these children are suffering numerous and severe insults to their central nervous system, such as intraventricular hemorrhage. At this time, it is unclear what the ultimate outcome and prognosis will be for many of these children. The issue of prematurity is an area of increasing concern to many developmental specialists.

Postnatal Etiologies

Infections acquired after birth, particularly during infancy, can potentially be a cause of severe developmental delay and eventual mental retardation. However, such infections usually must have devastating effects on the central nervous system to cause mental retardation. Agents known to potentially cause such damage include several viral agents (for example, herpes) and bacteria that lead to meningitis and encephalitis.

Head trauma, particularly that resulting from motor vehicle accidents, is an important and potentially preventable cause of loss of intellectual skills or potential in children. With new seat belt laws being enacted and enforced, the hope is that eventually this will become a negligible cause of such problems.

The last postnatal factor that can contribute to mental retardation is the environment of the child. A concrete example is mental retardation resulting from ingestion of lead. Lead is a central nervous system toxin that, if ingested in sufficient quantities, can lead to severe effects on central nervous system growth and development. Thus inquiry into a child's home environment must always be made, particularly with reference to age of the building, the presence of lead-based paint, and other factors such as supervision of the children.

A less concrete example of an environmental factor contributing or causing developmental delay is the psychosocially deprived environment. It is clear that children who have severe levels of deprivation and neglect can suffer significant developmental delay and stunted intellectual growth. It is unclear whether such developmental consequences are always reversible, and if there is a "dose-response" relationship between the severity of deprivation and neglect and the level of developmental retardation.

GENETIC-BIOLOGICAL-ENVIRONMENTAL INTERACTIONS

Although numerous potential etiologies for mental retardation have been presented, it should be noted that single factors rarely operate in isolation from other influences. For example, even in a child with a known genetic condition such as Down syndrome, it is important to inquire about maternal medication and alcohol ingestion, since such information can often contribute to one's understanding of the current condition of the child as well as the prognosis. It is also quite likely that, just as unfavorable environmental circumstances can negatively affect intellectual development, favorable developmental circumstances can greatly improve the prognosis of many mentally retarded children.

PSYCHIATRIC CONSIDERATIONS

Family Reactions

The range of parental reactions to a diagnosis of mental retardation in their child can include obvious grief, denial, anger, or even relief. The factors that determine the parental reaction include the age at which the child is diagnosed, the severity of the developmental disability, the parents' previous understanding of the meaning of mental retardation, and the parents' premorbid psychological functioning. The role of the mental health professional often includes providing supportive therapy and intervention for families of children with developmental problems.

Attention must always be given to the siblings of the mentally retarded child as well. Depending on the ages of the siblings, their reactions can include feelings of embarrassment, shame, and neglect as attention is drawn away from them because of medical or other problems of their developmentally disabled sibling.

Psychiatric and Behavior Problems in Mentally Retarded Individuals

It is known that individuals with mental retardation have a higher rate of psychiatric and behavioral problems than the nonretarded population. Although the precise reasons for this increased rate of psychopathology are unclear, some hypotheses have been put forward. An important concept in this regard is the acknowledgment that, in order to produce mental retardation, some level of developmental deviation or damage must have occurred to the central nervous system of the affected individual. Therefore, if brain systems subserving intellectual function have been affected by a specific pathological process (such as an infection or genetic abnormality), this would increase the possibility of damage to brain systems involved with functions such as motor behavior, sensory modulation, and control of emotion. An example of this principle would be the effects of the rubella virus during the first or second trimester of development. Although many children who suffer from congenital rubella syndrome are mentally retarded, these children also have a variety of other psychiatric and developmental abnormalities that reflect damage to other brain systems, such as sensorineural hearing loss and autistic behavior.

TABLE 19–7.   Diagnostic Criteria for Attention-Deficit Hyperactivity Disorder

Note: Consider a criterion met only if the behavior is considerably more frequent than that of most people of the same mental age.
A. A disturbance of at least six months during which at least eight of the following are present:
    (1) often fidgets with hands or feet or squirms in seat (in adolescents, may be limited to subjective feelings or restlessness)
    (2) has difficulty remaining seated when required to do so
    (3) is easily distracted by extraneous stimuli
    (4) has difficulty awaiting turn in games or group situations
    (5) often blurts out answers to questions before they have been completed
    (6) has difficulty following through on instructions from others (not due to oppositional behavior or failure of comprehension [e.g., fails to finish chores])
    (7) has difficulty sustaining attention in tasks or play activities
    (8) often shifts from one uncompleted activity to another
    (9) has difficulty playing quietly
    (10) often talks excessively
    (11) often interrupts or intrudes on others, e.g., butts into other children's games
    (12) often does not seem to listen to what is being said to him or her
    (13) often loses things necessary for tasks or activities at school or at home (e.g., toys, pencils, book assignments)
    (14) often engages in physically dangerous activities without considering possible consequences (not for the purpose of thrill-seeking) e.g., runs into street without looking
Note: The above items are listed in descending order of discriminating power based on data from a national field trial of the DSM-III-R criteria for Disruptive Behavior Disorders.
B. Onset before the age of seven
C. Does not meet the criteria for a Pervasive Developmental Disorder

Reprinted with permission from the *Diagnostic and Statistical Manual of Mental Disorders, Third Edition, Revised*. Copyright 1987 American Psychiatric Association.

Commonly Associated Conditions

One of the most common syndromes in mentally retarded children consists of problems with attention, distractibility, impulsivity, and hyperactivity. The current DSM-III-R diagnostic criteria for the diagnosis of attention-deficit hyperactivity disorder (ADHD) are listed in Table 19–7. It should be noted that these criteria include the point that the observed degree of attention deficit should be greater than that expected for the developmental age of the child (or adult) in question. Although children with mental retardation and ADHD have historically been reported to be less responsive to treatment with standard stimulant medication, recent studies have indicated that at least 50 percent of such children do have a favorable response to medications. With improvements in attention and decreased hyperactivity within the classroom setting and in the home, mentally retarded children can often work to their highest potential to achieve academic and social success.

Another neuropsychiatric syndrome that is increased in the mentally retarded population is pervasive developmental disorder. This category includes the diagnosis of autistic disorder, which is outlined in Table 19–8. It is noteworthy that certain conditions such as fragile X syndrome or congenital rubella syndrome are particularly likely to be associated with autistic behavior in the affected mentally retarded child. The presence of autistic disorder accompanying mental retardation significantly increases the degree of adaptive behavior deficits occurring in the affected individual.

At one time it was thought that mentally retarded individuals did not suffer from affective disorders. Although this issue is not completely resolved, it does appear that the manifestation of affective disorders may be different in retarded individuals as opposed to nonretarded individuals. In making the diagnosis of affective disorder in the mentally retarded individual, it is most useful to concentrate on alterations in primary biological functions such as sleep, appetite, activity level, and social behavior.

Another common problem seen in mentally retarded children and adults is stereotypic behavior. Table 19–9 shows the DSM-III-R criteria for stereotypy-habit disorder. Numerous hypotheses have been proposed to explain the occurrence of these behaviors in mentally retarded individuals. One popular hypothesis is that behavior such as hand flapping or rocking represents a disruption of normal biological modulation of motor and sensory processing, which is then reinforced by intrinsic (self-stimulatory) influences or environmental factors.

TABLE 19–8. Diagnostic Criteria for Autistic Disorder

At least eight of the following sixteen items are present, these to include at least two items from A, one from B, and one from C.

Note: Consider a criterion to be met only if the behavior is abnormal for the person's developmental level.

A. Qualitative impairment in reciprocal social interaction as manifested by the following:
   (1) marked lack of awareness of the existence or feelings of others (e.g., treats a person as if he or she were a piece of furniture; does not notice another person's distress; apparently has no concept of the need of others for privacy)
   (2) no or abnormal seeking of comfort at items of distress (e.g., does not come for comfort even when ill, hurt, or tired); seeks comfort in a stereotyped way (e.g., says "cheese, cheese, cheese" whenever hurt)
   (3) no or impaired imitation (e.g., does not wave bye-bye; does not copy mother's domestic activities; mechanical imitation of others' actions out of context)
   (4) no or abnormal social play (e.g., does not actively participate in simple games; prefers solitary play activities; involves other children in play only as "mechanical aids")
   (5) gross impairment in ability to make peer friendships (e.g., no interest in making peer friendships; despite interest in making friends, demonstrates lack of understanding of conventions of social interaction, for example, reads phone book to uninterested peer)
B. Qualitative impairment in verbal and nonverbal communication, and in imaginative activity as manifested by the following:
   (1) no mode of communication, such as communicative babbling, facial expression, gesture, mime, or spoken language
   (2) markedly abnormal nonverbal communication, as in the use of eye-to-eye gaze, facial expression, body posture, or gestures to initiate or modulate social interaction (e.g., does not anticipate being held, stiffens when held, does not look at the person or smile when making a social approach, does not greet parents or visitors, has a fixed stare in social situations)
   (3) absence of imaginative activity, such as playacting of adult roles, fantasy characters, or animals; lack of interest in stories about imaginary events
   (4) marked abnormalities in the production of speech, including volume, pitch, stress, rate, rhythm, and intonation (e.g., monotonous tone, questionlike melody, or high pitch)
   (5) marked abnormalities in the form or content of speech, including stereotyped and repetitive use of speech (e.g., immediate echolalia or mechanical repetition of television commercial); use of "you" when "I" is meant (e.g., using "You want cookie?" to mean "I want a cookie"); idiosyncratic use of words or phrases (e.g., "Go on green riding" to mean "I want to go on the swing"); or frequent irrelevant remarks (e.g., starts talking about train schedules during a conversation about sports)
   (6) marked impairment in the ability to initiate or sustain a conversation with others, despite adequate speech (e.g., indulging in lengthy monologues on one subject regardless of interjections from others)
C. Markedly restricted repertoire of activities and interests as manifested by the following:
   (1) stereotyped body movements, (e.g., hand-flicking or -twisting, spinning, head-banging, complex whole-body movements
   (2) persistent preoccupation with parts of objects (e.g., sniffing or smelling objects, repetitive feelings of texture of materials, spinning wheels of toy cars) or attachment to unusual objects (e.g., insists on carrying around a piece of string)
   (3) marked distress over changes in trivial aspects of the environment (e.g., when a vase is moved from usual position)
   (4) unreasonable insistence on following routines in precise detail (e.g., insisting that exactly the same routine always be followed when shopping)
   (5) markedly restricted range of interests and a preoccupation with one narrow interest (e.g., interested only in lining up objects, in amassing facts about meteorology, or in pretending to be a fantasy character)
D. Onset during infancy or childhood.
   Specify if childhood onset (after 36 months of age).

Reprinted with permission from the *Diagnostic and Statistical Manual of Mental Disorders, Third Edition, Revised*. Copyright 1987 American Psychiatric Associaton.

INTERVENTION

Prevention

Primary prevention refers to interventions that decrease the incidence of a medical condition by preventing its occurrence. With respect to mental retardation, such interventions would include prepregnancy testing and immunization of women at risk of contracting the rubella virus, genetic counseling of couples who could potentially pass on a genetic trait to their

---

TABLE 19–9. Diagnostic Criteria for Stereotypy/Habit Disorder

---

A. Intentional, repetitive, nonfunctional behaviors, such as hand-shaking or -waving, body-rocking, head-banging, mouthing of objects, nail-biting, picking at nose or skin.
B. The disturbance either causes physical injury to the child or markedly interferes with normal activities, e.g., injury to head from head-banging; inability to fall asleep because of constant rocking.
C. Does not meet the criteria for either a Pervasive Developmental Disorder or a Tic Disorder.

Reprinted with permission from the *Diagnostic and Statistical Manual of Mental Disorders, Third Edition, Revised*. Copyright 1987 American Psychiatric Associaton.

child (for example, fragile X syndrome), and programs to educate nonpregnant women on the effects of alcohol on the developing fetus.

Secondary prevention refers to procedures that decrease the morbidity resulting from a condition by intervening in the early stages of its course. An example of secondary prevention would be detection of phenylketonuria by screening in early infancy and placing the affected child on a special diet. If followed diligently, such diets have been shown to greatly decrease the severity of cognitive disability resulting from this metabolic disorder. Other examples of secondary prevention would include removing lead-based paint from a home in which a child has already shown elevated blood lead levels, an educational program targeting infant nutrition, and prenatal testing (that is, amniocentesis and chorionic villus sampling) for pregnant women at risk of having a child with a genetic condition.

The final category of prevention is referred to as tertiary prevention. Such interventions are designed to decrease the disability resulting from an already established condition. The most important example of tertiary prevention is special education for children with mental retardation. Educational programs for the mentally retarded are often highly specialized and designed to help the child attain the highest level of achievement of which he is capable, without causing stress through inappropriate expectations.

Psychiatric Treatment

Treatment of psychiatric and behavioral problems in the mentally retarded child often produces highly successful results that have a significant impact on the psychosocial functioning of the patient and family.

Psychotherapeutic interventions can be utilized in a variety of different contexts. In particular, behavioral therapy is often very useful in the treatment of problematic behaviors in the lower functioning child. These include self-injury (for example, head banging), aggressive behavior, enuresis or encopresis, social dysfunction, or motor stereotypies. Behavior therapy for these problems would consist of a careful analysis of environmental factors that may be contributing to the maintenance of maladaptive behaviors and intervention in the form of developing a specific treatment plan to decrease their occurrence and reinforce an alternate repertoire of more adaptive behaviors. Family ther-

apy can also be of great benefit at numerous points in time. Supportive and educational counseling of the parents and siblings of the newly diagnosed mentally retarded child can potentially prevent misconception and misunderstanding with respect to issues of etiology and prognosis. Family intervention can also help speed the process of acceptance of the diagnosis in parents who demonstrate a greater degree of denial. Individual psychotherapy with mildly mentally retarded children may also be beneficial in some cases, particularly in older children in whom some degree of insight into their own behavior and its psychosocial consequences is present.

Biological interventions, particularly psychotropic medications, have been utilized as a form of treatment for the mentally retarded for many years. Unfortunately, there is a sizable proportion of mentally retarded children who, once given medication, receive poor clinical monitoring or follow-up. This can lead to negative consequences for some of these children, such as the development of disfiguring and disabling tardive dyskinesia after long-term treatment with neuroleptic medication. However, when used properly and monitored closely for adverse and therapeutic effects, medication can often serve as a highly useful adjunct in the overall treatment plan of the mentally retarded child. Stimulant medication such as dextroamphetamine and methylphenidate can decrease the severity of attentional deficit and hyperactivity so as to enable the child to benefit socially and educationally from home and school environments. Identification and pharmacological treatment of an underlying affective disorder in a mentally retarded child can potentially decrease the frequency and severity of social withdrawal and irritability. There is evidence that medications such as lithium, carbamazepine, and propranolol may be useful in the treatment of disorders of impulse control, such as episodic aggression or severe affective lability.

There are rarely cases in which a single treatment modality is sufficient in providing an optimal treatment plan for the mentally retarded child. The mental health professional must take a flexible approach in developing treatment strategies for mentally retarded patients. Factors considered in the development of a comprehensive treatment plan should include information in the scientific literature, information and recommendations derived from a multidisciplinary evaluation, and a healthy respect for one's own abilities and limitations. In many cases, it is not unusual for professionals from several different disciplines (mental health, education, speech and language, and so forth) to be directly involved in the planning and implementation of a treatment plan. The ultimate goal of any treatment plan for the mentally retarded child relates directly to the definition of mental retardation given at the beginning of this chapter. The two goals are, thus, to improve intellectual functioning and to increase the level of adaptive functioning in the child's environment.

BIBLIOGRAPHY

Abel, E.L., Sokol, R.: Incidence of fetal alcohol syndrome and economic impact of FAS-related anomalies. Drug Alcohol Dependence 19:51-70, 1987.

Akesson, H.O.: The biological origin of mild mental retardation. Acta Psychiatr. Scand. 74:3-7, 1986.

Moser, H.W., Ramey, C.T., Leonard, C.O.: Mental retardation, in A.E. Emery and D.L. Rimoin (eds.), Principles and Practice of Medical Genetics, New York, Churchill Livingstone, 1983.

Munro, J.D.: Epidemiology and the extent of mental retardation. Psychiatr. Clin. North Am. 9:591-624, 1986.

Payton, J.B., Burkhart, J.E., Hersen, M., Helsel, W.J.: Treatment of ADDH in mentally retarded children: A preliminary study. J. Am. Acad. Child Adolesc. Psychiatry 28:761-767, 1989.

Reiss, A.L., Freund, L.F.: Fragile X syndrome. Biol. Psychiatry 27:223-240, 1990.

Rutter, M., Schopler, E.: Autism and pervasive developmental disorders: Concepts and diagnostic issues. J. Autism Devel. Disorders 17:159-186, 1987.

Part IV
Mental Disorders

Chapter 20

Phenomenology of Mental Disorders

Arthur Rifkin, M.D.

Phenomenology is the description of the formal structure of phenomena based on their interpretation or evaluation. The phenomenology of mental disorders is equivalent to the physical diagnosis of physical disorders. It is an extraction from the numerous ways that a person may be described by objective findings that are useful in the diagnosis of disorder. This definition should be noted for what it does not include, that is, aspects of the person that may be important in other contexts but that are irrelevant to the diagnosis of a physical or mental disorder. Character, intelligence, and attractiveness may be among these aspects irrelevant to a strictly phenomenologic description.

There is more to the practice of medicine than making a diagnosis. Judgments about a person's qualities not directly related to his or her medical condition may be crucial to a physician's ability to help that person. The restriction of phenomenology to the relatively few items needed for diagnosis should not be thought of as limiting the field of what is relevant to fully understand someone. Once a diagnosis is made

and the appropriate treatment planned, the art of medicine is required to apply this diagnosis and treatment plan to a particular person, in a particular family, in a particular ethnic or socioeconomic group, and so forth.

The trend in psychiatric diagnosis is toward the use of atheoretical descriptions of a combination of symptoms and their history, for example, the presence of certain symptoms and their duration and relationship to other symptoms. These symptoms are currently described in language that makes few or no assumptions about how the mind works.

This method contrasts with earlier methods of diagnosis. At the opposite extreme is the psychodynamic approach, in which postulated unconscious mechanisms are central. In such a schema, the person might be characterized by his or her state of resolution of an oedipal conflict, or by oral fixation. Such diagnostic categorization has much greater explanatory power than atheoretical descriptions based on unambiguous observations. Contemporary psychiatric practice tends to sacrifice greater explanatory reach to obtain greater validity and reliability. The weakness of the psychodynamic approach is its lack of proven validity, so that its acceptance has not been universal. Psychiatrists are frequently classified by "schools" according to allegiance to theoretical positions. This heterogeneity indicates that no theory of the mind, or of psychopathology, has compelled belief by scientific experiment. The current view of diagnosis removes it from the arena of competing theories by focusing on noncontroversial descriptions of symptoms, without any attempt to look "behind" them.

The science of psychiatry begins with clear descriptions of psychopathology and proceeds to test treatments by objective, empirically testable hypotheses. This science, which is now only in its second century, has brought great advances; however, what has been left out of this science should not be forgotten.

Phenomenology in psychiatry used to be much more complex than its present form. As understanding grows about what is relevant to diagnosis, the number of important symptoms decreases. In the past, the evidence for almost all diagnoses was limited to anecdotal descriptions, and assertions about response to treatment and general prognosis were nothing stronger than personal opinions based upon anecdotal experience. Therefore, a bewildering accumulation of phenomenologic descriptions attached to a host of different disorders. The advance of scientific understanding usually, but not always, results in simplification of former beliefs.

The predominant influence in psychiatry during the 19th and early 20th centuries was German. Emil Kraepelin divided psychiatric disorders into two major categories (excluding those with known physical etiology): dementia praecox (schizophrenia) and manic-depressive illness (currently called mood disorder). Prior to this, a great many distinctions were considered important, often based upon minute dissections of phenomenologic states, such as dividing delusions and hallucinations into many subcategories. The trend since Kraepelin has been to eliminate many of these distinctions because they are not empirically verifiably important. The apotheosis of this German tradition was Karl Jasper's *Textbook of General Psychopathology*. The reduction of relevant phenomenologic terms from about 1900 to now may be dramatically seen by comparing Jasper's book to the revised third edition of the *Diagnostic and Statistical Manual of Mental Disorders* (DSM-III-R), published by the American Psychiatric Association.

Without knowledge of phenomenology, the physician cannot apply understanding of psychiatry to the patient. It is fine to know what symptoms constitute the diagnosis of schizophrenia and to be up to date in the treatment of it, but if the physician cannot recognize correctly the symptoms of schizophrenia, such knowledge is wasted.

The phenomenology of mental disorders is thought frequently to be less precise, to be more vague, than the phenomenology of other fields. The usual hierarchical order would place physics first, then biology, then psychology; that is, reading the dial of a pH meter is thought to be more exact than karyotyping chromosomes, which in turn is thought to be more precise than describing a delusion. Such a hierarchy is not supportable, either conceptually or empirically. The value of any measure, whether it be reading a dial or listening to a person's description of his or her mental state, is its validity; that is, does this measure enable something to be done, and if so, with how much accuracy? A pH meter is extremely accurate and helpful in some situations, but the situation must be carefully described and the generalizations limited by those conditions. There is much more to the use of a pH meter than reading the dial; a calibrated instrument and certain conditions are required. When the pH meter is used in a system that is well defined as relevant and by a person with an understanding of that system, it produces results that are objectively reproducible and valid in that they enable someone to usefully apply that information.

This applies equally to a skilled person karyotyping chromosomes or describing delusions. The source of the data is not relevant to the accuracy of the data. For example, assume that there is a weak correlation between the blood pH and prognosis in a person with symptoms of fear, but a higher correlation between prognosis and the type of fear. In this instance, the skilled observer of the patient's mental state would be a more accurate predictor of this patient's prognosis than the skilled operator of the pH meter. Roughly speaking, the use of mental phenomenology to diagnose and treat mental disorders is as accurate and helpful as physical diagnosis with laboratory findings is in diagnosing physical disorders.

To accurately describe symptoms of mental disorder, certain terms are used in a specific sense that may or may not agree with their use in common speech. Jargon is the unnecessary use of a technical term when common speech would be as, or more, accurate. Appropriate use of technical terminology, or terms defined more strictly than in common speech, is justified if common speech would be less accurate. However, technical terms in psychiatry are needed less than they are used. The few that are justified should be used within the limits of their definitions. By and large, it is best to use common speech to describe, as carefully as one can, what one observes.

The following terms are relevant to making diagnoses. The reader is also referred to the Glossary of Technical Terms in the DSM-III-R.

GENERAL APPEARANCE AND GROOMING

Few technical terms are used in this category, and common sense is quite adequate. Although general appearance is not used often as a criterion in diagnosis and is often neglected in descriptions, one is sensitive to a person's general appearance more than one is probably aware. Much may be learned from a person's posture, gesture, dress, and grooming about his or her attitude toward the physician and the surroundings, and even his or her sense of reality. It is remarkable how rapidly people recognize someone who deviates from norms of behavior or dress. Grossly bizarre behavior or dress usually indicates a severe mental disorder.

MOOD AND AFFECT

Mood is a pervasive and sustained emotion that, in the extreme, markedly colors a person's conception of the world. Mood is to affect as climate is to weather. Common examples of mood include depression, elation, anger, and anxiety.

Affect is an immediately expressed and observed emotion, or a person's "emotionality." A feeling state becomes an affect when it is observable, for example, as overall demeanor or tone and modulation of voice.

The range of affect may be described as broad (normal), restricted (constricted), blunted, or flat.

- Restricted affect is characterized by a clear reduction in the expressive range and intensity of affects.
- Blunted affect is marked by a severe reduction in the intensity of affective expression.
- Flat affect shows a lack of signs of affective expression; the voice may be monotonous and the face immobile.

A common error is to mistake depressed mood for blunted or flat affect. The difference may be

crucial in diagnosis and treatment. Someone who is sad has a low voice, long silences, and engenders a feeling of sadness in the observer—one of the best guides to a person's affect. This is not blunted affect. Such a person is showing intense affect. Blunted and flat affects are noticeable by the absence of intensity.

Inappropriate affect is present if a person's ideas are discordant with affect. This is a feature of schizophrenia. While smiling and giggling, a person may describe a very frightening belief, such as strange beings taking over his or her body and devouring him or her. Inappropriate affect is not present when the affect is inappropriate to the situation. For example, some pupils might laugh while a teacher scolds them about poor behavior. Here, the discordance is between the pupils' affect and the situation, not between the pupils' affect and their ideas. The laughing pupils find the situation comical for some reason; the teacher would like them to have a different idea about the seriousness of their misconduct, but there is agreement between their ideas and their affects. This distinction may appear to be nit-picking, but it is important. Inappropriate affect often is a symptom of psychosis, whereas inappropriate behavior need not be.

Inappropriate affect must not be mistaken for cultural differences or a lack of understanding of the nature of the situation. A person who seems too calm for his or her ideas may be holding back his or her affect out of embarrassment or because he or she thinks it is not appropriate to show strong feelings when with a doctor. The interviewer should create an atmosphere that will reduce such restrictions. Cultural and ethnic differences must be taken into account in all judgments of affect, whether it is appropriateness or intensity of the affect. What seems at first to be an abnormal affect may fit into a person's accepted cultural patterns. If a patient's affect seems somewhat odd to a physician because of cultural differences, it is probable that the physician's affect seems just as odd to the patient.

ANXIETY

Anxiety, also known as apprehension, tension, nervousness, and uneasiness, is most commonly the emotion that accompanies thoughts of anticipated danger or unpleasantness. The feeling is the same whether the source of danger is known or unknown, although a distinction can be made between fear as anticipation of a known danger and anxiety as anticipation of an unknown danger. Common symptoms of anxiety fall into four categories:

1. Motor tension, such as shakiness, inability to relax, and restlessness.
2. Autonomic hyperactivity, such as sweating, palpitations, light-headedness, and diarrhea.
3. Apprehension, such as irony and fear.
4. Hypervigilance, such as distractibility, difficulty concentrating, impatience, and insomnia.

DEPRESSION

Depression is a common affect. When severe, it is described as a feeling of sadness or hopelessness, or colloquially as being "blue." The physician should not be deceived when a person who appears to be very sad says that he or she is not. Some severe types of depression are not felt to be similar to what one normally feels when sad, as when one grieves over a death or some less severe precipitant. Instead, the depression is felt as something different, and other words may be used to express it, such as emptiness, aloneness, or loneliness.

IRRITABILITY

Irritability ranges from mild annoyance to rage. It is important to specifically inquire about this, since many people feel anger without showing it. It may be important in differential diagnosis to know if some behavior is associated with anger. A child with attention deficit disorder may act destructively and be disobedient, as many children do with conduct disorder, but in the former there is more of a sense of innocence; the child does not mean to anger the teacher by walking around the classroom, and did not mean to break the vase—it was just a matter of not being able to restrain his or her impulse to quickly change activities when distracted by something new.

THINKING

It is in the area of phenomenology of mental symptoms that common speech is least helpful, and technical terms, or more precise definitions of common language, are needed most. The examination of thought disorder is commonly divided into two components: the process of thinking and its content. Speech is the major means by which one knows someone else's thoughts. If the person's ability to say what he or she thinks is impaired, it makes examination of this thinking difficult. If a person has aphasia, it may not be possible to judge the logic of his or her thinking, unless he or she can use language in some areas (for example, someone who cannot speak well may be able to write). The following discussion of the phenomenology of thought assumes a nonaphasic person.

The process of thinking may be disrupted in many ways. The speed of thinking is affected differentially in some disorders. A person with depression may think and speak slowly. A person with mania may think and speak so quickly that he or she is difficult to understand. If extreme, this rapidity is called flight of ideas: a nearly continuous flow of accelerated speech with abrupt changes from topic to topic, usually based on understandable associations, distracting stimuli, or play on words. If severe, the thread of understandability may be lost altogether, which is incoherence.

Speech may be normal in its rapidity but lack much meaning: the person who says a lot of words but expresses few ideas or imparts little information. This is called poverty of content. It is one of the more difficult disorders of thought to detect because the fluency is normal, the connections among the ideas are normal, there are no abnormalities of grammar, but after a while the listener feels that something is wrong.

The term *thought disorder* or *formal thought disorder* is used commonly to describe disturbances in the form of thought as distinguished from the content of thought. (A disorder of thought content would be, for example, a delusion or obsession; unfortunately, this thought content term is very broad and covers many types of disturbances that are better described separately, rather than gathered beneath one heading.) Formerly, thought disorder was considered pathognomic for schizophrenia, and distinguishing the varieties of it was not considered important for diagnosis or treatment. It is now being learned that thought disorder is present in many disorders and that distinguishing among the types may be important in differential diagnosis. The major distinctions are as follows.

Loosening of Associations

Ideas shift from one subject to another without a clear relationship between them and without the speaker's awareness of this lack of connection. For example, "I went to the movies yesterday and my mother's headaches are so bad—I don't know if I should have eaten that fish for lunch."

Incoherence

Incoherent speech is not understandable because of lack of meaningful connections, excessive use of incomplete ideas, irrelevancies, idiosyncratic use of words, or distorted grammar.

Neologisms

New words are invented by the speaker, words are distorted, or standard words are used in an idiosyncratic manner. Judgment is required to distinguish neological speech that is poetical, rich in metaphor, properly and imaginatively inventive—so that it makes language richer and more communicative—from language that is idiosyncratic and impedes understandability. This may be a function of place.

Perseveration

This phenomenon involves the persistent repetition of words, ideas, or subjects; for example, "I think I'll put on my hat, my hat, my hat, my hat." Not included as perseveration are repetitive phrases commonly used in normal speech such as "you know" and "like."

Blocking

Interruption of a train of speech before the thought has been completed is known as blocking. Upon inquiry, the person says that he or she cannot recall what he or she was saying or meant to say. This disturbance of thought is frequently overdiagnosed. Blocking does not include the pause, no matter how long, between ideas—a much more common disorder seen in slow thinking; blocking is present only if the speaker pauses in midthoughts and say that he or she has lost the idea.

Echolalia

Echolalia consists of a person's echoing someone's words, usually persistently.

Clanging

Clanging denotes speech in which sound rather than meaning seems to determine choice of word; for example, rhyming or punning: "To be or not to be, are you a bee or am I a bee?"

Poverty of Content

As previously discussed, this type of thought disorder occurs in a person whose speech is fluent and coherent but imparts little information.

DELUSIONS

A delusion is a false belief, sustained despite what others believe and despite evidence to the contrary. Not included are culturally accepted beliefs that others may consider false; supernatural religious ideas are a common example. Also not included are poor judgments, unless they are beyond any reasonable belief. An example of nondelusional poor judgment is the frequent belief among adolescents (and others) that they are too fat, to a degree that is not in accordance with usual norms of attractiveness. This may become a delusional conviction in persons with anorexia nervosa, who believe, despite emaciation, that a small amount of food would make them fat. Delusions are commonly categorized as follows.

Delusion of Control

In a delusion of control, some external force is felt to be controlling the person's thoughts, feelings, or actions. This does not include the belief that the person is influenced by some person, idea, or God if the external influence is not thought to be directing the person without his or her control.

Bizarre Delusion

A bizarre delusion is so clearly untrue that it has no possible basis in fact. Some delusions are clearly false, yet remotely possible; for example, "The CIA wants to find me because they think Castro told me when he will attack Miami." Although it is unlikely, it is factually possible for that assertion to be true; therefore, it is not a bizarre delusion. However, if the person says that the CIA wants to find him or her because of secrets given him or her by Martians, that belief, not being factually possible, is a bizarre delusion.

Grandiose Delusion

A grandiose delusion concerns exaggerated importance, power, knowledge, or identity; examples include "I am the Messiah" and "I can kill people by looking at them."

Mood-Congruent Delusion

The mood-congruent delusion is consistent with either a depressed or manic mood. In a depressed person, examples are: "I am the reason why the Germans attacked Poland" (guilt); "My insides are rotting away and I will soon die"; "The police are after me because when I worked as a telephone operator, I allowed my friends sometimes to make free calls." Delusions of guilt are closely connected to mood. In a manic person, mood-congruent delusions involve inflated worth, power, knowledge, or identity; that is, grandiose delusions.

Mood-Incongruent Delusion

The mood-incongruent delusion is not linked with a depressed or manic mood.

Persecutory Delusion

The persecutory delusion involves being attacked, harassed, cheated, persecuted, or conspired against. The term "paranoid delusions" is often used as a synonym, but this is not exact because paranoid schizophrenia is characterized by delusions of either a persecutory or grandiose nature. Ideas of grandiosity and persecution are often closely related. The man who believes he was responsible for the German invasion of Poland must believe he is a very special person; and the man who believes he is the secret power behind the President may easily believe that he has enemies who want to displace him from this position.

Delusion of Reference

A delusion of reference involves the belief that certain things or people have a particular and unusual significance, usually of a negative or pejorative nature; for example, the belief that a television show is directed personally to someone to tell him or her to act in a certain way. It is important to exclude referential ideas that are not delusional. In many mental disorders, people think that they are the object of attention when that is probably an exaggerated idea. A person with a phobia of elevators may think that the other people in the elevator notice his or her discomfort; this is a nondelusional idea or reference. For the idea to be delusional, there must be a gross distortion of reality, such as thinking that when the man in the elevator touched his tie, it was a message that he knew the person was very anxious and a signal for him or her never to ride the elevator again.

Somatic Delusion

A somatic delusion is about a person's own body; for example, "Ants are eating my brain." Distorted judgments must not be considered delusional unless they are grossly untrue. The conviction of being ugly is not a delusion unless there is a clear distortion of reality; for example, "My head comes to a point."

HALLUCINATION, HYPOCHONDRIASIS, ILLUSION

A hallucination is a sensory perception without external stimulation of the relevant sensory organ. It has the immediate sense of reality of a true perception. Perceptions associated with dreaming, falling asleep (hypnogogic), or awakening (hypnopompic) are not considered hallucinations.

An auditory hallucination may be of voices or other sounds. Visual hallucinations may be of realistic images or designs. Gustatory and olfactory hallucinations are usually of unpleasant tastes or odors. Somatic hallucinations are a perception of a physical experience localized with the body; commonly, this is restricted to a perception with a delusional misinterpretation. The distinction here between a delusion and a hallucination becomes difficult. If a person reports a gnawing pain in his or her head, this would not be considered a hallucination any more than a man having a myocardial infarction reporting that he felt his chest was being squeezed in a vise. However, if the person reports that bugs are eating at his brain and means that as a statement of actual truth, that is a somatic hallucination (with a delusion).

People with hypochondriasis are preoccupied with their physical symptoms and may describe vague symptoms that are not characteristic of a known physical disorder, such as "I hurt all over." These symptoms are not somatic hallucinations. Hypochondriasis is the unrealistic interpretation of physical signs or sensations as abnormal, leading to a preoccupation with the fear or belief of having a disease. This is a disorder of judgment, not a hallucination of sensation with delusional misinterpretation. As usually interpreted, somatic hallucinations are extremely unusual and grossly unrealistic perceptions.

An illusion is a misperception of a real external stimulus; for example, a shadow is considered to be a man lurking in the alley. The distinction between an illusion and a hallucination is important because the latter, but not the former, is considered a psychotic symptom. Considered with other positive symptoms, the presence of a visual hallucination would indicate that a person has schizophrenia; the presence of an illusion (and no hallucination) would not be enough to make such a diagnosis. "Illusion" in common speech means being deceived, either by a misperception or by a false idea. In this wider sense, it overlaps into the area of delusion. As a technical term, "illusion" is applied only to a perception.

ORGANIC MENTAL DISORDER

Some mental symptoms are associated commonly with a known dysfunction of the brain, that is, an organic mental disorder. Perseveration and echolalia are common mental symptoms in an organic mental disorder; two others are attention disturbance and disorientation.

Attention Disturbance

Attention is the ability to focus in a sustained manner on one task or activity. Persons with a disturbance of attention appear distracted, do not complete tasks, and may report difficulty concentrating.

Disorientation

Orientation is the awareness of one's relation to time, place, and person. Being in a hospital, away from usual sources of information, often results in difficulty in keeping track of days. A small error is not considered disorientation.

INTELLECTUAL FUNCTIONING

Examination of intellectual functioning is important in the diagnosis of dementia and some other disorders. Intellectual functioning includes memory, judgment, abstract thought, arithmetic calculations, and similar functions.

Memory

Memory is divided into recent (short-term) and remote (long-term). The person with memory impairment may misplace objects and forget appointments. Short-term memory may be tested by asking the patient to remember three objects early in the interview and questioning him or her later, usually 5 minutes or so after naming the objects.

Abstract Thought

Abstract thought, the ability to appreciate ideas from multiple frames of reference, may be tested by asking the meaning of proverbs. Difficulty in abstracting may be evident in an answer that does not recognize that the proverb is meant to be a specific instance of a general rule. For example, to the proverb "People who live in glass houses should not throw stones," a nonabstract answer would be, "Because the walls would break." Some answers are deviant because, although they are abstract, they show a thought disorder—disturbance in the form of thinking, such as loose association, incoherence, illogicality, or clanging.

Amnesia

Amnesia is abnormal forgetting. When forgetting crosses from normal to abnormal is a matter of judgment.

Confabulation

Confabulation is the fabrication of facts or events in response to questions about situations or events that are not recalled because of memory impairment. For example, the patient may never have seen the physician before, but he or she may say that he or she has and provide fabricated details. This is confabulation when the patient cannot really remember. If the patient's memory is normal and he or she consciously decides to fabricate, that is lying. Confabulation is important in the diagnosis of organic amnestic syndrome (formerly called Korsakoff's syndrome).

Conversion

Conversion is a loss or alteration of physical function that suggests a physical disorder but is rather an expression of a psychological need or conflict. Conversion must be differentiated from malingering because it is not under voluntary control. Common examples are paralysis and blindness. It is difficult at times to determine that a symptom is not under voluntary control.

ANXIETY DISORDERS

Of the many mental disorders, a few of the more common are described in the following sections. The criteria given here are not exhaustive. The reader should consult the DSM-III-R for more detailed descriptions of these and other disorders.

Nervousness is so common that patients and physicians may take it for granted, as merely background for some other symptoms that are the foreground. Often this is true. The level of anxiety of patients in an oncologist's waiting room may be very high and, at that time, is not the predominant concern (although it should not be neglected).

Within the general anxiety in which people live, some constellations of symptoms stand out because they have not only differing descriptive features but also differing prognoses and responses to treatment.

Panic Disorder

Panic disorder is characterized by discrete attacks of severe anxiety, usually described as a feeling of impending doom. Associated symptoms are headache, sweating, difficulty breathing, chest pain, "butterflies" in the stomach, trembling, hot or cold flashes, and tingling. The attack lasts minutes to hours and thereafter is dreaded. The person often comes to associate the attacks with certain situations, such as buses, subways, tunnels, crowded stores or theaters, or being alone and becomes phobic of these situations (agoraphobia). The common denominator of these situations appears to be difficulty in leaving it and obtaining help should a panic attack occur. In other phobias, the person is fearful

of the situation, such as heights, elevators, or spiders; in agoraphobia, the person fears that a panic attack may occur and is fearful of the situation in which he or she may get a panic attack. A major aspect of panic disorder is generalized anxiety; compared to panic anxiety, generalized anxiety is of longer duration, usually waxes and wanes according to the nearness of the feared situation, and is less intense.

Phobia

A phobia is a persistent, irrational fear of a specific object or situation. This fear is excessive and unreasonable and compels the person to avoid what is feared. This is diagnosed as a disorder only if this fear and avoidance are of more than trivial distress and alter functioning to some significant extent. Probably everyone has phobias to some degree. Yet such dislike and avoidance are a minor part of most persons' lives and do not merit a diagnosis of mental disorder. Phobias are classified into three types:

1. *Agoraphobia*. This phobia is discussed above, under the heading "Panic Disorder."
2. *Social phobia*. This phobia consists of a fear of and compelling desire to avoid situations in which the person is exposed to possible scrutiny by others, in which he or she fears acting in a manner that will be embarrassing.
3. *Simple phobia*. This is a residual category for other phobias. Common examples are fear of dogs, snakes, claustrophobia (fear of closed places), and acrophobia (fear of heights).

Obsessive Compulsive Disorder

Obsessions are persistent ideas or images that are experienced as unwanted and involuntary but cannot be suppressed or ignored. Compulsions are repetitive acts that seem purposive and realistic but that are done excessively and felt to be forced upon the person. Compulsive hand washing and other types of cleaning are common compulsions. True obsessions and compulsions should be distinguished from brooding and indecisiveness mainly by the latter twos' lacking the quality of being forced upon the person.

Generalized Anxiety Disorder

Persons with persistent, severe anxiety who do not fit into other categories are assigned to this residual group.

SCHIZOPHRENIA

This severe mental disorder occurs in about 1 percent of persons. Both sexes are equally affected. It is only one of several disorders in which psychotic symptoms are prominent. Psychotic symptoms are delusions, hallucinations, thought disorder, and bizarre behavior. Much controversy exists over the limits of schizophrenia and the other psychotic disorders.

According to DSM-III-R, the criteria for schizophrenia require:

1.   Certain types of psychotic symptoms during the active phase, such as (a) at least two of the following: (i) delusions, (ii) hallucinations, (iii) incoherence or marked loosening of association, (iv) catatonia, (v) flat or inappropriate affect; (b) bizarre delusions; or (c) hallucinations of a voice not related to sadness or elation, or of two or more voices speaking to each other.

2.   Impairment of functioning.

3.   No mood disorder present concomitantly.

4.   Continuous signs of illness for at least 6 months, consisting of an active phase or perhaps a prodromal or residual phase involving symptoms such as social withdrawal, blunted affect, odd beliefs, and marked lack of interest.

A couple of aspects of this definition of schizophrenia are important.

1.   The long list of possible symptoms and other criteria—not all are included in the brief summary above—indicates that precise knowledge of the disorder is lacking. For now, physicians must settle for a complex definition that will certainly be modified.

2.   The criteria are carefully constructed to avoid misclassifying someone with another type of psychotic disorder, especially those associated with mania and manic depression. If symptoms of these disorders are present, schizophrenia should not be diagnosed unless the symptoms of the affective disorder clearly came after the symptoms of schizophrenia or were of brief duration. When the distinction is very difficult, the term schizoaffective disorder is used. Whether this is a separate disorder is still unclear.

MAJOR DEPRESSION

The essential feature of major depression is a dysphoric mood, or loss of interest or pleasure in all or almost all activities; this mood is prominent and persistent. Delusions or hallucinations may be present, but are mood-congruent. Other common symptoms are:

- Poor appetite
- Insomnia or hypersomnia
- Psychomotor agitation or retardation
- Loss of interest
- Fatigue
- Feelings of worthlessness or guilt
- Diminished ability to concentrate
- Recurrent thoughts of death or suicide
- Attempted suicide

Major depression is more common in women (incidence 15 to 20 percent) than in men (10 percent). About 15 percent of persons with the disorder die by suicide. Yet, it is one of the more responsive disorders to treatment, both of the acute episode and prophylaxis. The main problem is that only a small percentage of persons with the disorder receive appropriate treatment, either because the diagnosis is not made or treatment is not adequate. All physicians, not just psychiatrists, should become familiar with the diagnosis of this disorder and its treatment.

Notably, there is nothing in the diagnostic criteria about whether there is a reason for the sad mood. It is a common mistake to neglect the diagnosis because the symptoms seem "appropriate" to the situation, such as a severe disappointment. Awareness of such a disappointment may be important in counseling the patient, but it is not relevant to the diagnosis or somatic treatment. An exception to this is bereavement, in which instance a full depressive syndrome may be a normal reaction. But symptoms of worthlessness, marked psychomotor retardation, and functional impairment suggest that major depression is present.

Many persons are sad but do not reach the criteria for major depression. This condition is called dysthymic disorder. Much less is known about its epidemiological features and its treatment.

BIBLIOGRAPHY

American Psychiatric Association: Diagnostic and Statistical Manual of Mental Disorders, ed. 3, rev. Washington, D.C., The Association, 1987.

Jaspers, K.: General Psychopathology, J. Hoenig and M.W. Hamilton (trans.). Manchester, England, Manchester University Press, 1963.

Chapter 21

DSM-III-R Classification of Mental Disorders

Howard Klar, M.D.

USING THE DSM-III-R

The *Diagnostic and Statistical Manual of Mental Disorders*, published by the American Psychiatric Association, first appeared in 1952. It has become the standard manual for the classification of mental disorders throughout North America and has been translated into many languages. The most recent version is the revised third edition, known as the DSM-III-R.

Definition of Mental Disorder

Although the DSM-III-R provides a classification of mental disorders, it makes no claim to define "mental disorder" in a general sense. Instead, each mental disorder is conceived as a clinically significant behavioral or psychological syndrome or pattern that has symptoms, impairments, or risk of death, pain, disability, or loss of freedom. The condition qualifies as a disorder only when it is produced by a dysfunction, which may be behavioral, psychological, or biological.

Mental disorders are not visualized as having sharp boundaries, either between themselves or between disorder and lack of disorder. Classifying mental disorders does not classify people, and people with the same mental disorder may have nothing else in common. For these reasons, people are not described, for example, as "alcoholics" or "schizophrenics" but rather as "people with alcohol dependence" or "people with schizophrenia."

Descriptive Approach

Since the etiology for most mental disorders is unknown, the DSM-III-R takes on a theoretical approach with regard to etiology and pathophysiologic process, except in conditions where these are known with reasonable certainty. A descriptive approach is taken, usually limited to descriptions of clinical features. When possible, these clinical features consist of easily and reliably identified behavioral signs or symptoms. The same approach is used for grouping the disorders into diagnostic classes.

For each disorder, the DSM-III-R describes the following: essential features, associated features, age at onset, course, impairment, complications, predisposing factors, prevalence, sex ratio, familial pattern, and differential diagnosis.

Cautions

The compilers of the DSM-III-R caution readers that its criteria are simply guidelines for clinical diagnoses and that special training in the field is needed for their use. They point out that its classification of mental disorders is not fixed or all-inclusive.

Multiaxial Evaluation

A multiaxial evaluation means that each case is measured against several different sets of information, or "axes." This avoids oversights, which might occur when a case is looked at from a single viewpoint. The DSM-III-R uses five axes. The first three are used in actual diagnosis; the other two provide supplemental information.

Axis I: Clinical Syndromes and V Codes. All the mental disorders classified belong on either axis I or II. The V codes refer to conditions not attributable to a mental disorder that are a focus of attention or treatment. Axis I disorders are clinical syndromes generally associated with adult life that usually are episodic.

Axis II: Developmental Disorders and Personality Disorders. Axis II disorders generally begin in childhood or adolescence and persist into adult life and remain more-or-less stable throughout a person's life. It is possible for an individual to have disorders on both axes I and II simultaneously.

Axis III: Physical Disorders and Conditions. Any physical disorder or condition of the patient that may be relevant to his or her mental state is noted in this axis.

Axis IV: Severity of Psychosocial Stressors. Axis IV consists of a scale with which to measure the severity of recent psychosocial stressors that may have caused the occurrence of a new mental disorder, the recurrence of an earlier one, or the exacerbation of an already existing one.

Axis V: Global Assessment of Functioning. Axis V consists of another scale, the global assessment of functioning (GAF) scale. The GAF scale allows the clinician to make an overall assessment of a person's psychological, social, and occupational functioning.

Multiple Diagnoses and Diagnostic Overlap

Patients can have more than one diagnosis on axis I or axis II, and patients can have diagnoses on both axis I and II. For example, on axis I a patient can be diagnosed as bipolar affective disorder, manic, and alcohol dependence and on axis II be diagnosed as borderline personality disorder. Within axis II only it is quite common for patients to be diagnosed as having several personality disorders concurrently. As clinicians have gained experience with the multiaxial system, they have become increasingly aware of the tendency of specific disorders to overlap with greater frequency than one might expect by chance. The concept of *comorbidity* has become increasingly important in psychiatric diagnosis.

The frequent concordant diagnoses of axis I, major depressive disorder, and axis II, borderline personality disorder, have spurred considerable important research into possible vulnerabilities that might underlie both disorders and that, if understood, might yield more specific and coherent approaches to treatment and perhaps prevention. Comorbidity studies are a direct result of the greater clarity and consistency of diagnosis provided by the multiaxial approach in DSM-III-R.

CLASSIFICATION OF MENTAL DISORDERS

The DSM-III-R organizes mental disorders into the following 19 diagnostic categories:

1. Disorders usually first evident in infancy, childhood, or adolescence
2. Organic mental disorders
3. Psychoactive substance use disorders
4. Schizophrenia
5. Delusional (paranoid) disorder
6. Psychotic disorders not elsewhere classified
7. Mood disorders
8. Anxiety disorders (or anxiety and phobic neuroses)
9. Somatoform disorders
10. Dissociative disorders (or hysterical neuroses, dissociative type)
11. Sexual disorders
12. Sleep disorders
13. Factitious disorders
14. Impulse control disorders not elsewhere classified

15. Adjustment disorder
16. Psychological factors affecting physical condition
17. Personality disorders
18. V codes for conditions not attributable to a mental disorder that are a focus of attention or treatment
19. Additional codes

These diagnostic classes are often subdivided; for example, personality disorders are subdivided into clusters A, B, and C. The individual mental disorders are each assigned a five-digit number; for example, 307.10 anorexia nervosa, 307.51 bulimia nervosa. For simplicity, these codes are not given in this chapter.

Some of the mental disorders are illustrated by vignettes to give the reader an idea of what a clinician might expect to see. However, for clarity, these case studies have been kept uncomplicated—more so than cases are likely to be in real life.

DISORDERS USUALLY FIRST EVIDENT IN INFANCY, CHILDHOOD, OR ADOLESCENCE

No sharp age boundaries set off the disorders classified here, and many disorders can extend into early adulthood. These disorders should be the first to be considered in the examination of a child or adolescent.

Developmental Disorders (Axis II)

Disturbance is in the acquisition of cognitive, language, motor, or social skills.

* *Mental Retardation (Axis II):* Subaverage intellectual functioning, accompanied by impaired adaptive functioning, with onset before age 18.
* *Pervasive Developmental Disorders:* Impairments in reciprocal social interaction, in verbal and nonverbal communication skills, and in imaginative activity. Activities and interests are often restricted. Autistic disorder is a severe form.
* *Specific Developmental Disorders (Axis II):* Impairment of academic, language, speech, and motor skills not caused by other disorders.
* *Other Developmental Disorders (Axis II):*

Developmental disorders that do not fit in the above categories.
* *Disruptive Behavior Disorders:* Socially disruptive behavior, including attention-deficit hyperactivity disorder, oppositional defiant disorder, and conduct disorder (see Table 21–1).
* *Anxiety Disorders of Childhood or Adolescence:* Disorders in which anxiety is the chief feature.
* *Eating Disorders:* Gross disturbances in eating behavior, including anorexia nervosa, bulimia nervosa, pica, and rumination disorder of infancy.
* *Gender Identity Disorders:* Disorders in which the person is confused as to which sex he or she belongs, including transsexualism.
* *Tic Disorders:* Three disorders in which tics are symptomatic. Tourette's disorder, chronic motor or vocal tic disorder, and transient tic disorder.
* *Elimination Disorders:* Inappropriate, involuntary or rarely voluntary voiding of feces (functional encopresis) or inappropriate, involuntary or voluntary voiding of urine (functional enuresis).
* *Speech Disorders Not Elsewhere Classified:* Cluttering and stuttering.
* *Other Disorders of Infancy, Childhood, or Adolescence:* Various disorders, including elective mutism and undifferentiated attention-deficit disorder.

ORGANIC MENTAL SYNDROMES AND DISORDERS

Psychological or behavioral abnormalities associated with transient or permanent dysfunction of the brain. The syndromes form a group without regard to etiology; the etiology is known or presumed for those grouped as disorders.

Organic Mental Syndromes

Organic mental syndromes are divided into six categories:

1. Delirium and dementia
2. Amnestic syndrome and organic hallucinosis
3. Organic delusional syndrome, organic mood syndrome, and organic anxiety syndrome
4. Organic personality syndrome
5. Intoxication and withdrawal

TABLE 21-1.   Diagnostic Criteria for Conduct Disorder

A.   A disturbance of conduct lasting at least six months, during which at least three of the following have been present:

   (1)   has stolen without confrontation of a victim on more than one occasion (including forgery)
   (2)   has run away from home overnight at least twice while living in parental or parental surrogate home (or once without returning)
   (3)   often lies (other than to avoid physical or sexual abuse)
   (4)   has deliberately engaged in fire-setting
   (5)   is often truant from school (for older person, absent from work)
   (6)   has broken into someone else's house, building, or car
   (7)   has deliberately destroyed others' property (other than by fire-setting)
   (8)   has been physically cruel to animals
   (9)   has forced someone into sexual activity with him or her
  (10)   has used a weapon in more than one fight
  (11)   often initiates physical fights
  (12)   has stolen with confrontation of a victim (e.g., mugging, purse-snatching, extortion, armed robbery)
  (13)   has been physically cruel to people

   Note: The above items are listed in descending order of discriminating power based on data from a national field trial of the DSM-III-R criteria for Disruptive Behavior Disorders.

B.   If 18 or older, does not meet criteria for Antisocial Personality Disorder.

Criteria for Severity of Conduct Disorder:

   Mild: Few if any conduct problems in excess of those required to make the diagnosis, **and** conduct problems cause only minor harm to others.

   Moderate: Number of conduct problems and effect on others intermediate between "mild" and "severe."

   Severe: Many conduct problems in excess of those required to make the diagnosis, **or** conduct problems cause considerable harm to others, e.g., serious physical injury to victims, extensive vandalism or theft, prolonged absence from home.

Reprinted with permission from the *Diagnostic and Statistical Manual of Mental Disorders, Third Edition, Revised.* Washington, D.C., American Psychiatric Association, 1987

---

6.   Organic mental syndrome not otherwise specified

Organic Mental Disorders

Organic mental disorders are divided into three categories:

1.   Those associated with aging
2.   Those associated with psychoactive substances
3.   A miscellaneous group.

• *Dementias Arising in the Senium and Presenium:* Senile and presenile dementias, including those of the Alzheimer type.
• *Psychoactive Substance-Induced Organic Mental Disorders:* Organic mental disorders caused by the direct effects of psychoactive substances on the nervous system. The substances are classified as alcohol, amphetamine and similarly acting sympathomimetics, caffeine, cannabis, cocaine, hallucinogens, inhalants, nicotine, opioids, phencyclidine (PCP) or similarly acting arylcyclohexylamines, and sedatives, hypnotics, or anxiolytics.

• *Organic Mental Disorders Associated with Axis III Physical Disorders or Conditions, or Whose Etiology Is Unknown:* Examples of these include delirium associated with pneumonia and dementia associated with brain tumor.

PSYCHOACTIVE SUBSTANCE USE DISORDERS

These disorders consist of symptoms and maladaptive behavioral changes associated with more or less regular use of psychoactive substances that affect the central nervous system. Continued use of the substance despite the problems it causes the individual constitutes the disorder and is distinguished from moderate use of a substance or use for appropriate medical purposes. The fact that these disorders refer to behavior associated with regular use distinguishes them from psychoactive substance-induced organic mental disorders, which describe the direct acute or chronic effects of such substances on the central nervous system. Nearly always, an individual who has the substance use disorder also has the substance-induced organic mental disorder; for example, an individual with a cocaine dependence disorder usually has a cocaine intoxication and/or withdrawal disorder.

Two broad categories exist: psychoactive substance dependence (Table 21–2) and psychoactive substance abuse. Abuse is often distinguished from dependence by its lack of regularity. A diagnosis of abuse is more likely to be made for those who have just started taking psychoactive substances and is more likely to involve substances without strong withdrawal symptoms. Weekend drug binges and repeated drunk driving are examples of abuse.

Nine types of substances are associated with both abuse and dependence: alcohol; amphetamine or similarly acting sympathomimetics; cannabis; cocaine; hallucinogens; inhalants; opioids; phencyclidine (PCP) or similarly acting arylcy-

clohexylamines; and sedatives, hypnotics, or anxiolytics. Dependence (but not abuse) is seen with nicotine because nearly everyone who uses nicotine-containing substances in a maladaptive way—for example, exacerbating a condition by episodic smoking—is dependent on nicotine.

Use of multiple substances is frequent, and in these cases multiple diagnoses are made.

SCHIZOPHRENIA

Schizophrenia is characterized by symptoms of psychosis during its active phase, by reduced ability to function, and by a time length of at least 6 months during which other typical symptoms may also be present. Delusions, hallucinations, or other typical distortions of thought or emotion nearly always occur in this illness.

TABLE 21–2.   Diagnostic Criteria for Psychoactive Substance Dependence

A. At least three of the following:

(1) substance often taken in larger amounts or over a longer period than the person intended

(2) persistent desire or one or more unsuccessful efforts to cut down or control substance use

(3) a great deal of time spent in activities necessary to get the substance (e.g., theft), taking the substance (e.g., chain smoking), or recovering from its effects

(4) frequent intoxication or withdrawal symptoms when expected to fulfill major role obligations at work, school, or home (e.g., does not go to work because hung over, goes to school or work "high," intoxicated while taking care of his or her children), or when substance use is physically hazardous (e.g., drives when intoxicated)

(5) important social, occupational, or recreational activities given up or reduced because of substance use

(6) continued substance use despite knowledge of having a persistent or recurrent social, psychological, or physical problem that is caused or exacerbated by the use of the substance (e.g., keeps using heroin despite family arguments about it, cocaine-induced depression, or having an ulcer made worse by drinking)

(7) marked tolerance: need for markedly increased amounts of the substance (i.e., at least a 50% increase) in order to achieve intoxication or desired effect, or markedly diminished effect with continued use of the same amount

Note: The following items may not apply to cannabis, hallucinogens, or phencyclidine (PCP):

(8) characteristic withdrawal symptoms (see specific withdrawal syndromes under Psychoactive Substance-induced Organic Mental Disorders)

(9) substance often taken to relieve or avoid withdrawal symptoms

B. Some symptoms of the disturbance have persisted for at least one month, or have occurred repeatedly over a long period of time.

Criteria for Severity of Psychoactive Substance Dependence:

Mild: Few, if any, symptoms in excess of those required to make the diagnosis, and the symptoms result in no more than mild impairment in occupational functioning or in usual social activities or relationships with others.

Moderate: Symptoms or functional impairment between "mild" and "severe."

Severe: Many symptoms in excess of those required to make the diagnosis, and the symptoms markedly interfere with occupational functioning or with usual social activities or relationships with others.[1]

In Partial Remission: During the past six months, some use of the substance and some symptoms of dependence.

In Full Remission: During the past six months, either no use of the substance, or use of the substance and no symptoms of dependence.

---

[1]Because of the availability of cigarettes and other nicotine-containing substances and the absence of a clinically significant nicotine intoxication syndrome, impairment in occupational or social functioning is not necessary for a rating of severe Nicotine Dependence.
Reprinted with permission from the *Diagnostic and Statistical Manual of Mental Disorders, Third Edition, Revised.* Washington, D.C., American Psychiatric Association, 1987

Schizophrenia is not diagnosed when the disturbance has an organic cause or is a result of mood disorder or schizoaffective disorder.

Schizophrenia is divided into five types:

1. Catatonic type
2. Disorganized type (Table 21–3)
3. Paranoid type (Table 21–4)
4. Undifferentiated type
5. Residual type

DELUSIONAL (PARANOID) DISORDER

The presence of a persistent, nonbizarre delusion that is not due to any other mental disorder. The diagnosis is made only when it cannot be established that an organic factor initiated and maintained the disturbance.

Aside from the delusion, the behavior of an individual with this disorder is not strikingly odd. When used with this disorder, the term *paranoid* does not have its usual connotations; the delusions tend to be erotomanic, grandiose, jealous, persecutory, or somatic.

PSYCHOTIC DISORDERS NOT ELSEWHERE CLASSIFIED

Four specific disorders and one miscellaneous group are placed in this diagnostic class:

1. Brief reactive psychosis
2. Schizophreniform disorder
3. Schizoaffective disorder
4. Induced psychotic disorder
5. Psychotic disorder not otherwise specified (atypical psychosis)

MOOD DISORDERS

Mood consists of prolonged emotion, usually either depression or elation. Mood disorders are mood disturbances not having some other identifiable cause. Mood disorders are also known as affective disorders.

Mood disorders are divided into bipolar disorders and depressive disorders.

Bipolar Disorders

Manic or hypomanic episodes, usually with a history of major depressive episodes, are characteristic of bipolar disorders. Two disorders are placed in this category: bipolar disorder and cyclothymia. In bipolar disorder, one or more manic episodes occur, usually with one or more major depressive episodes. In cyclothymia, numerous hypomanic episodes occur, with numerous periods of depressive symptoms.

- *Manic Episode:* A period in which the predominant mood is elevated, expansive, or ir-

---

TABLE 21–3. Diagnostic criteria for Schizophrenia, Disorganized Type

A type of Schizophrenia in which the following criteria are met:
A. Incoherence, marked loosening of associations, or grossly disorganized behavior.
B. Flat or grossly inappropriate affect.
C. Does not meet the criteria for Catatonic Type.

Reprinted with permission from the *Diagnostic and Statistical Manual of Mental Disorders, Third Edition, Revised*. Washington, D.C., American Psychiatric Association, 1987

TABLE 21–4. Diagnostic criteria for Schizophrenia, Paranoid Type

A type of Schizophrenia in which there are:
A. Preoccupation with one or more systematized delusions or with frequent auditory hallucinations related to a single theme.
B. *None* of the following: incoherence, marked loosening of associations, flat or grossly inappropriate affect, catatonic behavior, grossly disorganized behavior.
Specify stable type if criteria A and B have been met during all past and present active phases of the illness.

Reprinted with permission from the *Diagnostic and Statistical Manual of Mental Disorders, Third Edition, Revised*. Washington, D.C., American Psychiatric Association, 1987

ritable to such an extent that functioning and social activities are impaired; the individual may need hospitalization to avoid harm to self or others.

- *Hypomanic episode:* Similar to a manic episode, except that the symptoms are less severe and delusions never occur.
- *Major Depressive Episode:* A depressed mood or loss of interest in life, occurring for most of the day, nearly every day, for a period of at least 2 weeks.

Depressive Disorders

One or more periods of depression, without a history of manic or hypomanic episodes, are characteristic of depressive disorders. Two disorders are placed in this category: major depression and dysthymia (or depressive neurosis). Major depression may be single-episode or recurrent. In dysthymia the depressed mood has occurred most days for at least 2 years (Table 21–5).

ANXIETY DISORDERS (OR ANXIETY AND PHOBIC NEUROSES)

Anxiety disorders are typified by symptoms of anxiety and avoidance behavior. These are probably the most commonly occurring mental disorders and are divided into eight categories:

1. Panic disorder with and without agoraphobia
2. Agoraphobia without history of panic disorder
3. Social phobia
4. Simple phobia
5. Obsessive compulsive disorder (or obsessive compulsive neurosis)
6. Posttraumatic stress disorder
7. Generalized anxiety disorder
8. Anxiety disorder not otherwise specified

SOMATOFORM DISORDERS

Individuals with somatoform disorders have *physical* symptoms without a known physical cause but that are likely due to psychological causes. Unlike factitious disorders, the symptoms are never intentionally produced. Six disorders and a miscellaneous group are placed in this diagnostic class:

1. Body dysmorphic disorder (dysmorphophobia) (Table 21–6)
2. Conversion disorder (or hysterical neurosis, conversion type)
3. Hypochondriasis (or hypochondriacal neurosis)
4. Somatization disorder
5. Somatoform pain disorder
6. Undifferentiated somatoform disorder
7. Somatoform disorder not otherwise specified

DISSOCIATIVE DISORDERS (OR HYSTERICAL NEUROSES, DISSOCIATIVE TYPE)

Dissociative disorders consist of a disturbance or change in the normally integrative functions of identity, memory, or consciousness. Multiple personality and amnesia are the most widely known of these disorders.

1. Multiple personality disorder
2. Psychogenic fugue
3. Psychogenic amnesia
4. Depersonalization disorder (or depersonalization neurosis)
5. Dissociative disorder not otherwise specified

SEXUAL DISORDERS

Sexual disorders are divided into three broad categories:

1. Paraphilias
2. Sexual dysfunctions
3. Other sexual disorders

Paraphilias

Recurrent intense sexual urges and sexually arousing fantasies involving nonhuman objects, suffering or humiliation (not simulated) of oneself or one's partner, or children or other non-

TABLE 21–5.   Diagnostic criteria for Dysthymia

A. Depressed mood (or can be irritable mood in children and adolescents) for most of the day, more days than not, as indicated either by subjective account or observation by others, for at least two years (one year for children and adolescents)
B. Presence, while depressed, of at least two of the following:
    (1) poor appetite or overeating
    (2) insomnia or hypersomnia
    (3) low energy or fatigue
    (4) low self-esteem
    (5) poor concentration or difficulty making decisions
    (6) feelings of hopelessness
C. During a two-year period (one-year for children and adolescents) of the disturbance, never without the symptoms in A for more than two months at a time.
D. No evidence of an unequivocal Major Depressive Episode during the first two years (one year for children and adolescents) of the disturbance.

    Note: There may have been a previous Major Depressive Episode, provided there was a full remission (no significant signs or symptoms for six months) before development of the Dysthymia. In addition, after these two years (one year in children or adolescents) of Dysthymia, there may be superimposed episodes of Major Depression, in which case both diagnoses are given.

E. Has never had a Manic Episode or an unequivocal Hypomanic Episode.
F. Not superimposed on a chronic psychotic disorder, such as Schizophrenia or Delusional Disorder.
G. It cannot be established that an organic factor initiated and maintained the disturbance, e.g., prolonged administration of an antihypertensive medication.

Specify primary or secondary type:

    Primary type: the mood disturbance is not related to a preexisting, chronic, nonmood, Axis I or Axis III disorder, e.g., Anorexia Nervosa, Somatization Disorder, a Psychoactive Substance Dependence Disorder, an Anxiety Disorder, or rheumatoid arthritis.

    Secondary type: the mood disturbance is apparently related to a preexisting, chronic, nonmood Axis I or Axis III disorder.

    Specify early onset or late onset:

    Early onset: onset of the disturbance before age 21.
    Late onset: onset of the disturbance at age 21 or later.

Reprinted with permission from the *Diagnostic and Statistical Manual of Mental Disorders, Third Edition, Revised*. Washington, D.C., American Psychiatric Association, 1987

TABLE 21–6.   Diagnostic Criteria for Body Dysmorphic Disorder

A. Preoccupation with some imagined defect in appearance in normal-appearing person. If a slight physical anomaly is present, the person's concern is grossly excessive.
B. The belief in the defect is not of delusional intensity, as in Delusional Disorder, Somatic Type (i.e., the person can acknowledge the possibility that he or she may be exaggerating the extent of the defect or that there may be no defect at all).
C. Occurrence not exclusively during the course of Anorexia Nervosa or Transsexualism.

Reprinted with permission from the *Diagnostic and Statistical Manual of Mental Disorders, Third Edition, Revised*. Washington, D.C., American Psychiatric Association, 1987

consenting persons. The diagnosis is made only if the individual has acted upon these urges or is markedly distressed by them. Paraphilias are also known as sexual deviations. Eight disorders and a miscellaneous group are placed in this category:

1. Exhibitionism
2. Fetishism
3. Frotteurism
4. Pedophilia
5. Sexual masochism
6. Sexual sadism
7. Transvestic fetishism
8. Voyeurism
9. Paraphilia not otherwise specified

Sexual Dysfunctions

Inhibitions that interfere with normal sexual response. This diagnosis is usually made only when the sexual dysfunction is a major part of the clinical picture, although it need not be part of the dominant disturbance. This diagnosis is not made if the sexual dysfunction is caused wholly by organic factors, such as a physical disorder or medication, or by another Axis I mental disorder. This category is divided into sexual desire disorders, sexual arousal disorders, orgasm disorders, and sexual pain disorders.

Other Sexual Disorders

These include sexual disorders that do not belong in the above categories.

SLEEP DISORDERS

This diagnostic class encompasses disorders of sleep that are chronic, that is, of at least a month's duration. When some other mental disorder causes the disturbance of sleep, a sleep disorder will be diagnosed also only when it is the major complaint. Sleep disorders are divided into dyssomnias and parasomnias.

Dyssomnias

Disturbance in the amount, quality, or timing of sleep. Three groups of disorders are placed in this category:

1. Insomnia disorders
2. Hypersomnia disorders
3. Sleep-wake schedule disorder

Parasomnias

Sleep disturbance caused by an abnormal event that takes place during sleep or between wakefulness and sleep. The parasomnias comprise three groups:

1. Dream anxiety disorder (nightmare disorder)
2. Sleep terror disorder
3. Sleepwalking disorder
4. Parasomnia not otherwise specified

FACTITIOUS DISORDERS

Factitious disorders are those intentionally produced or feigned. They qualify as a mental disorder because they result from compulsive behavior, being thus under the individual's control only to a certain extent. They are distinguished from malingering, that is, the simulation of a condition with the deliberate goal of avoiding something. Two kinds exist: factitious disorder with physical symptoms and factitious disorder with psychological symptoms.

IMPULSE CONTROL DISORDERS NOT ELSEWHERE CLASSIFIED

This diagnostic class contains five disorders of impulse control and a miscellaneous group that do not fit into previous diagnostic classes:

1. Intermittent explosive disorder
2. Kleptomania
3. Pathological gambling
4. Pyromania
5. Trichotillomania
6. Impulse control disorder not otherwise specified

ADJUSTMENT DISORDER

An adjustment disorder consists of a maladaptive reaction to a psychosocial stressor that takes place within 3 months after onset of the stressor and that persists for longer than 6 months. Symptoms vary, and the nine types correspond to the symptoms; for example, adjustment order with anxious mood.

PSYCHOLOGICAL FACTORS AFFECTING PHYSICAL CONDITION

These include psychological factors that contribute to the initiation or exacerbation of a physical condition, for example, vomiting.

PERSONALITY DISORDERS

A personality disorder is diagnosed only when personality traits are so inflexible or maladaptive that they affect functioning or produce distress. These disorders often become evident during adolescence and persist in the adult; frequently they become milder in middle or old age.

Personality disorders are divided into three clusters—A, B, and C—and a miscellaneous category.

Cluster A

People with cluster A personality disorders often appear odd or eccentric. Three disorders are included: paranoid personality disorder, schizoid personality disorder (Table 21–7), and schizotypal personality disorder.

Cluster B

Those with cluster B personality disorders often appear dramatic, emotional, or erratic. Included here are antisocial personality disorder, borderline personality disorder, histrionic personality disorder, and narcissistic personality disorder.

Cluster C

Persons with cluster C personality disorders often appear anxious or fearful. Included here are avoidant personality disorder, dependent personality disorder, obsessive compulsive personality disorder, and passive aggressive personality disorder.

V CODES FOR CONDITIONS NOT ATTRIBUTABLE TO A MENTAL DISORDER THAT ARE A FOCUS OF ATTENTION OR TREATMENT

V precedes the numeric code assigned to these conditions. Examples are borderline intellectual functioning, malingering, and marital problem.

ADDITIONAL CODES

These categories apply when a diagnosis cannot be made or has been deferred.

CLINICAL CASE STUDIES

Case Study 1: Schizophrenia

John, 18 years old, was brought to the Student Health Services doctor by his student residence advisor. He had spent the last week sitting in his room, refusing to leave; he had spent many of the last 24 hours on his knees praying. When his roommates asked him what was wrong, he called them devil-worshipers. They said that John, since his arrival in college, 4 months previously, had become increasingly withdrawn and remote; he had also begun to look at them in an odd way. They summoned the advisor when John began throwing things at them and talking to the television.

At the clinic, John appeared disheveled and bleary-eyed; he seemed remote and aloof and made no eye contact with the physician. When asked what was troubling him, he fell to his knees and prayed. When the physician questioned why he was praying during an interview,

---

TABLE 21–7.   Diagnostic Criteria for Schizoid Personality Disorder

A.   A pervasive pattern of indifference to social relationships and a restricted range of emotional experience and expression, beginning by early adulthood and present in a variety of contexts, as indicated by at least *four* of the following:
   (1)   neither desires nor enjoys close relationships, including being part of a family
   (2)   almost always chooses solitary activities
   (3)   rarely, if ever, claims or appears to experience strong emotions, such as anger and joy
   (4)   indicates little if any desire to have sexual experiences with another person (age being taken into account)
   (5)   is indifferent to the praise and criticism of others
   (6)   has no close friends or confidants (or only one) other than first-degree relatives
   (7)   displays constricted affect, e.g., is aloof, cold, rarely reciprocates gestures or facial expressions, such as smiles or nods
B.   Occurrence not exclusively during the course of Schizophrenia or a Delusional Disorder.

Reprinted with permission from *Diagnostic and Statistical Manual of Mental Disorders, Third Edition, Revised*. Washington, D.C., American Psychiatric Association, 1987

John became agitated and began to pray frantically. At this point, the physician suggested to him that he might be better off in the hospital. He continued to pray.

John's family was contacted. They gave the history of a young man who had always been rather aloof and distant but had managed to function socially. Shortly before his departure for college, they noticed that he became intensely interested in philosophy—particularly in the rather obscure works of certain esoteric theologians. His family explained this simply as anxiety about going to college.

His family history included an uncle who had been in and out of institutions all of his life and a grandmother who his mother described as a "weirdo," always talking about conspiracies and strange experiences. His parents, sister, and brother had never had any psychiatric problems.

John was tested at the hospital over the next 3 days, without receiving medication. His physical and neurological examinations proved normal; his urine toxicology was negative. On the ward, he continued to behave bizarrely, praying on occasion, talking to the ceiling, and quickly turning about to mutter to people who appeared to him but not the hospital staff.

This is a case of schizophrenia. The significant clinical feature of this case is the length of the prodrome of isolation, withdrawal, and reclusiveness, which are then followed by an acute episode of psychosis. Psychosis is evidenced in this case by the delusions and bizarre behavior. Schizophrenia is often a disease of young adults that becomes apparent during their first separation from home.

Case Study 2: Depression

Adelle Dawson, a 64-year-old woman was brought to the family doctor by her husband. The doctor, who knew Mrs. Dawson well, noticed that she looked markedly different than before. Her face was expressionless, and her appearance, which had always been crisp and even a trifle provocative, was now dour and gray. She gave him one-word answers. Her husband said that, over the past week, she had become increasingly withdrawn, had much difficulty sleeping—frequently waking after 4 in the morning and not getting back to sleep. The husband had become particularly concerned that evening when he saw her fiddling for some time with the gas stove. When he asked her about it, she said, "I just want to make sure it's working." This was when he decided to bring her to see the doctor.

They had been married for 40 years and had two children, both now married and doing well. Her husband had recently retired, and the couple was planning to live in a sunny, more easy-going climate. He said she had lost about 9 pounds in the last 2 weeks. She had not shown any interest in her reading group, which in the past she had been passionate about, and was also unwilling to play golf with him, which had been a favorite pastime of theirs. She seemed bored and unmoved when her children called—even when she spoke to her grandchildren, previously very precious to her.

Her husband said that she had never had any psychiatric difficulties, although she had always been a person who had kept her emotions to herself. "She isn't a big talker," he said. Her brother had committed suicide at the age of 71; apart from that, there was nothing of relevance in her family history. Her physical examination revealed mild osteoarthritis in her hands and an old appendectomy scar. Her lab test results, including thyroid function, were normal.

The family doctor referred Mrs. Dawson to a psychiatrist, who made a diagnosis of depression, based on pervasive loss of interest, energy, and enthusiasm, in concert with the vegetative symptoms of weight loss, loss of libido, loss of interest in her usual activities, and sleep disturbance.

Case Study 3: Obsessive Compulsive Disorder

Ben was a 26-year-old veteran who was brought to the emergency room of a city hospital by the police. He was noticed standing in the aisle of a supermarket for more than an hour. When the manager asked him to leave, Ben said he couldn't decide what to eat and refused to leave the store. When the police came, he left without a struggle.

On evaluation at the hospital, his body was found to be wasted from malnourishment. He spoke coherently and logically but sat rather rigidly in his chair. He tended to answer questions either "Yes, sir" or "No, sir," as if he were still in the army, which he was discharged from only 3 months before. When asked why he had lost so much weight, he answered, "I can't figure out what to eat."

Further investigation revealed that his deterioration began shortly after his army discharge. He found decisions about food overwhelming. To some extent, he was afraid of being poisoned by impurities. Every food he looked at seemed to be potentially contaminated. When he could find no acceptable foods, he drank water. Ben stated that he knew many of the foods he refused to eat were probably fine, but he felt the need to constantly read and reread label after label, never being reassured that he had noticed all the potential contaminants he might ingest.

When offered food at the hospital, he sat and stared at it. He asked question after question about its purity, preparation, care, and so on. His hospital room was meticulous. His shirts were placed in an exact order, and his two pairs of shoes were carefully aligned. The staff noticed that, at times, it took Ben 30 to 40 minutes to brush his teeth; only when they insisted that he do so could he be motivated to leave the bathroom.

His physical examination was unremarkable, other than the signs of malnutrition. He had no history of developmental problems, a good army record, and no family history of psychiatric problems.

This is a case of obsessive compulsive disorder. The diagnosis was made on the basis of the patient's obsessive checking of labels, obsessive slowness, and compulsion to read and reread labels. There are two parts to this disorder: the obsessions, which are intrusive thoughts; and the compulsions, which are irresistible, often distressing actions. Many patients deny the extent to which these rituals or intrusive thoughts interfere with their functioning; for example, Ben saw no problem in taking 40 minutes to brush his teeth—that way he could be sure he was doing it right. People with varying degrees of this disorder can indeed function despite it, or can be so impaired by it that they are mistakenly diagnosed as chronic schizophrenics.

Case Study 4: Dementia

A neighbor brought Mr. Warner, a 73-year-old retired schoolteacher, to the emergency room after he burned his fingers while cooking soup. She was in the habit of looking in on him every day. Although the soup he had been cooking had evaporated, the stove heat was still on beneath the pan. His home looked uncared for. She also noticed that lately his shirts were often not properly buttoned, as if he was having difficulty dressing himself. She thought maybe this was due to arthritis from getting old. All the same, there was no denying he was "different" from what he used to be. At times, he even seemed surprised when she showed up.

The burns were not serious. After his fingers

had been dressed, the physician—whom he struck as being confused and irritable—asked him some questions. He avoided questions about orientation and calculation that he could not answer. When asked the difference between an apple and an orange, he said simply that they were alike. When asked the date, he answered, "Oh, you know the date." When asked to count backward from 100 by threes—something he might be expected to be able to do, since he had been a math teacher—he stared blankly and said, "Don't bother me." He could not name any public figures in the news of late. When asked if he knew his own name, he replied, "Of course"—then began to stammer.

This is a case of primary degenerative dementia of the Alzheimer type (commonly called Alzheimer's disease or senile dementia), an organic mental disorder. It is remarkable for its cognitive impairments, memory deficit, and difficulty in getting dressed (dressing apraxia). A CAT scan of Mr. Warner's head revealed frontal cortical atrophy and widened cerebral sulci.

Case Study 5: Mania

A 28-year-old physician, Dr. Jeffers, was brought to the emergency room by a colleague who had noticed him, over the past 3 days, to be increasingly irritable and euphoric, with grandiose ideas. Dr. Jeffers' secretary mentioned that he had been phoning patients and strangers all over the world, claiming to have a cure for leukemia. He had been in this condition three times previously and had been hospitalized briefly each time. He was being treated with lithium but complained bitterly about needing this "crutch." Mostly he functioned quite well, although there were periods when he felt pessimistic, useless, and lethargic.

He had two siblings, who were doing well; his father committed suicide when he was 7. When his girlfriend arrived at the emergency room, she said that he had not slept for the past two nights, constantly requiring or demanding sex; that day he had phoned her at work to demand that they meet in a church to have "a hot time in the eyes of God."

This is a case of mania, and the symptoms include grandiosity, logorrhea, hypersexuality, insomnia, and euphoria. Manic patients are often hospitalized because their grandiosity and agitation bring them into conflict with others or with the authorities. Severe mania almost always requires in-patient hospital treatment.

Case Study 6: Panic Disorder with Agoraphobia

Dr. Williams, a 39-year-old pediatrician, sought psychiatric care because of debilitating anxiety attacks. He had always been "a little nervous." He was 25 when he had his first major anxiety attack; he suffered tachycardia and shortness of breath and feared he was having a heart attack—until a physical examination showed otherwise. Since that time, he had suffered a number of similar anxiety attacks. Of late, he had been restricting his activities because of them; for example, he was no longer willing to go sailing on his own, a favorite pastime of his, for fear he would be seized by anxiety and be unable to get back to shore.

He was happily married, with two children; no specific family problems brought on any of the anxiety attacks. He neither drank nor abused drugs and had no family history of serious psychiatric problems, although his mother was "a bit nervous."

This is a case of panic disorder with agoraphobia (or developing agoraphobia), one of the anxiety disorders.

Case Study 7: Borderline Personality Disorder

Nineteen-year-old Sandy came alone to the emergency room after having cut one wrist with a razor blade. She said, "I was so pissed off with my boyfriend, I couldn't stand it anymore. So I showed him." Her boyfriend of 4 months had announced that he was leaving her, saying he had had enough of her temperamental behavior.

Sandy had a history of tumultuous relationships from early in her adolescence, when she had an affair with a high school teacher and informed everyone of this affair when the teacher broke up with her. Shortly after that, she began drinking heavily and smoking marijuana and started having numerous affairs with older men in her community. She continued to do reasonably well in high school and even won a music scholarship to a local university. However, drinking and convictions for driving while in-toxicated had prevented her from starting classes the previous fall.

She said her mother had been hospitalized a number of times for depression, and her father was "nowhere to be found." She claimed that she often felt as if she were living in a test tube, and had made similarly self-destructive gestures previously "to get rid of the feeling."

This is a case of borderline personality disorder, a cluster B personality disorder. Such patients are notable for their quicksilver moods, intense interpersonal relationships, manipulative suicide attempts, self-destructive behavior, drinking and drug abuse, and contentious behaviors.

Case Study 8: Alcohol Amnestic Disorder

Slim Callahan, the 57-year-old retired major league baseball player, was hospitalized following a car accident in which he had been severely intoxicated. In the ensuing 2 weeks, he was treated for alcohol withdrawal. His symptoms cleared quickly; however, he remained somewhat confused. Physicians treating him noticed that he could not recall their names and appeared to be "out of it" on occasion. He was seen by a psychiatric consultant for memory impairment.

Slim, a happy-go-lucky sort of guy, could recall the batting averages of many of the most famous players of his era but was unable to give the date or time and could not remember the names of three objects for 5 minutes.

This is a case of alcohol amnestic disorder due to thiamine deficiency (also known as Korsakoff's syndrome), which is an alcohol-induced organic mental disorder, following an acute episode of Wernicke's encephalopathy, a neurologic disease manifested by confusion, ataxia, and nystagmus. This two-part disease is also known as Wernicke-Korsakoff syndrome. It is probably most common in men 40 to 60 years old. The prognosis is poor. Thiamine is the best treatment; it prevents progression but does not necessarily yield improvement. Recovery can occur over a period of months.

Chapter 22

Delirium and Dementia

Kenneth L. Davis, M.D., and Thomas B. Horvath, M.D.

A number of disorders of human experience and behavior are associated with abnormalities of the brain. These dementias and delirious states typically afflict the elderly and patients with multiple medical disorders. The numbers of such patients are increasing, leading to major public health problems.

Delirious states and dementias result from the temporary or permanent impairment of the function or structure of a significant number of neurons. Neurons are sensitive to reductions in energy supply or to any interference with the enzymes or cofactors in the oxidative cycle. The glial cells are essential for membrane transport and some metabolic pathways; changes in blood flow or cerebral edema can interfere with these functions. The electrical functions of the neuron depend on the excitability of the cell membrane, which is affected by energy supply, osmolality, electrolyte concentrations, and acid-base balance. The continuing disruption of the chemical milieu of the neuron, or the degeneration of its protein structure, will eventually lead to cell death.

Table 22–1 presents the abnormalities of the internal milieu that most commonly lead to neuronal dysfunction. In clinical situations multiple metabolic abnormalities are not uncommon.

DELIRIUM

Delirium is characterized by the rapid evolution of impaired attention and a fluctuating

TABLE 22–1. Physiological Abnormalities Leading to Neuronal Dysfunction

Oxygen, glucose, or blood-flow reduction
Thiamine, nicotinic acid, B_{12}, or folic acid deficiency
Water-electrolyte imbalance
Acidosis and carbon dioxide retention
Internal toxins, due to organ failures
External toxins, due to iatrogenic and industrial effects
Trauma
Immune reactions
Neuronal protein structural degeneration
Neurotransmitter disturbances

TABLE 22–2.   Diagnostic Criteria for Delirium

A. Reduced ability to maintain attention to external stimuli (e.g., questions must be repeated because attention wanders) and to appropriately shift attention to new external stimuli (e.g., perseverates answer to a previous question).

B. Disorganized thinking, as indicated by rambling, irrelevant, or incoherent speech.

C. At least two of the following:
   (1) reduced level of consciousness, e.g., difficulty keeping awake during examination
   (2) perceptual disturbances: misinterpretations, illusions, or hallucinations
   (3) disturbance of sleep-wake cycle with insomnia or daytime sleepiness
   (4) increased or decreased psychomotor activity
   (5) disorientation to time, place, or person
   (6) memory impairment, e.g., inability to learn new material, such as the names of several unrelated objects after five minutes, or to remember past events, such as history of current episode of illness

D. Clinical features develop over a short period of time (usually hours to days) and tend to fluctuate over the course of a day.

E. Either (1) or (2):
   (1) evidence from the history, physical examination, or laboratory tests of a specific organic factor (or factors) judged to be etiologically related to the disturbance
   (2) in the absence of such evidence, an etiologic organic factor can be presumed if the disturbance cannot be accounted for by any nonorganic mental disorder, e.g., Manic Episode accounting for agitation and sleep disturbance

---

Reprinted with permission from the *Diagnostic and Statistical Manual of Mental Disorders, Third Edition, Revised*. Copyright 1987 American Psychiatric Association.

state of awareness. The patient's perception, thinking, and memory are all disturbed to varying degrees. Delirium often presents with a disturbance of the wake-sleep cycle, with daytime drowsiness and nocturnal agitation. Later on, illusions and hallucinations develop in the waking state. Delusions are usually secondary to illusions and hallucinations and represent attempts to make sense of confusing and bizarre mental experiences. Some patients exhibit psychomotor overactivity and autonomic arousal, whereas others show stupor, apathy, and somnolence and progress toward a coma. Table 22–2 gives the diagnostic criteria for delirium.

Delirium is primarily a disturbance of the polysynaptic reticular formation and related structures subserving arousal and attention. Increasing evidence exists that reticular formation and hippocampal cholinergic transmission are impaired first in the course of many metabolic encephalopathies. The dorsal tegmental pathway from the mesencephalic reticular formation to the tectum and thalamus seems to be the site of action. Acetylcholine synthesis is easily disrupted by anoxia and related conditions. Physostigmine can improve the mental state in some deliria. Delirious states associated with alcohol withdrawal are complicated by a rebound hyperactivity of the locus coeruleus. Table 22–3 summarizes the predisposing causes of delirium, and Table 22–4 describes the precipitating causes.

TABLE 22–3.   Conditions that Predispose to Delirium

Advancing age and Alzheimer's changes
Brain injury, strokes, and trauma
Alcoholism: toxic, nutritional, traumatic, and hepatic problems
Diabetes: metabolic, osmolar, and vascular changes
Cardiac disease: cardiac failure, arrhythmia, medications
Cancer: metastases, endocrine, metabolic, and immune changes
Psychiatric illness: drug and overdose effects

TABLE 22–4.   Clinical Conditions that May Precipitate Delirium

---

Organ failures: respiratory, cardiac, hepatic, renal
Intoxication with, and withdrawal from, sedative drugs and alcohol
Systemic and intracranial infections
Head injury and its aftereffects
Endocrine disorders
Malnutrition

DEMENTIA

Dementia develops insidiously, often without a clear event marking the end of normal mental function. The person becomes forgetful and has difficulty coping with novel tasks. The person's emotional controls may be impaired, social judgment may be reduced, and personality changes may occur.

TABLE 22–5.   Diagnostic Criteria for Dementia

A. Demonstrable evidence of impairment in short- and long-term memory. Impairment in short-term memory (inability to learn new information) may be indicated by inability to remember three objects after five minutes. Long-term memory impairment (inability to remember information that was known in the past) may be indicated by inability to remember past personal information (e.g., what happened yesterday, birthplace, occupation) or facts of common knowledge (e.g., past Presidents, well-known dates).

B. At least one of the following:
   (1) impairment in abstract thinking, as indicated by inability to find similarities and differences between related words, difficulty in defining words and concepts, and other similar tasks
   (2) impaired judgment, as indicated by inability to make reasonable plans to deal with interpersonal, family, and job-related problems and issues
   (3) other disturbances of higher cortical function, such as aphasia (disorder of language), apraxia (inability to carry out motor activities despite intact comprehension and motor function), agnosia (failure to recognize or identify objects despite intact sensory function), and "constructional difficulty" (e.g., inability to copy three-dimensional figures, assemble blocks, or arrange sticks in specific designs)
   (4) personality changes, i.e., alteration or accentuation of premorbid traits

C. The disturbance in A and B significantly interferes with work or usual social activities or relationships with others.

D. Not occurring exclusively during the course of Delirium.

E. Either (1) or (2):
   (1) there is evidence from the history, physical examination, or laboratory tests of a specific organic factor (or factors) judged to be etiologically related to the disturbance
   (2) in the absence of such evidence, an etiologic organic factor can be presumed if the disturbance cannot be accounted for by any nonorganic mental disorder, e.g., Major Depression accounting for cognitive impairment

Criteria for severity of Dementia:

Mild: Although work or social activities are significantly impaired, the capacity for independent living remains, with adequate personal hygiene and relatively intact judgment.

Moderate: Independent living is hazardous, and some degree of supervision is necessary.

Severe: Activities of daily living are so impaired that continual supervision is required, e.g., unable to maintain minimal personal hygiene; largely incoherent or mute.

Reprinted with permission from the *Diagnostic and Statistical Manual of Mental Disorders, Third Edition, Revised*. Copyright 1987 American Psychiatric Association.

Failure in cognitive performance often results in anxiety, which in turn evokes a range of conscious coping strategies and unconscious psychological defense mechanisms. Common coping strategies include the avoidance of novelty, the restriction of activities, and the simplifications of complex tasks and performances. When these strategies fail to prevent failure, the defenses of denial, rationalization, projection (with paranoid ideas and delusion formation), and obsessions come into play.

Demented patients have a variable and incomplete perception of their cognitive failure. Some may show only shallow emotional responses to grave defects. In other patients the anxiety breaks through despite all the coping and defensive maneuvers. They manifest the familiar "fight-or-flight" response, with panic, agitation, or rage. If both flight and fight prove ineffective, the patient becomes hopeless or helpless, depressed, and immobile.

These reactions depend to some extent on the premorbid personality of the patient. Favorite character traits may be overemphasized; previously successful coping strategies are overused,

and often a caricature of the premorbid personality develops. However, in patients with lesions of the frontal and temporal lobes, radical personality alterations are seen that are the direct effect of the lesion on the biological substrates of planning, motivation, and emotional responsiveness.

Delusions are poorly organized and represent the patient's attempt to make some order among his or her conflicting and incoherent memories. Delusions of jealousy, with accusations of infidelity, are common; neighbors, relatives, and even family physicians may figure prominently in some delusional systems. If the disorder worsens, the delusions often become more fragmentary and disappear with the dissolution of other higher mental functions. The formal diagnostic criteria for dementia appear in Table 22–5.

Dementia is a failure of cortical and subcortical integrative mechanisms. At times, dementia is due to a patchwork of many small infarcts or the toxic effects of external poisons (alcohol, heavy metals) or internal metabolites (liver failure), but most commonly it is due to an idiopathic degeneration of neurons, often including, but not limited to, deterioration of the cholinergic neurons originating in the nucleus basalis. Table 22–6 lists the causes of dementia.

ALZHEIMER'S DISEASE

Alzheimer's disease, also termed senile dementia of the Alzheimer's type (SDAT), is the most common cause of dementia and the source of most rapid increases in knowledge in the last few years. Macroscopic examination of Alzheimer's disease brains shows ventricular dilation and cortical atrophy with widening of the sulci. Microscopic examinations show a characteristic combination of neural degeneration with neurofibrillary tangles, senile plaques, and granulovacuolar degeneration of some neurons.

The neurofibrillary tangles are twisted helical protein filaments, and their presence indicates disruption of distal axonal transport. They occur not only in Alzheimer's disease but also in the punch-drunk syndrome, Parkinson's-dementia syndrome of Guam, Pick's disease, and progressive supranuclear palsy.

Plaques, containing large quantities of amyloid-related protein, appear to be the debris produced by distal degeneration of neurons (terminal axons, synaptosomes), surrounded by microglia, astrocytes, and perivascular amyloid. Plaques are also seen in aged normal individuals, in middle-aged Down's syndrome patients, and in mice with scrapies (a viral disorder). The hippocampal Purkinje cells show a form of granulovacuolar degeneration. Plaques are most common in the hippocampus and are frequent in the neocortex. There is a good correlation between plaque density and intellectual decline.

These pathologic changes are quite different from those in other degenerative diseases leading to dementia. In Pick's disease, there are inclusion bodies in neurons from the frontal cortex. In Creutzfeldt-Jakob's disease, there is spongiform degeneration of neurons and swelling astrocytes. In Parkinson's disease and Huntington's chorea, the primary damage is to the basal ganglia: intracytoplasmic inclusion bodies and loss of dopamine neurons in the substantia nigra in the former, and neuronal loss in the caudate and putamen in the latter. Extrinsic metabolic disorders (anoxia and so on) lead to diffuse neuronal swelling.

In aging brains, atrophy is common but not inevitable. There is an age-related neuronal loss, but it is most prominent in the cerebellum, then in the caudate nucleus, and then in the inferior

TABLE 22–6.	Common Causes of Dementia
Degenerative	Alzheimer's disease
	Huntington's disease
	Parkinson's disease
Vascular	Multi-infarct dementia:
	Cortical distribution
	Sub-cortical lacunar syndrome
	Vascular imflammatory disease
Mechanical	Traumatic cerebral atrophy
	Normal pressure hydrocephalus
	Chronic subdural hematoma
Metabolic	Hypothyroidism
	Hypoglycemia
	Postanoxic encephalopathy
	Chronic hepatic encephalopathy
	Uremia
	Nonmetastatic effects of carcinoma
	B_{12} deficiency
Toxic	Alcoholic cerebral atrophy
	Chronic sedative intoxication
	Heavy metals
	Organic compounds
	Carbon monoxide
Infectious	Neurosyphilis
	Chronic meningitis
	AIDS encephalopathy
Neoplastic	Metastatic tumor
	Meningioma
	Glioma
	Pituitary tumor

olive. There is no age correlation with neurofibrillary tangles or granulovacuolar degeneration. The accumulation of lipofuscin is an age-related change, but it has no correlation with intellectual decline.

CAT Deficiency

Considerable neurochemical evidence indicates that Alzheimer's disease can be characterized as a primary degenerative condition of cholinergic terminals in the hippocampus and cortex. This defect is manifested in a marked loss of choline acetyltransferase (CAT) but relatively normal muscarinic receptor binding. CAT is an enzyme that assists in the manufacture of the neurotransmitter acetylcholine, which is important in memory and learning.

CAT deficiency has been positively correlated with mental test scores and senile plaque formation. Recent studies have indicated noradrenergic (locus coeruleus) and serotonergic (raphe nucleus) degeneration in a subpopulation of Alzheimer patients with a younger age of onset. Somatostatin and corticotropin releasing factor concentrations are also reduced in Alzheimer's disease. However, the vast majority of neurotransmitters and neuromodulators studied to date are apparently unchanged.

Cholinergic nerve terminals throughout the cortex and hippocampus have their cell bodies in the nucleus basalis, close to the septum. Consequently, it is not surprising that post mortem examination of late-stage patients with Alzheimer's disease often shows decreased numbers of cholinergic cells in the nucleus basalis. Cholinergic fibers also travel in the septohippocampal pathway. In the hippocampus, these interact with GABA and glutamate neurons. In turn, the cholinergic cells receive some input from noradrenergic locus coeruleus cells. Abnormalities in these neurotransmitter systems could obviously influence cholinergic transmission and possibly the symptoms of drug responsivity of the patient with Alzheimer's disease. For further information on neurotransmitters, see Chapter 8: Neurophysiological and Neurochemical Basis of Behavior. See also Chapter 9: Neurotransmitter Receptor Function.

The most consistent and persuasive evidence for a change in a neurotransmitter or neuromodulator in Alzheimer's disease is for acetylcholine. The central finding is a marked deficiency in CAT activity in the autopsied brains of patients with carefully diagnosed Alzheimer's disease. Numerous studies, including hundreds of patients, have all confirmed this abnormality. In part, the significance of a CAT deficiency is based on the fact that CAT is localized in cholinergic neurons and, as such, is a marker for the cholinergic neuron. Hence, a loss of CAT activity suggests a loss of cholinergic neurons.

General agreement exists that the most substantial reductions in CAT activity occur in the frontal and temporal cortex, as well as in the amygdala and hippocampus. These brain areas have been linked to learning and memory, suggesting a functional significance to the CAT deficiency in Alzheimer's disease. Equally important in implicating diminished CAT activity in the pathophysiology of Alzheimer's disease is the high correlation between a brain area's loss of CAT and the extent of its neurofibrillary tangles and senile plaques. Similarly, there is a significant correlation between CAT activity and mental test scores. Correlations between other post mortem neurotransmitter deficits and either histopathologic measurements or psychological assessment parameters have not yet been so robustly established.

Pharmacologic Studies

Pharmacologically induced alterations in central cholinergic activity produce profound changes in learning and memory. Substances that promote the activity of acetylcholine as a transmitter may positively affect performance in areas negatively affected by Alzheimer's disease. Conversely, substances that block acetylcholine as a transmitter may produce a condition similar to Alzheimer's disease.

Both scopolamine and atropine are antagonistic to the muscarinic cholinergic receptors of acetylcholine, and thus their presence interferes with acetylcholine's activity as a neurotransmitter. The cognitive effects of scopolamine have been studied by a number of investigators. Inevitably, the first cognitive effect noted after the administration of scopolamine is an inability to learn new information and encode it into long-term memory. Atropine had cognitive effects that closely resembled those of scopolamine. Scopolamine produces memory deficits in normal young subjects that did not significantly differ from those of a group of Alzheimer patients between the ages of 65 and 85. Thus, blocking central muscarinic cholinergic transmission produces one of the core symptoms of Alzheimer's disease—a difficulty in learning new information. However, scopolamine does not produce other of the cardinal symptoms of Alzheimer's disease, such as the aphasia, disorientation, or apraxia, as readily as it affects new learning, suggesting that the symptoms of Alzheimer's disease cannot be explained solely as a manifestation of a hypocholinergic state. See Chapter 2: Learning and Memory.

Very low doses of cholinergic agents that increase cholinergic activity—either the acetylcholinesterase inhibitor physostigmine or the muscarinic receptor agonist arecoline—also enhance the ability of normal young subjects to learn new information. Hence, cholinomimetics and anticholinergic agents, in a narrow dose range, have opposite effects upon learning of information that exceeds short-term memory.

Animal Studies

Data on the effects of cholinergic compounds upon cognitive performance in nonhuman primates are consistent with those of human studies. Scopolamine produced a specific inability of the monkeys to learn new material. This deficit could be corrected by physostigmine but not by amphetamine. Indeed, amphetamine worsened the performance of scopolamine-treated monkeys. Most noteworthy is the fact that whereas young monkeys consistently respond to a specific dose of physostigmine with an enhancement of learning, the response of aged monkeys is far less predictable. Although physostigmine generally improves performance on various learning tasks in aged monkeys, the doses that produce this effect vary from animal to animal.

The induction of a hypocholinergic state in rodents by a specific lesion of the nucleus basalis with an excitotoxin has been readily accomplished. Such animals display a problem in learning and retaining new information, although they appear relatively normal in most other behaviors. To the degree that Alzheimer's disease is a hypocholinergic condition, the animal with a nucleus basalis lesion is a useful model.

Summary

The following is the evidence that a cholinergic deficit is pathophysiologically involved in Alzheimer's disease.

1. There is undoubtedly a CAT deficit in the brains of patients with Alzheimer's disease.
2. The CAT deficit includes brain areas involved in the behavioral disturbances associated with Alzheimer's disease.
3. The CAT deficit correlates with the histopathologic and psychological changes in Alzheimer's disease.
4. A pharmacologically induced diminution in central cholinergic activity produces a learning deficit that is similar to the learning deficit in Alzheimer's disease.
5. Cholinomimetic agents enhance learning in young normal subjects.

Although other neurotransmitters or neuromodulators are deficient in some patients with Alzheimer's disease—particularly norepinephrine, somatostatin, serotonin, and corticotropin releasing factor—none have yet been implicated so extensively in the symptoms of the illness as acetylcholine. It would seem extremely likely that any pharmacotherapy of Alzheimer's disease would have to attempt to increase cholinergic activity, although the ultimate pharmacotherapy for the disease will undoubtedly have to reverse other deficits as well, some of which at this point may be unknown.

THERAPEUTIC STRATEGIES IN ALZHEIMER'S DISEASE

Despite the clear direction to future pharmacological studies provided by the neurochemical, pathological, and pharmacological investigations reviewed above, the development of potential therapeutic agents for Alzheimer's disease is substantially impaired by the paucity of cholinomimetic agents for human use. Basically, there are three approaches to enhancing central cholinergic activity:

Approach	Site
Increasing synthesis and release of acetylcholine	Presynaptic cholinergic neuron
Inhibiting breakdown of acetylcholine	Synapse
Stimulating the cholinergic receptor	Postsynaptic receptor

A strategy to increase cholinergic activity that relies exclusively upon presynaptic cholinergic neurons is likely to be limited by the progressive degeneration and subsequent loss of these neurons in Alzheimer's disease. Unless remaining cholinergic neurons have a substantial ability to compensate for the loss of surrounding cholinergic neurons, a therapeutic intervention dependent upon intact and functioning cholinergic neurons can be flawed. Thus, this approach would seem best suited for patients with early, mild to moderate Alzheimer's disease.

Increasing Synthesis and Release of Acetylcholine

Attempts to enhance cholinergic activity and improve the symptoms of Alzheimer's disease through the administration of the acetylcholine precursors choline and phosphatidylcholine have not been particularly successful. Attention has shifted to the use of releasing agents, of which 4-aminopyridine is the prototype. Trials of this agent in patients with Alzheimer's disease have not yet yielded impressive results, although hints of clinical improvement have been reported. The possibility has been raised that the combination of cholinergic precursors with releasing agents may prove more efficacious than either alone, since precursors are best able to increase cholinergic activity under conditions in which the cholinergic neuron is rapidly firing. Such a circumstance of enhanced firing could be envisioned following the administration of a releasing agent like 4-aminopyridine.

Inhibiting Breakdown of Acetylcholine

Inhibition of the breakdown of synaptic acetylcholine is the second basic approach to augmenting central cholinergic activity. This approach, like the presynaptic strategy, is dependent on an intact presynaptic neuron. However, unlike the precursor approach, the acetylcholinesterase inhibitor does not require the presynaptic neuron to augment the synthesis of acetylcholine, a condition that may not readily be attained. Furthermore, acetylcholinesterase inhibition has the benefit of increasing activity at both nicotinic and muscarinic cholinergic receptors. Since there is some evidence implicating nicotinic activity in cognition, there is an obvious advantage to a nonspecific agent.

Experimental alterations of cholinesterase activity always occur in the direction of diminishing kinetics, that is, no interventions are capable of increasing the activity of this extraordinarily efficient enzymatic system. Thus, interventions employ anticholinesterase compounds that covalently interact with the enzyme, much like acetylcholine, in a reversible or irreversible way. Characteristic pharmacological effects of these inhibitors are due primarily to the prevention of acetylcholine hydrolysis at cholinergic sites. The prototype carbamate, physostigmine, is representative of reversible inhibitors, which have had the most extensive clinical evaluation in movement disorders and neuropsychiatric syndromes, including Alzheimer's disease. However, physostigmine's relatively short duration of action in humans renders it less desirable therapeutically in the long-term treatment of nonfluctuating clinical conditions such as Alzheimer's disease.

Tetrahydroaminoacridine (THA) is a competitive acetylcholinesterase inhibitor with a longer half-life than intermediate physostigmine. The major advantages of THA are that it exists in an oral preparation and produces minimal peripheral side effects at doses that are centrally active. However, aminoacridines are associated with hepatotoxicity, a problem that can substantially diminish their utility.

The synaptic approach to the potential therapeutics of Alzheimer's disease has been a difficult one to test. Physostigmine has been far more extensively studied than the aminoacridines. Results with physostigmine indicate that a proportion of patients have a modest, but clinically significant, improvement on the drug. However, erratic plasma levels, secondary to hydrolases that destroy physostigmine, have undoubtedly contributed to lack of efficacy in some patients.

The effects of THA on patients with Alzheimer's disease are now under intensive investigation.

Stimulating the Cholinergic Receptor

The third approach to augmenting central cholinergic activity is by direct stimulation of the postsynaptic cholinergic receptor. Since muscarinic receptor binding sites are not reduced in patients with Alzheimer's disease beyond what apparently occurs in normal aging, this at first seems to be a particularly promising option. However, closer examination reveals potential problems. It is unclear whether cholinergic agonists would produce an effect that is physiologically equivalent to the effect of acetylcholine released by a functionally intact cholinergic neuron. Thus, if the basis of cholinergic transmission is episodic or phasic, it is uncertain if the tonic effects of pharmacologically induced cholinergic agonism would be at all equivalent.

Yet other problems exist with the receptor agonist strategy. Five distinct subtypes of muscarinic receptors have been identified through molecular techniques. At present, pharmacological agonists do not have as much specificity as exists on a molecular level in the brain. Until more precise pharmacological probes are available, existing cholinergic agonists may stimulate receptors that will either not enhance or perhaps adversely affect cognitive functioning.

Finally, there is the conceptual problem of "receptor mismatches." In the case of peptidergic neurotransmitters, it is clear that receptors exist in areas not innervated by presynaptic sites releasing such neurotransmitters. Possibly a similar situation exists for cholinergic receptors; if such is the case, cholinergic receptors would exist that, under normal conditions, would not be stimulated. However, with the administration of a cholinergic agonist, these otherwise inactive receptors become stimulated, with unpredictable effects on behavior.

Perhaps these difficulties with the postsynaptic strategy account for the fact that trials with cholinergic agonist have not produced very robust effects in patients with Alzheimer's disease. Trials with bethanechol, administered through an intraventricular shunt, and the study of oxotremorine and RS86 have produced discouraging results.

Future Strategies

Alzheimer's disease is much more than simply a cholinergic deficit. Deficiencies in corticotropin releasing factor and somatostatin seem to be rather common, and abnormalities in concentrations of serotonin and norepinephrine, particularly in younger patients, are frequently encountered. The net effect on behavior that these various neurotransmitter and neuromodulator deficits produce has not been determined. Furthermore, there is a very real possibility that the efficacy of a cholinergic approach can be substantially altered by the addition of another deficient neurotransmitter. For example, performance deficits produced in rodents after a lesion of the nucleus basalis are reversed to a level of performance equivalent to that of nonlesioned animals by a variety of cholinergic drugs. Yet the addition of a locus coeruleus lesion to the nucleus basalis lesion virtually eliminates the efficacy of a cholinergic approach. When a noradrenergic agent is added to a cholinergic drug in animals with lesions of both the nucleus basalis and locus coeruleus, the animals' behavior is once again normalized. It would not be surprising if a similar circumstance exists in the Alzheimer's patient with a noradrenergic problem in addition to the cholinergic deficit. If this is so, an important future direction for the therapeutics of Alzheimer's disease will be the administration of multiple drugs to reverse more than simply the cholinergic deficit.

Trophic factors are a series of peptides that have the capacity to enhance growth in various tissues. Nerve growth factor has a particular predilection for enhancing the activity of cholinergic neurons; it has been isolated from a number of locations and has profound effects on cells in the nucleus basalis and in the septum. Since these cell groups are undoubtedly affected in Alzheimer's disease, it has been suggested that a derangement in trophic factor metabolism may contribute to Alzheimer's neuropathology. Nerve growth factor and related compounds also provide an alternative approach to the therapeutics of Alzheimer's disease. Animal models suggest that the behavioral and neurochemical consequences of lesions in the septal hippocampal region or the nucleus basalis can be partially reversed by treatment with nerve growth factor. This work may be extended to humans in the future.

MULTIINFARCT DEMENTIA

After Alzheimer's disease, multiinfarct dementia is the second most common cause of dementia. It not uncommonly coexists with Alzheimer's disease. Like Alzheimer's disease, it follows an inevitable downhill course, often ending in a vegetative state.

Multiinfarct dementia is differentiated from Alzheimer's disease by its history and concomitant symptoms. Symptoms of vascular disease, both within and outside the brain, are a usual aspect of multiinfarct dementia. Patients may have focalizing neurological signs, a past or recent history of transient ischemic episodes, hypertension, and cerebrovascular disease. The Hachinski scale is often used to facilitate the diagnosis of multiinfarct dementia. The scale is a categorization of those symptoms and signs whose presence increases the confidence a clinician can have in the diagnosis of multiinfarct dementia.

No therapeutic interventions for the treatment of multiinfarct dementia have proven efficacious. However, the vascular nature of this condition leads to a number of theoretical implications. For example, if the predisposing conditions leading to cerebral infarcts can be diminished, it is conceivable that the progression of dementia can be slowed, if not stopped. Thus, one looks forward to carefully designed studies to determine if antihypertensives, aspirin, or other pharmacological agents that can enhance cerebrovascular circulation or decrease the propensity for thrombotic or embolic episodes will alter the course of this disease.

FOCAL NEUROPSYCHOLOGICAL SYNDROMES

Amnestic Syndrome

Amnestic syndrome was first described by S.S. Korsakoff in malnourished alcoholics and is characterized by an inability to retain new memories for longer than a few minutes. Other cognitive functions are surprisingly well preserved, but patients appear to lack initiative or personal depth. Confabulations have been traditionally regarded as an important part of the syndrome and arise both from attempts to fill the gaps in memory and from faulty temporal sequencing of recalled memories. Perceptual changes, mild cognitive difficulties, and temporal disorientations may occur, and the patient's mood is often apathetic.

The amnestic syndrome is an excellent example of neurological localization. The common denominator is the bilateral interruption of the hippocampal-fornix-septal-mammillo-thalamic Papez or Vinogradia circuit. Common causes are thiamine deficiency, head injury, vertebrobasilar ischemia, and viral encephalopathy.

Organic Personality Syndrome

Alterations in personality style pose some of the most difficult diagnostic dilemmas. The subject frequently remains oblivious to behavioral changes and responds angrily to the complaints of family members. A careful history obtained from several reliable sources is more revealing than a mental-state examination. Diagnostic features include loss of emotional control, impaired foresight, and coarsening of social instincts. Frontal lobe lesions are associated with the loss of planning ability, loss of emotional control, and loss of social judgment. Temporal lobe irritative lesions seem to deepen emotional responses of all kinds and lead to strong mystical or religious feelings.

The organic personality syndrome at times represents the earliest presentation of other mental syndromes, and, with time, other neurological defects develop; this may be the case with general paresis, alcoholism, and Pick's disease, and with space-occupying lesions. For physicians the main danger is to interpret the personality change in entirely psychodynamic terms and thus miss an early diagnosis of a potentially reversible lesion.

Organic Delusional Syndrome

The mental state of some organic patients can be consistent with the presentation of schizophrenia, but their family history is negative for schizophrenia, and the premorbid personality and social adjustment are usually quite normal. These phenocopies of schizophrenia had dopamine hyperactivity or nucleus accumbens limbic overactivation or both as their common denominator.

Organic Affective Syndrome

Depressive moods commonly accompany all types of organic and functional mental disorders and represent an understandable response to the loss of mental capacities. In a number of cases the dysphoric mood and the associated symptoms of weight loss, sleep disturbances, and so forth develop in a clear relationship to an organic disturbance of brain function. Often there is no significant cognitive impairment. The syndrome is to be distinguished from the so-called depressive pseudodementia, in which the mental state appears to show cognitive deterioration, as well as depression, but in which medical investigation fails to locate an organic abnormality, and the mental state improves upon the treatment of the depression.

Organic affective syndromes emphasize the correlation between vegetative symptoms in affective disorders and hypothalamic malfunction.

TABLE 22–7. Common Causes of Organic Brain Syndromes with Selective Psychological Deficits

Amnestic syndrome	Wernicke-Korsakoff syndrome
	Bilateral hippocampal infarction
	Trauma to base of brain
	Subarachnoid hemorrhage with basal organization
	Tuberculous meningitis
	Carbon monoxide poisoning
	Herpes simplex encephalitis
	Tumors of third ventricle
	Early Alzheimer's disease
	Transient global amnesia
Hallucinosis	Psychedelic drug ingestion and "flashbacks"
	Chronic alcoholic auditory hallucinosis
	Brain tumor, especially in occipital and temporal areas
	Epilepsy
	Sensory deprivation
	Deafness and/or blindness
Organic personality syndrome	Early manifestation of a dementia, especially alcoholic, GPI, Pick's
	Frontal lobe tumors or injury
	Temporal lobe epilepsy
	Pseudobulbar syndrome
Organic delusional syndrome	Amphetamine psychosis
	Multiple drug abuse
	Temporal lobe epilepsy (especially in interictal period)
	Any cause of delirium or dementia
Organic affective syndrome	Cushing's syndrome, excessive steroids
	Amphetamine and cocaine withdrawal
	Reserpine, alpha-methyldopa
	Systemic viral illness, especially hepatitis
	Pancreatic carcinoma
	Any cause of delirium or dementia

They also draw attention to certain noradrenergic, medial forebrain bundle–related reinforcement and reward areas.

Table 22–7 lists the common causes of organic
brain syndromes with selective psychological
deficits.

Focal Cognitive or Psychomotor Defects

The apraxias, agnosias, and dysphasias traditionally belong to neurology. A psychiatric assessment needs to include them, however, for
two reasons: (1) they appear in advanced dementias, and (2) they may be mistaken for hysterical conversion reactions or for bizarre
psychotic behaviors. Occasionally a focal neurological sign can also be used as a sensitive
index of a generalized metabolic disturbance, as
when the severity of constructional apraxia indicates the extent of early hepatic encephalopathy. For information on apraxias, agnosias, and
aphasias, see Chapter 4: Higher Cortical Processes.

BIBLIOGRAPHY

Cummings, J.L., Benson, D.F.: Dementia: A Clinical Approach, Boston, Butterworths, 1983.
Horvath, T.B.: Organic brain syndromes, in Psychiatry for
the Primary Care Physician, Baltimore, Williams & Wil-
kins, 1979.
Horvath, T.B., et al.: Organic mental syndromes and disorders, in Comprehensive Textbook of Psychiatry, ed. 5,
H.I. Kaplan, B.J. Sadock (eds.). Baltimore, Williams &
Wilkins, 1989.
Katzman, R., Terry, R.: The Neurology of Aging. Philadelphia, F.A. Davis, 1983.
Lipowski, Z.J.: Delirium: Acute Brain Failure in Man. Philadelphia, F.A.Davis, 1988.
Mc Candless, D.W.: Cerebral Energy Metabolism and Metabolic Encephalopathy. New York, Plenum Press, 1985.
Mohs, R.C., Davis, K.L.: The experimental pharmacology
of Alzheimer's disease and related dementias, in Psycho-
pharmacology: The Third Generation of Progress, H.Y.
Meltzer (ed.). New York, Raven Press, 1987.
Perl, D.B., Pendlebury, W.W.: Neuropathology of Alzheimer's disease and related dementias, in Psychopharmacology: The Third Generation of Progress, H.Y. Meltzer
(ed.). New York, Raven Press, 1987.
Perry, E.K.: Cortical neurotransmitter chemistry in Alzheimer's disease, in Psychopharmacology: The Third Generation of Progress, H.Y. Meltzer (ed.). New York, Raven
Press, 1987.
Terry, R.D.: Aging and the Brain. New York, Raven Press,
1988.

Chapter 23

Pathophysiology of Pain

Philip Kanof, M.D., Ph.D.

Pain is more than a simple perception of an unpleasant or noxious sensory stimulus. The experience of pain may be divided into three parts: (1) nociception—the recognition and signaling of a deleterious stimulus (for example, tissue injury); (2) pain—the conscious awareness of the nociceptive event; and (3) suffering—the emotional and behavioral sequelae of pain.

NEUROANATOMY OF PAIN PERCEPTION

The perception of pain begins with its own sensory apparatus. Finely branched free nerve endings are present in the skin as well as in the tissues of many internal organs. These nerve endings are supplied by a nerve cell body located in the dorsal root ganglion of the spinal cord. A single dorsal root ganglion cell may supply the pain sensory fibers covering several square millimeters of skin. When the nerve endings are excited, impulses are sent along the sensory axon and enter the dorsal horn of the spinal cord through the posterior root.

Pain fibers are composed of two morphologically distinct types: A-delta fibers and C-fibers (Fig. 23–1).

A-Delta Fibers

A-delta fibers are 6 to 8 μm in diameter, are myelinated, and conduct impulses at 5 to 30 m/s. They enter the spinal cord primarily through the medial aspect of the dorsal root. Some fibers project to the ventral root, where they mediate certain spinal reflexes associated with pain. Most fibers synapse onto the cell bodies of secondary sensory cells located in the dorsal horn of the spinal cord, and some ascend in the posterior column of the spinal cord to synapse in the medulla. A-delta fibers are thought to mediate sharp, prickly pain.

C-Fibers

C-fibers are to 2 to 4 μm in diameter, are unmyelinated, and conduct impulses at 0.5 to

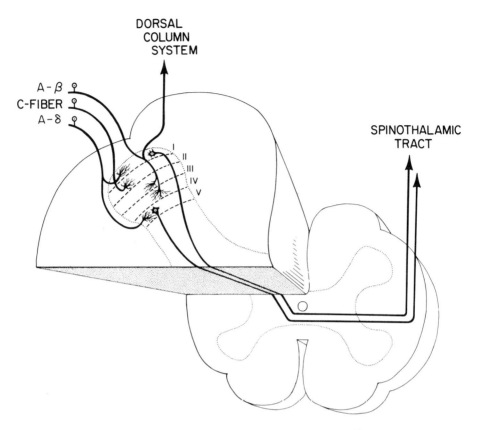

FIGURE 23–1. Dorsal root nociceptive afferents. (From Maciewicz, R., Fields, H.L.: Pain pathways, in *Diseases of the Nervous System: Clinical Neurobiology*, A.K. Asbury, G.M. McKhann, and W.I. McDonald (eds.). Philadelphia, Saunders, 1986)

2 m/s. They enter the spinal cord primarily through the lateral aspect of the posterior root. Most fibers travel through the substantia gelatinosa and synapse on the cell bodies of secondary sensory neurons in the dorsal horn; some are also involved in spinal reflexes. C-fibers are thought to mediate slow burning pain.

Lateral Neospinothalamic Tract

The cell bodies of secondary sensory neurons lie in the dorsal horn of the spinal cord and give rise to two ascending pain pathways: the lateral neospinothalamic tract and the paleospinothalamic tract.

In the lateral neospinothalamic tract, cell bodies in the dorsal horn send out axons, most of which decussate and ascend in pathways on the contralateral side. These axons give off collateral projections throughout the medulla, pons, and midbrain but terminate mainly in the ventral posterolateral nucleus of the thalamus (Fig. 23–2). From these thalamic nuclei, tertiary neurons project to the parietal cortex (mainly the secondary sensory cortex). The lateral neospinothalamic tract is thought to provide information concerning pain localization and intensity.

Paleospinothalamic Tract

The paleospinothalamic tract is a more primitive pain pathway. Cell bodies in the dorsal horn send out axons that also decussate and ascend on the contralateral side. These axons give off collateral projections to the reticular activating system in the midbrain and terminate mainly in the intralaminar and parafascicular nuclei of the thalamus. From these thalamic nuclei, there are tertiary projections to the limbic system. The paleospinothalamic tract is thought to be involved in arousal and in the emotional responses to pain.

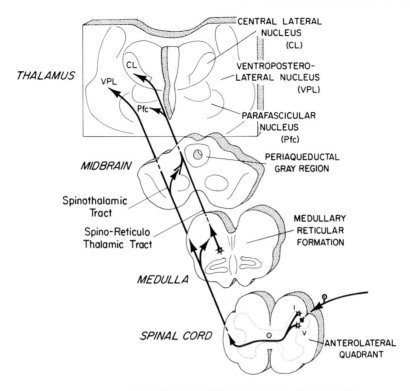

FIGURE 23–2.   Ascending nociceptive pathways. (From Maciewicz, R., Fields, H.L.: Pain pathways, in Diseases of the Nervous System: Clinical Neurobiology, A.K. Asbury, G.M. McKhann, and W.I. McDonald (eds.). Philadelphia, Saunders, 1986)

CHEMICAL MEDIATORS OF PAIN

The finely branching nerve endings present in the skin and internal organs "sense" pain when tissue injury is produced. A wide variety of chemical mediators may be released in tissue injury. These include prostaglandins, histamine, and bradykinin. These mediators depolarize the nerve endings, leading to the generation of an action potential along the axon of the primary sensory afferent neuron. Subcutaneous injection of any of the above putative mediators is perceived as pain. The analgesic actions of acetylsalicylic acid and other nonsteroidal antiinflammatory drugs may be due to their ability to inhibit the enzyme prostaglandin synthetase, thus blocking the ability of prostaglandins to be produced in response to tissue injury. Injection of high concentrations of potassium ion also depolarizes the nerve endings of pain fibers and is perceived as pain. This may be of physiological relevance; when severe tissue injury occurs, cells are destroyed, and the high concentrations of potassium that exist intracellularly leak out and are available to depolarize nerve endings.

Some afferent pain fibers synapsing onto cells in the dorsal root of the spinal cord use substance P as the neurotransmitter. Substance P is a peptide containing 11 amino acids. When afferent pain fibers are activated, substance P is released and depolarizes the cell bodies in the dorsal horn of the spinal cord, giving rise to the ascending spinothalamic pain tracts. Intrathecal injection of the neurotoxin capsaicin into animals causes degeneration of the neurons containing substance P. This results in a significant increase in the pain threshold observed in these animals. A selective antagonist of substance P at its receptor sight might be of great clinical value as an analgesic agent. See also Substance P in Chapter 10: Neuropeptides.

MODULATORY PATHWAYS AFFECTING PAIN PERCEPTION

It is well known that the perception of pain can be influenced by a wide variety of experiences, including affective state, stress, and the experience of pain in other parts of the body.

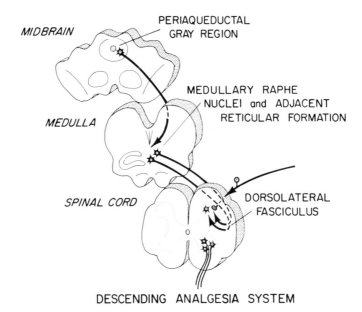

FIGURE 23–3..   Descending analgesia system. (From Maciewicz, R., Fields, H.L.: Pain pathways, in Diseases of the Nervous System: Clinical Neurobiology, A.K. Asbury, G.M. McKhann, and W.I. McDonald (eds.). Philadelphia, Saunders, 1986)

The anatomy and physiology of descending pathways involved in the modulation of pain perception have been clarified recently.

Periaqueductal Gray Matter

The periaqueductal gray matter in the midbrain is a key area for pain control. Electrical stimulation of this area in animals or humans specifically produces an analgesic effect, without altering the perception of other types of sensation, motor function, arousal, or motivation (Fig. 23–3). In humans, analgesia does not occur until 5 to 15 minutes after the onset of stimulation; however, analgesia may be long lasting, persisting up to 24 hours after stimulation is stopped.

The observation that the opiate antagonist naloxone blocks the analgesia produced by periaqueductal gray matter stimulation strongly indicates that endogenous opiates are involved in this process. The periaqueductal gray matter is known to have a high concentration of opiate receptors and of endogenous opiates. Enkephalins are present in small interneurons in this region (Fig. 23–4), while β-endorphin is present in nerve endings that originate from cells in the arcuate nucleus of the hypothalamus. Stimulation of the periaqueductal gray matter causes the release of these endogenous opiates locally

(where they may act as neurotransmitters), as well as into the cerebrospinal fluid (where, by diffusion, they may exert effects on distant neurons, thus acting as neuromodulators). One important site of action of the endogenous opiates is the nucleus raphe magnus. Cell bodies of this nucleus give rise to a descending serotonergic pathway. The axons of this pathway go through the dorsolateral funiculus and end on enkephalinergic interneurons present in the substantia gelatinosa. This descending pathway appears to mediate analgesia produced by periaqueductal gray matter stimulation. Impairing its function (either by surgical transection of the dorsolateral funiculus or by causing depletion of serotonin levels through the use of the tryptophan hydroxylase inhibitor parachlorophenylalanine) greatly attenuates the degree of analgesia produced by periaqueductal gray matter stimulation.

See Serotonin in Chapter 8: Neurophysiological and Neurochemical Basis of Behavior.

Enkephalins

The enkephalinergic interneurons in the substantia gelatinosa terminate on the presynaptic nerve terminals of the afferent primary sensory neurons. When this interneuron fires (perhaps after an excitatory stimulus from the seroto-

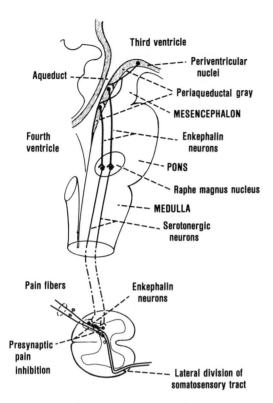

FIGURE 23–4. Analgesia system of brainstem and spinal cord, showing inhibition of incoming pain signals at cord level. (From Guyton, A.C.: Basic Neuroscience: Anatomy and Physiology. Philadelphia, Saunders, 1987)

nergic pathway originating in the nucleus raphe magnus), enkephalins are released and act at opiate receptors present on the substance P–containing presynaptic nerve terminal. The net functional effect of the enkephalin is to decrease the amount of substance P released from the afferent sensory nerve terminal.

Thus, the release of substance P may be governed by two distinct factors: (1) the intensity of the original stimulus (as coded for by the frequency of action potential firing along the pain afferent sensory fiber) and (2) the degree of presynaptic inhibition of substance P release by enkephalin (governed in part by the descending modulatory pain pathways). Therefore, a lowering of the perception of pain may result either from a decrease in the pain stimulus intensity (proportional to the action potential frequency of the afferent sensory fibers) or by an increase in the inhibitory tone of the descending modulatory pathways.

The actions of these modulatory pathways explain in part the analgesic actions of two other classes of drugs: opiates and antidepressants.

Opiates

Exogenous opiates act at several loci involved in pain perception. Through their activation of opiate receptors on the presynaptic nerve terminals of the substance P–containing afferent sensory fibers, opiates decrease the amount of substance P released per nerve impulse. Opiates also act at receptors in the periaqueductal gray matter, activating the descending serotonergic pathway involved in modulating synaptic function in the dorsal horn of the spinal cord. In addition, opiates act at receptor sites in the limbic system and may be involved in altering the affective and behavioral responses to pain.

Tricyclic Antidepressant Drugs

Certain tricyclic antidepressant drugs, such as amitriptyline, are effective in the treatment of certain chronic pain syndromes. One biochemical action of these drugs is their ability to potentiate the synaptic actions of serotonin by blocking its reuptake into the presynaptic nerve terminal. Thus, in the presence of amitriptyline, released serotonin stays in the vicinity of the synaptic cleft longer than usual and may produce greater excitation of enkephalinergic interneurons, leading to a decrease in substance P release.

DIFFERENT PAIN TYPES

The enormous variety of ways in which patients describe pain clearly indicates that it is a mistake to think of pain as a single sensation with a single neuroanatomical or neurochemical basis. It is clinically useful to distinguish between two types of pain: pain resulting from tissue injury and deafferentation pain.

Tissue Injury Pain

Pain resulting from tissue injury may have diverse clinical characteristics, ranging from sharp, knifelike pain to dull aches or burning sensations (Fig. 23–5). The way this pain is perceived depends on the types of receptors located in the organ injured, the type of injury, the time course of production of the injury, and the types of chemical mediators involved. The anatomical and neurochemical basis of this type of pain was outlined above. As one would predict, this pain may be abolished by section of the posterior

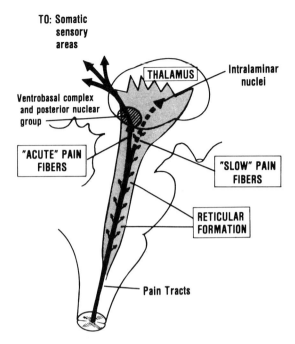

FIGURE 23–5. Transmission of pain signals into hindbrain, thalamus, and cortex via "pricking pain" pathway and "burning pain" pathway. (From Guyton, A.C.: Basic Neuroscience. Anatomy and Physiology. Philadelphia, Saunders, 1987)

nerve roots involved or by stereotaxic lesions of the neospinothalamic tracts. Lesions of the ventral posterolateral nucleus of the thalamus cause loss of cutaneous sharp touch or pinprick on the contralateral side but leave deep pain unaffected. Lesions of the intralaminar nuclei of the thalamus relieve chronic deep pain effectively without impairing sharp touch or pinprick. Pain resulting from tissue injury can often be blocked almost completely by periaqueductal gray matter stimulation or by administration of adequate doses of narcotic analgesics. Tricyclic antidepressants are also useful as an adjunct to other analgesics. Clearly, the clinician has many options for relieving pain, no matter how severe, when it results from tissue injury.

Deafferentation Pain

Deafferentation pain is often described as an episodic, sharp, lancinating, radiating pain that is associated with a chronic injury to the primary sensory afferent nerve. Examples include phantom limb pain, postherpetic neuralgia, and the pain of tic douloureux. The course of an episode of pain is unpredictable. This type of pain is sometimes precipitated by a trivial stimulus (for example, touching the injured area precipitates an attack of pain lasting for hours) and is sensitive to affective state (for example, it may be aggravated by fatigue or anxiety). Electrophysiological studies in nerve trunks from affected areas suggest that this pain may be associated with spontaneous electrical discharges in injured sensory afferents. This may be one reason that antiepileptic drugs, such as diphenylhydantoin or carbamazepine, are often quite effective in treating this type of pain.

The anatomical and neurochemical basis of deafferentation pain is poorly understood. In contrast to pain due to tissue injury, this type of pain is only partially responsive to narcotic analgesics and is not relieved by periaqueductal gray matter stimulation. Tricyclic antidepressants are ineffective. Lesions of the ventral posterolateral or intralaminar nuclei of the thalamus are also ineffective. However, lesions of the posteromedial and pulvinar nuclei of the thalamus, as well as to certain parts of the limbic system (amygdala, cingulate cortex), have been helpful. In fact, relief of severe intractable deafferentation pain is one of the few accepted indications for the psychosurgical procedure of cingulotomy (the bilateral destruction of the anterior portions of the cingulate gyrus and bundle). Patients who have undergone this procedure often report that they still feel the pain but that their degree of suffering is greatly diminished. Pain threshold has been shown to be unaltered in patients following cingulotomy. Deafferentation pain is a common type of pain seen in patients with a variety of chronic pain syndromes, and the clinician's options in treating such patients remain limited.

BIBLIOGRAPHY

Basbaum, A.I., Fields, M.L.: Endogenous pain control systems: Brainstem spinal pathways and endorphin circuitry. Annu. Rev. Neurosci. 7:309-338, 1984.
Davar, G., Maciewicz, R.J.: Deafferentation pain syndromes. Neurol. Clin. 7:289-304, 1989.
Hoffert, M.J.: The neurophysiology of pain. Neurol. Clin. 7:183-203, 1989.
Leah, J., Menetrey, D.: Neuropeptides in propriospinal neurons in the rat. Brain Res. 495:173-177, 1989.
Payne, R.: Cancer pain: Anatomy, physiology and pharmacology. Cancer 63:2266-2274, 1989.
Portenoy, R.K.: Mechanisms of clinical pain: Observations and speculations. Neurol. Clin. 7:205-230, 1989.
Watkins, L.R., Mayer, D.J.: Organization of endogenous opiate and nonopiate pain control systems. Science 216:1185-1192, 1982.

Chapter 24

Drug and Alcohol Dependency

Leonard Handelsman, M.D.

It has never been an easy matter for student physicians to develop an empathic and knowledgeable approach to patients with alcohol or drug dependency, even though physicians are often called on to care for such patients. The AIDS epidemic, which particularly affects intravenous drug users, only highlights this problem for physicians. In contrast to the situation with other disorders, attitudes toward addiction are often consolidated before medical training and may be influenced profoundly by the student's direct experience with addiction in his or her family, by religious and ideological beliefs, or by the student's own pattern of substance use.

As is the case with most chronic illnesses, it is difficult for the student physician training on acute care wards to grasp the long view of alcohol or drug dependency disorders. Faced with a patient whose disorder was self-initiated and whose daily behavior flies in the face of common sense, many physicians lapse into a moral, rather than a clinical, view of the problem. The moral view has two basic forms. The first labels the addict as an inferior patient; the second explains

away the addiction as an inevitable consequence of overwhelming psychosocial stress. Neither of these moral views addresses the core of the addictive process, which is the repetitive self-administration of psychoactive substances in the face of negative consequences.

This chapter provides an orientation to the phenomenology of addiction and to behavioral pharmacological concepts essential to understanding the rationale for pharmacological treatments. In doing so, this approach leaves aside artificially psychosocial concepts of pathogenesis and treatment. Certainly, addiction could not be maintained without suitable agricultural practices, complex marketing structures, or subcultural value systems; nor would it be possible to treat an addiction without an understanding of the patient's background or emotional makeup.

Figure 24–1 illustrates one scheme to incorporate the many biological and psychosocial factors contributing to the history of a drug dependency disorder. In this scheme, drug dependency is viewed as a series of vulnerabilities: to be exposed to the substance, to continue sub-

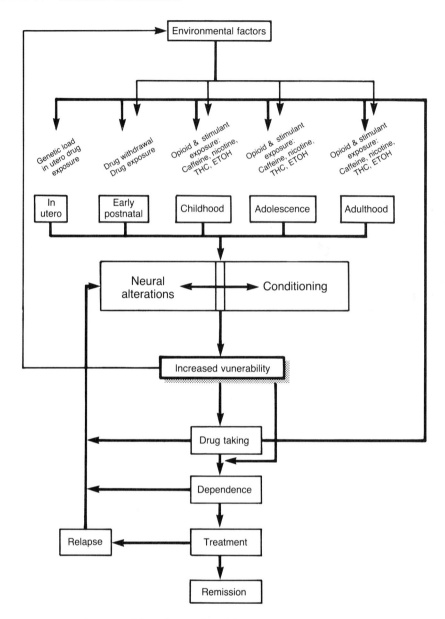

FIGURE 24–1. Development of drug abuse vulnerability. (Courtesy of Eliot L. Gardner, Albert Einstein College of Medicine)

stance exposure, to develop a dependency disorder, to fail to respond to treatment for the disorder, to respond to treatment but relapse. This model is in keeping with the medical model of other psychiatric disorders that incorporates the concept of multifactorial pathogenesis and multiple treatment outcomes. The older disease model of substance dependency posits a single downhill course to "rock bottom" and treatment as a single uphill course. This model has great historical importance in that it organized a complex set of biological and psychosocial phenom-

ena into a pathogenetic model. This model is still the mainstay of self-help groups and is useful for patient education.

Definition of the following terms is essential for an understanding of the discussion below.

• **Intoxication**: Maladaptive behavior or a substance-specific syndrome that are due to the recent ingestion of a psychoactive substance and that do not correspond to other specific organic mental syndromes such as delirium, delusional disorder, hallucinosis, mood syndrome, or anxiety syndrome.

- **Withdrawal**: A substance-specific syndrome that follows the cessation of or reduction in intake of a psychoactive substance that the person previously used regularly and that does not correspond to organic mental syndromes such as delirium, delusional disorder, hallucinosis, mood syndrome, or anxiety syndrome.
- **Tolerance**: Decrease or disappearance of a given effect upon repeated administration of a drug.
- **Sensitization**: Increase of a given effect or the onset of novel effects upon repeated administration of a drug.

DIAGNOSTIC SYSTEMS AND INDICES OF SUBSTANCE DEPENDENCE

Because symptomatology related to substance use is so complex and variable, no one classification system can adequately describe substance-related disorders. The approach to this problem in the revised third edition of the *Diagnostic and Statistical Manual of Mental Disorders* (DSM-III-R), published by the American Psychiatric Association, is to use two broad categories within the axis I disorders (all mental disorders except personality disorders and specific developmental disorders) in conjunction with the remaining four axes. The two categories are substance-related organic mental syndromes and psychoactive substance dependence disorders.

The substance-related organic mental syndromes must be considered in the differential diagnosis of any altered mental state. They are broadly divided into (1) symptoms typical of intoxication or withdrawal states (for example, cocaine intoxication or alcohol withdrawal) and (2) symptoms reflecting a particular psychopathological state (for example, alcohol delirium, alcohol amnestic disorder, cocaine delusional disorder, or cocaine affective disorder). Thus, the substance-related organic mental syndromes are clusters of response patterns to either the administration of a drug or its withdrawal over a brief or long period. Several of these disorders may pertain to an individual patient.

The psychoactive substance dependence disorders describe a cluster of symptoms and maladaptive and drug-seeking behaviors that derive from regular substance use. Often, it is difficult to draw a clear line between heavy, socially acceptable use and use that constitutes a disorder. A dependence disorder is defined by DSM-III-R as the presence of three or more of nine criteria; the disorder is further graded as mild, moderate, or severe, depending on the number of criteria fulfilled and the impact of drug taking on overall psychosocial function.

Criteria for Dependence and Abuse

The nine criteria for dependence include three representing the presence of physiological dependence (1 to 3) and six reflecting excessive drug taking (4 to 9):

1. Tolerance
2. Withdrawal
3. Drug taking to relieve withdrawal symptoms
4. Substance used in larger amount or for longer than intended
5. Persistent desire to use substance; inability to cut down or control use
6. A great deal of time spent in getting or taking the substance or in recovering from substance use
7. Intoxication or withdrawal symptoms when expected to meet important obligations
8. Important activities given up because of substance abuse
9. Continued substance use despite knowledge that substance use has a deleterious effect on health or functioning

A substance "abuse" disorder is defined by DSM-III-R as the presence of maladaptive substance use indicated by continued use despite knowledge of a recurrent problem due to that use or recurrent use that is physically hazardous, but the patient fails to meet at least three of the nine criteria required for the diagnosis of "dependence." In the cases of both dependence and abuse, the criteria must be present for at least 1 month or, if intermittent, for a longer period.

Unfortunately, DSM-III-R changed the definition of several commonly accepted terms. Previously, the term *abuse* referred to the phenomenon now described as *dependence,* with the exception of the three criteria referring to physiological dependence, whereas the previous definition of *dependence* coincided with the presence of tolerance or withdrawal, which is now called *physiological dependence*.

It is particularly important that the syndrome of dependence not be confused with physiological dependence. The presence of tolerance or withdrawal can be demonstrated after administration of many nonaddictive medications such as neuroleptics, betablockers, and nitroglycerin. Furthermore, the medically appropriate use of potentially addictive drugs may result in mild levels of tolerance or withdrawal but not the development of abuse or dependence. For example, discontinuation of postoperative opioid analgesics may induce mild symptoms of withdrawal without causing abuse or dependence. The confusion between physiological dependence and a dependence disorder contributes, on the one hand, to the unfortunate practice of prescribing insufficient doses of opioid analgesics and, on the other, to the inability of physicians to identify correctly a drug-dependence problem in the absence of signs of physiological dependence.

Psychoactive substance dependence disorders are often associated with other major psychiatric syndromes, serious personality disorders, medical illnessess, stressors, and maladaptive lifestyles, which may be classified according to DSM-III-R along axes I to V, respectively. These factors may contribute to the initiation and maintenance of substance use but may just as likely arise from the stubstance use or dependence itself.

Addiction Severity Index

Because of the complexity of factors associated with addiction, a multidimensional assessment must be made at the outset of the treatment of substance dependence. A particularly useful approach is incorporated in the Addiction Severity Index (ASI). This index is generated from a questionnaire that gathers information about medical, employment, drug and alcohol taking, social, legal, and psychiatric problems; each subscale has been shown to have external validity with other common scales used for the same specific purpose. Using the ASI, the physician can assess the patient's function in each dimension independently at the beginning of treatment and later after treatment interventions.

Patient Screening

There is often a need to screen a patient for the likelihood that he or she has a substance abuse or dependence disorder, rather than conduct a full-scale clinical interview. This screening is particularly important in the case of potential alcohol abuse or dependence. Because alcohol consumption is legal, it is often difficult to differentiate heavy drinking from abuse or

dependence in the medical history. Several checklists have been used for this purpose, each with a slightly different emphasis; however in each case, the most valid indicator of the presence of abuse or dependence is the total number of abnormal responses, rather than the response to any particular item on the scale. Thus it is the range of dysfunction that signals the presence of a substance dependence disorder.

EPIDEMIOLOGICAL CONSIDERATIONS

In the past 10 years, epidemiological studies of addiction have gained greater sophistication in describing the prevalence of psychoactive substance dependence disorders. The National Institute of Mental Health—Epidemiological Catchment Area study of the prevalence of DSM-III–defined disorders showed that alcohol abuse was the most prevalent psychiatric disorder among men, with a lifetime prevalence of 5 to 10 percent and a point prevalence of 5 percent. However, this study excluded homeless or transient people from the survey sample and thus does not reflect the prevalence of substance use or its consequences in that particularly problematic population.

Other approaches in the determination of prevalence of illegal substance use include:

- Survey of medical and psychiatric sequelae of use as reflected in emergency room presentations
- Survey of street market conditions of the drug
- Survey of number of students who have tried the drug
- Survey of number of admissions for treatment

Since all of these methods are incomplete, results from several types of studies must be considered together. These methods are particularly useful in determining episodic epidemics of drug use, for example, the epidemic of heroin addiction in the early 1970s, or the epidemic of cocaine addiction in the late 1970s and early 1980s. They also may identify pockets of intensive drug addiction.

Based on the composite results of recent epidemiological studies, it is believed that 2 million Americans have used heroin and that 500,000 are addicts. In 1987, cocaine overtook other drugs as the leading cause for drug-related emergency room presentations. Widespread experimentation with cocaine continues: a survey of 27-year-olds in 1985 who had been studied as high school seniors showed the lifetime prevalence of cocaine use to be 40 percent. With the introduction of cocaine in the form of "crack"—an inexpensive, highly potent, rapid-onset product—cocaine use has spread into groups that were previously unable to afford large quantities of the drug.

Epidemiological studies also provide clinically useful information about age of onset of addictive disorders; for example, heroin and cocaine addictions have been shown to begin during adolescence or early adulthood, whereas alcohol addiction can begin then and in middle and old age also.

BIOBEHAVIORAL PATHOGENETIC MECHANISMS

Like all psychoactive drugs, addictive drugs enter the central nervous system and produce their effects either through specific receptor mechanisms or by modifying cell membranes. It is thought that all significant aspects of acute and chronic drug administration are mediated within the central nervous system. However, effects on the peripheral nervous system or other organ systems may complicate central nervous system effects and thereby contribute to the maintenance of an addiction. For example, opioid-withdrawal diarrhea may be mediated by gastrointestinal mechanisms; however, the appearance of this diarrhea may be an important cue to the opioid-dependent addict to seek more narcotics.

The effects caused by the initial exposure to a psychoactive drug are mediated by defined pharmacological mechanisms but are not solely determined by the pharmacological activity of the drug. The effect also depends on the environmental conditions of the drug exposure and on the history of prior exposures to *other* drugs. For example, in squirrel monkeys trained to respond to terminate an electric shock, administration of pentobarbital increased the rate of responding. However, those monkeys which had been exposed briefly to morphine during the procedure in the past did not increase their rate of responding when challenged with pentobarbital. If the monkeys were first administered morphine before a shock-termination session and administered d-amphetamine before a subsequent shock-termination session, the effect of pentobarbital on responding for shock termination was restored. While the mechanism for such an effect is not clear, this example demonstrates that a brief drug exposure may modify

the effects of subsequent drug exposure, even when different classes of drugs are involved.

Tolerance and Sensitization

Exposure to a psychoactive drug not only produces an intoxication but modifies the nature of future intoxications to a given drug. Chronic drug exposure may induce tolerance or sensitization to a given effect, the overall outcome of chronic drug exposure being a complex expression of tolerance and sensitization to multiple drug effects. Exposure to a psychoactive drug may also induce withdrawal effects as early as the first dose. It is a useful clinical rule of thumb, but not a scientifically established fact, that the degree of tolerance to the major effects of a drug and the degree of withdrawal symptoms upon cessation of that drug are correlated.

As is the case for the initial exposure to a drug, the development of tolerance or sensitization depends both on neuroadaptational mechanisms and environmental factors. Neuroadaptation to chronic opioid and cocaine administration are discussed below. In general, studies of tolerance or sensitization have focused on regulation of receptor sensitivity or number or on neurotransmitter synthesis. More recent studies, using recombinant DNA methods, are examining the regulation of transcription and translation processes. Many animal experiments have now shown that there is an environmentally dependent process of conditioning that contributes to the development of both tolerance and sensitization. Thus, a constant environment, as opposed to the introduction of novel environmental stimuli, contributes to both tolerance and sensitization.

Reinforcing Effect of Addictive Drugs

At the core of most recent discussions of abuse liability of addictive drugs is the recognition that these psychoactive drugs are distinguished by their ability to stimulate particular reward circuitry in the brain without producing other significant aversive effects or impairing the organism's ability to seek the drug. Direct specific electrical stimulation of these reward circuits has a reinforcing effect; that is, it can be used to shape behavior and is thus analogous to food for the hungry animal or water for the thirsty animal. By and large, with the exception of hallucinogens such as LSD, all drugs abused by humans function as positive reinforcers in laboratory animals.

The structure and neurochemistry of the brain's reward circuitry are under study. The narrow view of such circuitry focuses on the mesolimbic or mesocortical dopaminergic system, while broader views include these pathways in addition to the hypothalamus, septum, and hippocampus. With the exception again of LSD, substances abused by humans have been shown to stimulate mesolimbic dopamine activity in studies using classical histochemistry or new in vivo electrochemical methods. For further discussion of the dopaminergic system, see Chapter 8: Neurophysiological and Neurochemical Basis of Behavior.

It is not clear whether the reinforcing effect of addictive psychoactive drugs is the same as their euphoric effect. In humans, administration of abused drugs under laboratory conditions produces a euphoric effect, and most drug-dependent patients report a euphoric effect when they began using drugs. However, chronic drug use is often associated with unpleasant effects or the feeling that the drug only eliminates unpleasant withdrawal effects without inducing euphoria. Since chronic drug dependence occurs often without the subjective feeling of euphoria, it is perhaps best to separate the ability of a drug to induce euphoria from its ability to gain control over behavior as a reinforcer.

COCAINE ABUSE AND DEPENDENCE

Cocaine is a reuptake blocker of dopamine, norepinephrine, and serotonin and a sodium-channel blocker. Its effects as an intoxicant and addictive drug are mediated primarily by its dopamine reuptake blockade action, while its peripheral cardiac inotropic and chronotropic and its vasopressor effects are mediated primarily by its norepinephrine reuptake blockade action. Although the indirect dopamine agonist effect of cocaine can be demonstrated in all dopaminergic pathways, the mesocortical and mesolimbic dopamine pathways have been shown to be the most important.

Repeated exposure to cocaine changes the nature of the intoxication in both humans and animals, through a process called "behavioral sensitization." Thus, an intoxication that once consisted of euphoria, hyperactivity, and garrulousness becomes a dysphoric, paranoid experience, the paranoia so severe as to mimic an acute psychotic episode of schizophrenia. Because cocaine has some proconvulsant activity, it was once thought that the underlying mechanism of behavioral sensitization resembled the "kindling" of seizure activity after repeated subconvulsant levels of electrical stimulation. Now it is believed that the behavioral sensitization is due mainly to the sensitization of dopaminergic transmission. Multiple studies of the phenomenon, however, have produced conflicting evidence as to whether dopaminergic sensitization is mediated pre- or postsynaptically.

For many years, the "physical" nature of cocaine addiction was in question because of the absence of significant tolerance to cocaine and because of the inconsistent features of the abstinence syndrome. In contrast to abstinence following chronic alcohol or opioid use, which is often marked by easily observable physical signs and symptoms, abstinence following chronic cocaine use is marked by a rather inconsistent pattern of anergy, anhedonia, and sleep disturbance, during which craving for cocaine may be rather low. Furthermore, "psychological" craving for cocaine and bouts of cocaine use are often triggered only by environmental conditions signaling the availability of cocaine.

Animal Self-administration Experiments

The discovery of endogenous brain reward circuits and the finding that many laboratory animals avidly learn to self-administer cocaine have led to an investigation of the physical basis of this behavior and to a revision of theories about the basic mechanisms of addiction. Many laboratory animals learn to bar-press for systemic cocaine administration on several schedules of reinforcement. On a fixed-ratio schedule (one dose of cocaine for a fixed number of bar presses), the rate of bar-pressing and the interadministration interval tend to be constant. This constancy is often observed in human cocaine abusers who self-administer cocaine every 15 to 20 minutes. This relationship between dose and interadministration interval applies to other self-administered drugs; however, it is tightest for cocaine. This regulated self-administration of cocaine is subserved by the mesolimbic or mesocortical dopamine systems and can be manipulated by dopamine agonists or antagonists. For example, administration of haloperidol increases the frequency of bar presses, while administration of a longer acting dopamine agonist decreases the frequency.

Animal models of cocaine administration have

provided other parallels to human cocaine addiction. Once trained to self-administer cocaine, an animal begins a chain of self-administration behavior in response either to the presentation of cocaine or to the presentation of an environmental cue signaling the availability of cocaine; in the absence of such a cue, the self-administration behavior does not occur. Self-administration behavior can be rapidly extinguished (after a brief burst of bar-pressing behavior) once cocaine is withdrawn. However, the self-administration behavior can also be easily reinstated upon a noncontingent administration of cocaine or the presentation of an environmental cue signaling the availability of cocaine. This is similar to the difficulty cocaine addicts (and some other addicts) face when they leave in-patient treatment: once they are reexposed to the environmental signals of drug availability, they experience a powerful resurgence of craving and relapse into drug-using routines.

Treatment with Dopamine Agonists and Antagonists

The knowledge that dopaminergic pathways are central to cocaine's addictive action has several consequences for the pharmacological management of cocaine addiction. The use of antipsychotic dopamine antagonists has been proposed, based on the rationale that they would block intoxication and thereby discourage use. Open trials of antipsychotic drugs have yielded equivocal results, but large doses for long durations of treatment have not yet been tried; in one report, neuroleptic treatment attenuated the paranoid psychosis associated with cocaine use but not craving, euphoria, or continued cocaine use.

A strategy using dopamine agonists such as amantadine or bromocriptine has also been proposed. One rationale for this strategy is that chronic cocaine use may deplete presynaptic dopamine stores and that cocaine craving arises from a hypodopaminergic state; there is little direct evidence to support or refute this position. Another rationale is that dopamine agonists decrease the frequency of self-administration in animals; thus, dopamine agonists may prevent a chain of cocaine self-administration from starting or brake the process once it has started. Pilot studies of dopamine agonist treatment of cocaine dependence in primary cocaine users and methadone-maintained (polydrug) cocaine users appear promising.

Preliminary studies also suggest that imipramine and desipramine are effective in reducing cocaine craving and use, even in the absence of major depression. The biological rationale for this effect is not established; however, it has been shown that chronic, but not acute, antidepressant administration in rats increases dopaminergic activity. This action is consistent with the strategy of using dopamine agonists.

OPIOID ABUSE AND DEPENDENCE

The impetus to understand narcotic addiction and pain management has led to the discovery of a series of endogenous peptides and a set of receptors that mediate their action both in the central nervous system and the periphery. The mechanisms and regulation of transcription, translation, posttranslational processing, and secretion of the endogenous opioids are under investigation. The endogenous opioids are derivatives of larger propeptides, which are cleaved by peptidase enzymes to generate the active opioid and, in some cases, other additional bioactive peptides, for example, the synthesis of both adrenocorticotropic hormone (ACTH) and β-endorphin from proopiomelanocortin in the anterior pituitary. Opioid peptides may also be cosecreted with other types of neurotransmitters. The following three categories of opioid peptides are thought to be the endogenous ligands for three receptor subtypes.

Opioid Peptide	Receptor Subtype
Beta-endorphin	Mu
Met- and leu-enkephalins	Delta
Dynorphin	Kappa

A fourth receptor type, the sigma opioid receptor, may be a phencyclidine receptor that modulates N-methyl-D-aspartate receptor activity. Though kappa agonists have analgesic properties and can induce tolerance and withdrawal syndromes, most addictive narcotics are mu and delta agonists. The pure opioid antagonists naloxone and naltrexone are considered mu (and, to a lesser degree, delta) receptor antagonists. For further information on receptors, see Chapter 9: Neurotransmitter Receptor Function.

Opioid receptors are widely distributed throughout the central and peripheral nervous systems. The major concentration of β-endorphin releasing neurons in the brain is located in the arcuate nucleus, while enkephalinergic neurons are widely scattered.

Opioids are thought to play a role in analgesia by gating nociceptive pain signals at three major sites: (1) the dorsal root ganglia and spinal cord, (2) the thalamus, and (3) the periaqueductal gray matter, which is known to be rich in opioid-releasing neurons. Electrical stimulation of the periaqueductal gray matter or microinjection of endogenous opioid peptides or narcotic analgesics into that area produces naloxone-reversible analgesia. For further information on pain transmission, see Chapter 23: Pathophysiology of Pain.

Opioid drugs are known to have a wide range of effects on motoric and affective function. Opioid-releasing neurons are associated with the forebrain dopaminergic pathways, both in the mesencephalon near dopaminergic cell bodies and in the limbic, striatal, and cortical dopamine projection areas. As such, opioid-releasing neurons are positioned to modulate or read out dopamine transmission; this may account for the reinforcing activity of opioids. As in the case of cocaine, many laboratory animals self-administer narcotics, though the rate of self-administration and the relationship between dosage and frequency of self-administration are more elastic for opioids than for cocaine. Rats self-administer opioid substances (endogenous or exogenous) in response to the microinjection of the drug directly into the ventral tegmental area (near the cell bodies of the mesolimbic and mesocortical dopamine neurons), but not when the drug is microinjected into the periaqueductal gray matter; conversely, microinjection of opioids into the ventral tegmental area fails to induce analgesia. Thus, the effects of opioids as analgesics and as reinforcers appear to be mediated at different anatomic locations. Microinjection of opioid substances into the ventral tegmental area also resembles systemic cocaine administration in that repeated drug administration produces sensitization of the dopamine system and concomitant behavioral sensitization of locomotor activity rather than tolerance.

Opioid Tolerance and Withdrawal

One of the traditional hallmarks of opioid addiction is the development of tolerance and withdrawal (that is, physiological dependence) after chronic, repeated opioid administration. From a clinical standpoint, tolerance is usually described with regard to the analgesic or euphorigenic effects of opioid drugs. A cluster of withdrawal symptoms—including opioid craving, nausea, vomiting, muscle aches, lacrimation, rhinorrhea, sweating, yawning, fever, and insomnia—is noted when, after heavy chronic

opioid administration, drug use ceases or the person is challenged with an opioid antagonist. Under laboratory conditions, however, tolerance and withdrawal can be demonstrated in a dose-dependent manner after the first administration of an opioid drug.

Although it is no longer believed that the avoidance of withdrawal symptoms is the major cause of opioid addiction, the subjective experience of opioid withdrawal, coupled with an urgent need to administer opioids, is reported widely by opioid addicts seeking drug treatment. Therefore, it is somewhat puzzling that, in a recent study of heroin addicts applying for treatment, there was no significant difference in withdrawal symptoms elicited by naloxone vs. saline placebo injection. This means that the complaints of opioid-dependent patients of spontaneous withdrawal symptoms cannot be explained simplistically by a model of naloxone-induced withdrawal.

The molecular basis of opioid tolerance and withdrawal has yet to be defined. In contrast to chronic naltrexone (antagonist) treatment, which induces behaviorally significant, postsynaptic mu-opioid receptor supersensitivity, chronic opioid (agonist) treatment has been shown to produce postsynaptic subsensitivity in only a small fraction of studies. In several cell models, chronic opioid administration (which inhibits guanosinetriphosphate-dependent cAMP synthesis) induces increased sensitivity to neurotransmitters that stimulate cAMP synthesis. This mechanism could explain both tolerance and the appearance of withdrawal symptoms upon the removal of opioids but is not consistent with other experimental findings. For information on the postsynaptic role of cyclic adenosine-monophosphate (cAMP), see under the heading "cAMP" in Chapter 8: Neurophysiological and Neurochemical Basis of Behavior.

The discovery that clonidine, an alpha-adrenergic agonist, can attenuate the opioid withdrawal syndrome led to the hypothesis that opioid withdrawal is mediated by the unbridled hyperactivity of central noradrenergic neurons. These noradrenergic neurons (primarily located in the locus coeruleus) are inhibited by the presynaptic activation of both opioids and alpha-adrenergic receptors. Thus, it was postulated that clonidine could reduce opioid withdrawal symptoms by inhibiting overactive noradrenergic neurons that were no longer inhibited by opioids. However, studies using neurotransmitter metabolite markers of central noradrenergic activity have not confirmed the noradrenergic hypothesis of opioid withdrawal.

The time frame for the emergence of the opioid withdrawal syndrome depends both on the duration of action of the opioid and a variety of host factors that are poorly understood. In general, the shorter the duration of action, the more rapid the onset and the resolution of the acute withdrawal syndrome. Many withdrawal phenomena, however, take far longer to resolve. Former opioid addicts often report sleep and mood difficulties for months after detoxification; this delayed withdrawal syndrome may also include the reemergence of an intense craving for narcotics, which is sometimes provoked by environmental factors associated with prior narcotics use. Opioid effects on gonadotropin-releasing factors also resolve slowly after the first phase of acute withdrawal.

Opioid Dependence Treatment

The first phase of opioid dependence treatment requires a decision whether to use substitute narcotics to stabilize opioid craving and suppress withdrawal or to detoxify the patient in preparation for "drug-free" management. Detoxification from physiological opioid dependence is accomplished by scheduled administration of decreasing doses of an opioid like methadone or by the administration of clonidine. In most cases, patients are offered "drug-free" treatment plans during their early presentations and offered substitute treatment after "drug-free" treatment fails; the vast majority of patients treated with "drug-free" modalities relapse within a year. In view of the high risk for HIV infection incurred by intravenous narcotics use, substitute treatment may be indicated at the first presentation for treatment.

"Drug-free" treatments are sometimes supplemented by naltrexone. Naltrexone, a long-acting oral opioid antagonist, blocks the effect of narcotics for 1 to 2 days, depriving the patient of the ability to get "high" and giving the patient with opioid craving some extra time to find psychosocial help for the continuation of abstinence. With the exception of the treatment of highly motivated professionals, naltrexone has not improved the success rate of "drug-free" treatment of opioid dependence.

Substitution treatment using oral methadone is the mainstay of most outpatient treatment programs. Methadone, like morphine or heroin, is a mu agonist with some additional kappa receptor activity. Because of its long duration of action, methadone need only be administered every 24 hours. Methadone maintenance is as-

sociated with high retention in treatment, successful repression of the use of illegal narcotics, and substantial gains in psychosocial function.

Unlike alcohol or stimulants, narcotics themselves have little intrinsic toxicity (aside from the risk of overdose). Furthermore, the tolerance that develops to opioids is far greater than the tolerance to other psychoactive substances. Thus, methadone administration causes virtually no "high" in the opioid-dependent patient but suppresses craving and withdrawal symptoms. At high doses, methadone induces complete tolerance to the euphoric effects of opioids, precluding the experience of any "high" after adminstration of illicit narcotics; this is called a "blocking" dose of methadone.

ALCOHOL ABUSE AND DEPENDENCE

Although alcohol abuse and dependence are the most common substance disorders, the least is known about the molecular basis for alcohol's addictive properties. Multiple neurotransmitter systems are affected by acute or chronic exposure to alcohol. Alcohol's action is mediated broadly by its action on membrane fluidity. Its activity may also be mediated by receptor-specific mechanisms. One such receptor site is in or near the GABA-benzodiazepine-chloride ionophore complex; this may explain the similarity of action of alcohol and benzodiazepines and crosstolerance between the two. A second receptor-specific mechanism may be the agonist activity of ethanol at the delta opioid receptor. Such activity may play some role in explaining the complex relationship between alcohol and narcotic consumption demonstrated in many animal experiments. A third receptor-specific mechanism may be indicated by binding at the N-methyl-D-aspartate (NMDA)-type glutamate receptor complex. This glutamate receptor has been implicated in a broad range of neurological phenomena including seizures, cell death, and learning. The activity of alcohol at the NMDA-type glutamate receptor may thus ultimately explain diverse effects of alcohol such as withdrawal seizures, dementia, and impaired memory formation.

Although the percentage of alcohol-dependent patients with physiological dependence is not known, it is important to suspect physiological dependence and manage detoxification carefully because cessation of alcohol intake can be associated with serious delirium, convulsions, and mortality. The crosstolerance to many of the sedative and anxiolytic effects between alcohol and benzodiazepines underlies the current practice of using decreasing doses of benzodiazepines to manage alcohol withdrawal in physiologically dependent patients.

The only pharmacological treatment available for alcohol abuse or dependence relies on the avoidance of a noxious event. Disulfiram irreversibly inhibits the action of the enzyme aldehyde dehydrogenase, causing an increase in plasma acetaldehyde levels after alcohol intake. This causes a range of symptoms from nausea and flushing to serious symptoms such as convulsions and cardiovascular collapse. To avoid this reaction, the patient must avoid alcohol intake. Most studies indicate a short-term improvement in treatment outcome through use of disulfiram; however, long-term efficacy has not been established. Disulfiram may be most useful in the early stages of treatment while the patient is becoming attached to a group like Alcoholics Anonymous or for the brief management of relapses.

Chronic alcohol use has been linked to both subacute and chronic encephalopathies caused by direct alcohol toxicity and by nutritional deficits commonly associated with alcohol dependence. Wernicke's encephalopathy results from acute thiamine deficiency and may be present in the classic form with short-term memory impairment, dyscoordination, and peripheral neuropathy or with a more global cognitive or depressive impairment. Chronic alcoholism may lead to either global dementia or a dementia of the Korsakoff type, in which short-term memory deficits, and thus impairment of new learning, are the most outstanding features.

Despite the relative paucity of specific information about the effects of alcohol on the nervous system, great headway has been made in the demonstration of a genetic component in the development of alcohol dependence. Children raised away from their biological parents have been shown to resemble them in their degree of problems arising from alcohol use. This discovery, together with the widespread clinical observation that alcoholism runs in families, led to a search for biological markers of vulnerability to the development of alcohol dependence. Preliminary research indicates that children of alcoholics are less sensitive to the aversive effects of alcohol and may be less able to perceive the effects of alcohol on their behavior. They also show neuroendocrine responses to ethanol that are blunted compared to normal controls. For a more detailed discussion of genetic factors, see under the heading Alcoholism in Chapter 3: Behavior Genetics.

DUAL DIAGNOSIS PATIENTS

Patients with a "dual diagnosis" are those with substance dependence disorders in addition to other major psychiatric disorders. It is not certain whether the number of such patients is on the rise or whether they are now being recognized for the first time. Systematic epidemiological studies to determine the prevalence of dual diagnosis patients in drug treatment programs and psychiatric programs are under way. There are indications that patients in drug treatment programs may have as much as twice the lifetime and point prevalence of affective and anxiety disorders of the general population. In some cases, the existence of unrecognized psychiatric disorders can explain the initiation of and loss of control over drug use, poor response to standard drug dependence treatments, and excessive relapses. Psychiatric illness might also modify the pharmacological effects of drugs. For example, minor tranquilizers are rated more positively reinforcing ("liked") by anxious patients than by normals.

Some physicians view drug use as a form of "self-medication" against unpleasant psychiatric symptoms; for example, cocaine might be used to relieve depression, or narcotics might be used to relieve anxiety. Such a view awaits empirical verification. In many drug treatment settings, however, many patterns of drug use may be associated with the same underlying psychiatric diagnosis.

The outcome of treatment of substance dependence disorders may be improved by the identification and treatment of other psychiatric disorders. In general, treatment of other disorders improves judgment and motivation to engage in drug treatment and often relieves the patient's guilt over past treatment failures.

BIBLIOGRAPHY

Bozarth, M. (ed.): Methods of Assessing the Reinforcing Properties of Abused Drugs. New York, Springer-Verlag, 1987.

Vaillant, G.E.: The Natural History of Alcoholism. Cambridge, Mass., Harvard University Press, 1983.

Chapter 25
Anxiety

Michael Murphy, M.D., Ph.D., and
Leonard Handelsman, M.D.

PATHOPHYSIOLOGY

The term *anxiety* is often used interchangeably with nervousness, tension, or fear. Additionally, health care professionals add an interpretation to the definition based upon personal experience, and a concept based upon consensus often is not readily available. Interestingly, specialized training in human behavior tends to confuse rather than clarify the issue. For example, psychoanalysts generally equate anxiety with fear in the absence of external threat, while behaviorists demand the presence of highly specific, but harmless, fear-provoking stimuli.

Even with agreement on a definition of anxiety, there may be markedly different opinions as to the psychopathological implication of its presence. Unlike many other medical disorders, some anxiety is usually regarded as adaptive, and pathology is defined in quantitative more than qualitative terms, that is, the relationship of anxiety to the stressor, the frequency of anxiety signs or symptoms, and the effect of anxiety upon ongoing activities.

Animal Models for Anxiety

A common concept of anxiety based upon operational definitions can be provided without controversy: Anxiety is the response of an organism, behaviorally expressed, to a neutral harmless stimulus that has been paired with a later noxious event. The neutral stimulus may be, for example, a ringing bell (for rats) or the announcement of a test (for medical students); the subsequent noxious stimulus in these examples can be an electric shock or a failing grade, respectively. If the behavioral response (which may be inactivity) to the neutral stimulus increases, then, by definition, anxiety increases. In contrast, environmental manipulations including drug use that selectively suppress this behavioral response are termed *anxiolytic*.

Three major types of paradigms have been developed to create an operationalized concept of anxiety in animals. One technique uses immediate punishment in the context of conflicted behavioral goals; for example, reward *and* punishment for the stimulus at the same time. A second technique focuses on variables that modify the uncertainty within an environment or allow greater control of aversive stimuli; for example, in humans with carbon dioxide–induced panic, an illusion of limiting carbon dioxide inhalation reduces panic symptoms. A third technique induces behavior indicative of anxiety (for instance, aversion) through chemical perturbations; for example, injection of anxiogenic compounds such as β-carbolines or pentylenetetrazol.

Neurophysiological Substrate for Anxiety

Although anxiety is a relatively nonspecific emotion that can be operationally defined in simplistic yet predictive animal models, it is mediated by an interconnected system of anatomy that defies comprehensive description. The output of this system, moreover, produces moods and behaviors that are both more subtle and different than those obtained by stimulation of any component part. Thus, manipulation of the amygdala, hypothalamus, and mesencephalon produces rage, fear, or a diffuse pain sensation, which are qualitatively different experiences from anxiety. Yet, each of these structures interacts with others to create a limbic system midbrain circuit mediating the experience and expression of anxiety.

Limbic System Midbrain Circuitry

Limbic system midbrain circuitry subserving anxiety exists in phylogenetically old neuroanatomy. These structures tend to be more medial and caudal to newer tissue that arrived by addition to, rather than transformation of, previously existing areas. In general, anatomy associated with pleasurable states facilitates goal-directed behavior, while other areas that mediate dysphoria suppress goal-directed activity in animal experiments. Thus, the limbic system midbrain circuit might be functionally divided into rewarding and nonrewarding components, each with different physiological and neurochemical properties. Rewarding and nonrewarding (aversive or punishing) structures could be classified as follows:

Rewarding	Punishing
Preoptic area	Dorsal portion of mesencephalic central gray substance
Septum	
Lateral hypo-thalamus	Posterior hypothalamus
Hippocampus	Some intralaminar thalamic nuclei
	Amygdala

As one component of the limbic system midbrain circuit is activated, the other component is inhibited. Rewarding and aversive structures thus produce reciprocal inhibition, and approach behavior may be the result of disinhibition of rewarding structures coupled to simultaneous suppression of a system mediating punishment. This speculated ebb and flow of rewarding and nonrewarding influences may be integrated within the hypothalamus. The hypothalamus is a natural target for limbic system output, since it exerts an extensive control over an organism's neuroendocrine and behavioral activity. Thus, a study of hypothalamic-pituitary function as a reflection of disturbed limbic system physiology would seem to have merit in anxiety states and affective disorders. See Chapter 12: Hypothalamic Control.

Neurochemical Basis of Anxiety

Behavior within approach-avoidance conflict paradigms is partially mediated through limbic system midbrain circuitry, and the neurochemistry of this area, particularly in reference to synaptic transmission, is known. Although there are a panoply of chemical neurotransmitters and neuromodulators that may be important in the mediation of anxiety, only norepinephrine, serotonin, and, more importantly, gamma-aminobutyric acid (GABA) provide a heuristically and clinically useful framework. Much of this information is obtained from perturbations of biochemistry and behavior, following parenteral, oral, or intraventricular administration of a variety of pharmacological agents.

Noradrenergic System

Relationships between stress responses and the noradrenergic system of the brain have been studied for decades. In general, stimulation of the locus coeruleus activates a major noradrenergic system within the central nervous system and produces stress reactions in mammals that resemble fear. Yohimbine, a drug that enhances noradrenergic output from the locus coeruleus, can provoke subjective states in humans described as increased paniclike anxiety. Withdrawal from the chronic use of alcohol or narcotics is also associated with increased noradrenergic activity and includes symptoms often indistinguishable from anxiety. Similarly, electrolytic destruction or pharmacological suppression of the locus coeruleus (for example, through benzodiazepines or narcotics) reduces naturally occurring fear reactions and is effective within animal models of anxiety previously described. Yet compounds reducing noradrenergic activity are not invariably anxiolytic within man (e.g., clonidine, propranolol). A modulating but not specific role for norepinephrine in the experience of anxiety is suggested.

For more information on the noradrenergic system, see under the heading Norepinephrine in Chapter 8: Neurophysiological and Neurochemical Basis of Behavior.

Serotoninergic System

With few exceptions, there is substantial evidence that the serotoninergic system is involved in stress. Brain serotonin levels tend to increase in stress, particularly within aversive structures of the mesencephalon. Punished behavior is also released from suppression following chemical depletion of serotonin, lesioning of serotoninergic pathways, or use of serotoninergic antagonists such as methysergide. Similarly, the anxiolytic properties of minor tranquilizers can be attenuated by procedures that augment serotoninergic activity. These same anticonflict effects of anxiolytics are associated with reduced serotonin turnover rates. Buspirone, an anxiolytic agent that may not cause physiological dependence, attenuates anxiety states through its action on a serotonin receptor.

For more information on the serotoninergic system, see under the heading Serotonin in Chapter 8: Neurophysiological and Neurochemical Basis of Behavior.

GABAergic System

The most comprehensive thesis for a neurochemical basis of anxiety involves GABA neurotransmission and identification of an allosterically linked receptor for anxiolytics. GABA receptors are located both presynaptically and postsynaptically within the central nervous system, but presynaptic innervation is predominant. GABA receptors are uniformly inhibitory, are present mainly within the cerebrum rather than the spinal cord, and decrease neuronal excitability by increasing chloride flux into the cell.

Electrophysiological and biochemical studies have suggested that benzodiazepine anxiolytics mediate effects through the GABAergic system. Because of the GABA innervation of various monoamine and cholinergic systems, modification of GABAergic activity by minor tranquilizers could result in extensive repercussions throughout the entire mammalian central nervous system, including changes in the synthesis of monoamines or of serotonin.

The receptor binding site for the benzodiazepine tranquilizers (for example, diazepam, alprazolam) is close to the binding site for GABA and the chloride ion channel. Benzodiazepines are thought to facilitate the effect of GABA on the chloride ion channel. Compounds such as the beta-carbolines can also bind at the benzodiazepine receptor but produce an anxiogenic, rather than an anxiolytic, effect; these agents are known as *inverse agonists*. A third kind of drug can bind to the benzodiazepine receptor and exert no net effect. This type of drug can displace a benzodiazepine drug and thus "antagonize" its effect. One such agent, flumazenil (R015-1788), may be available clinically to reverse benzodiazepine overdosage. Endogenous ligands for the benzodiazepine receptor, such as diazepam-binding inhibitor, have been identified, but their function is still uncertain.

Recent experiments indicate that the GABAergic system mediates distress behavior in infant rats when they are separated from their mother and that benzodiazepine tranquilizers attenuate this behavior. Some evidence in humans links the early expression of inappropriately severe separation anxiety and school phobias in young children with the subsequent development of panic anxiety in adulthood. It is possible that a GABAergic theory could explain the ontogenetic development of different forms of anxiety.

For more information on the GABAergic system, see under the heading GABA in Chapter 8: Neurophysiological and Neurochemical Basis of Behavior.

ANXIETY DISORDERS

The DSM-III-R groups the following disorders under the heading of anxiety disorders:

- Panic disorder
- Generalized anxiety disorder
- Phobic disorders
- Obsessive compulsive disorder
- Posttraumatic stress disorder

Anxiety and avoidance behavior are the symptoms typical of these disorders. Of all psychiatric disturbances, anxiety disorders are by far the most common. Simple phobia (one of the phobia disorders) is thought to be the most frequent disturbance in the general population; however, the most frequent disturbance among those seeking psychiatric treatment is panic disorder.

Panic Disorder

Unexpected panic attacks without an organic cause characterize this condition. These attacks are of short duration—usually minutes, only rarely hours—but their fear or discomfort is intense. See Table 25–1 for the diagnostic criteria for panic disorder.

Panic disorder is divided into two clinical conditions: panic disorder with agoraphobia and panic disorder without agoraphobia. The DSM-III-R defines agoraphobia as "the fear of being in places or situations from which escape might be difficult (or embarrassing) or in which help might not be available in the event of a panic attack." A person's panic attacks can become sensitized to a stimulus in the environment, with the result that the person can develop a phobia about the stimulus.

Some chemical conditions may sensitize people to panic disorder, for example, withdrawal from alcohol or drugs, particularly sedatives. A hyperadrenergic state within the locus coeruleus may contribute to this sensitization.

In people prone to panic disorder, a variety of chemical challenges can provoke a panic attack. Infusions of lactate, yohimbine, and caffeine, as well as hyperventilation with carbon dioxide–enriched air, all induce panic attacks. The mechanism of this effect is not certain, and people with panic disorder may be prone to induction by some agents but not others. Presynaptic receptors, normally reducing noradrenergic activity, may be subsensitive and thus permissive for a hyperactive noradrenergic state. This may explain a biological vulnerability to panic symptoms.

In contrast to the treatment of generalized anxiety disorder (see below), panic disorder responds to pharmacotherapy consisting of either tricyclic antidepressants (for example, imipramine) or MAO inhibitors (for example, phenelzine). As in the treatment of clinical depression, panic disorder responds to antidepressant med-

---

TABLE 25–1.   Diagnostic Criteria for Panic Disorder

A. At some time during the disturbance, one or more panic attacks (discrete periods of intense fear or discomfort) have occurred that were (1) unexpected, i.e., did not occur immediately before or on exposure to a situation that almost always caused anxiety, and (2) not triggered by situations in which the person was the focus of others' attention.

B. Either four attacks, as defined in criterion A, have occurred within a four-week period, or one or more attacks have been followed by a period of at least a month of persistent fear of having another attack.

C. At least four of the following symptoms developed during at least one of the attacks:
    (1) shortness of breath (dyspnea) or smothering sensations
    (2) dizziness, unsteady feelings, or faintness
    (3) palpitations or accelerated heart rate (tachycardia)
    (4) trembling or shaking
    (5) sweating
    (6) choking
    (7) nausea or abdominal distress
    (8) depersonalization or derealization
    (9) numbness or tingling sensations (paresthesias)
    (10) flushes (hot flashes) or chills
    (11) chest pain or discomfort
    (12) fear of dying
    (13) fear of going crazy or of doing something uncontrolled

    Note: Attacks involving four or more symptoms are panic attacks; attacks involving fewer than four symptoms are limited symptom attacks (see Agoraphobia without History of Panic Disorder).

D. During at least some of the attacks, at least four of the C symptoms developed suddenly and increased in intensity within ten minutes of the beginning of the first C symptom noticed in the attack.

E. It cannot be established that an organic factor initiated and maintained the disturbance, e.g., Amphetamine or Caffeine Intoxication, hyperthyroidism.

    Note: Mitral valve prolapse may be an associated condition, but does not preclude a diagnosis of Panic Disorder.

---

ication after 2 to 3 weeks of adequate therapy. Panic disorder also responds to high-potency benzodiazepine anxiolytics (for example, alprazolam), but these medications must be administered on a regular basis and may induce physiological dependence.

Panic disorder may be genetically determined and also may be associated with other medical conditions (see Generalized Anxiety Disorder). It also occurs frequently with major depression, in which case both disorders may be diagnosed.

Generalized Anxiety Disorder

Much less is known about this condition than panic disorder, and some question the consistency and validity with which a diagnosis can be made. The characteristic feature of generalized anxiety disorder is excessive anxiety over two or more life circumstances, with resulting physical symptoms typical of tension. Some symptoms of other psychiatric disorders often resemble those of this disorder.

Depressive disorder should be considered in patients who complain of chronic anxiety. If depression is diagnosed, the clinical presentations of anxiety and depression should be treated as a depressive disorder. Indeed, antidepressants acquire anxiolytic properties in animal models of anxiety if administered on a long-term basis. As is the case in all psychiatric disorders, the possibility of organic causes should be excluded; organic causes may include hyperthyroidism, hypercaffeinism, stroke, and pheochromocytoma. If behavioral or psychosocial treatments fail to resolve the generalized anxiety disorder, pharmacotherapy with benzodiazepine anxiolytics or buspirone may be used. Symptoms of anxiety generally respond within 1 to 2 weeks, and the clinical benefit within 2 weeks is highly predictive of the amount of benefit to be achieved within 6 weeks. Many patients confuse the rapid-onset muscle relaxant and sedative effect of benzodiazepines with anxiolytic effects. Tolerance to sedative effects but not anxiolytic effects occurs in both animals and man.

The development of physiological dependence on benzodiazepine tranquilizers is possible. Therefore, these medications are best used for a limited duration (1 to 2 months) or in an intermittent or pulsatile fashion. Few patients, however, develop drug-seeking behavior for benzodiazepines. Most vulnerable are patients with preexistent dependence on alcohol,

sedatives, and narcotics. The long-term use of benzodiazepines in patients with a history of substance use disorder is problematic.

Social Phobia

This disorder consists of a fear of being seen by others to act in a humiliating or embarrassing way. The phobia may involve any kind of social situation, such as eating in public. The person recognizes that his or her fear is unreasonable and yet may be unable to stop repetitive behavior reinforcing the phobia.

Simple Phobia

Simple phobia is the persistent fear of an object or situation, excluding the circumstances of panic disorder and social phobia. Phobias about butterflies, mice, blood, enclosed spaces (claustrophobia), heights (acrophobia), and air travel are all simple phobias. See Table 25–2 for the diagnostic criteria.

Pharmacotherapy for social or simple phobia when it is the primary diagnosis is singularly ineffective.

Obsessive Compulsive Disorder

Known also as obsessive compulsive neurosis, this disorder is marked by recurrent obsessions or compulsions severe enough to interfere with normal life. Obsessions can be defined as persistent illogical thoughts or impulses; the person recognizes them as such and tries to suppress them. Compulsions are the stereotyped behaviors that develop in response to attempted suppression of obsessions; when the person tries to resist the compulsion, tension builds. See Table 25–3 for the diagnostic criteria of obsessive compulsive disorder.

This disorder may be far more common than previously thought (1 to 3 percent lifetime prevalence) with an episodic (2 percent), continuous (84 percent), or deteriorating course (14 percent) described. Up to 4 percent of the cases may have clinically important features with comorbidity, especially major depression, commonly encountered. In a minority of cases, a history of organic neurologic insult will be discovered. About 25 percent of the cases also have tics or full-fledged Tourette's syndrome. Neuroimaging studies suggest neurological abnormalities in the frontal lobes, thalamus, and basal ganglia, but observations are not diagnostically useful.

Obsessive compulsive disorder responds to behavioral therapy, psychotherapy in intractable cases, and to pharmacotherapy with antidepressants that are *selective* serotonin uptake blockers (for example, fluoxetine or chlorimipramine).

However, the role of serotonin in the pathophysiology of this disorder is not understood. Obsessive compulsive disorder is within the category of anxiety disorders, but clinical and biological features may warrant its reclassification.

Posttraumatic Stress Disorder

This disorder is typified by the appearance of characteristic symptoms following a psychologically traumatic happening of an unusual kind. The event would be beyond the more familiar bereavement, marital discord, illness, or financial loss and would be recognized generally as a terrifying occurrence. The characteristic symptoms involve, in the words of DSM-III-R, "reexperiencing the traumatic event, avoidance of stimuli associated with the event or numbing of general responsiveness, and increased arousal."

The essential feature in posttraumatic stress disorder is the reexperiencing of trauma. Nonetheless, anxiety, depressive feelings, and social withdrawal may be prominent issues. The disorder may coexist with other psychiatric disorders, particularly major depression and substance dependence disorders, and may present for clinical attention only when the other disorders intensify. Treatment of the coexistent disorders is generally necessary to attain improvement in the posttraumatic stress disorder symptoms.

TABLE 25–2.   Diagnostic Criteria for Simple Phobia

A. A persistent fear of a circumscribed stimulus (object or situation) other than fear of having a panic attack (as in Panic Disorder) or of humiliation or embarrassment in certain social situations (as in Social Phobia).
   Note: Do not include fears that are part of Panic Disorder with Agoraphobia or Agoraphobia without History of Panic Disorder.
B. During some phase of the disturbance, exposure to the specific phobic stimulus (or stimuli) almost invariably provokes an immediate anxiety response.
C. The object or situation is avoided, or endured with intense anxiety.
D. The fear or the avoidant behavior significantly interferes with the person's normal routine or with usual social activities or relationships with others, or there is marked distress about having the fear.
E. The person recognizes that his or her fear is excessive or unreasonable.
F. The phobic stimulus is unrelated to the content of the obsessions of Obsessive Compulsive Disorder or the trauma of Post-traumatic Stress Disorder.

TABLE 25–3.   Diagnostic Criteria for Obsessive Compulsive Disorder

A. Either obsessions or compulsions:
   Obsessions: (1), (2), (3), and (4):
   (1) recurrent and persistent ideas, thoughts, impulses, or images that are experienced, at least initially, as intrusive and senseless, e.g., a parent's having repeated impulses to kill a loved child, a religious person's having recurrent blasphemous thoughts
   (2) the person attempts to ignore or suppress such thoughts or impulses or to neutralize them with some other thought or action
   (3) the person recognizes that the obsessions are the product of his or her own mind, not imposed from without (as in thought insertion)
   (4) if another Axis I disorder is present, the content of the obsession is unrelated to it, e.g., the ideas, thoughts, impulses, or images are not about food in the presence of an Eating Disorder, about drugs in the presence of a Psychoactive Substance Use Disorder, or guilty thought in the presence of a Major Depression
   Compulsions: (1), (2), and (3):
   (1) repetitive, purposeful, and intentional behaviors that are performed in response to an obsession, or according to certain rules or in a stereotyped fashion
   (2) the behavior is designed to neutralize or to prevent discomfort or some dreaded event or situation; however, either the activity is not connected in a realistic way with what it is designed to neutralize or prevent, or it is clearly excessive
   (3) the person recognizes that his or her behavior is excessive or unreasonable (this may not be true for young children; it may no longer be true for people whose obsessions have evolved into overvalued ideas)
B. The obsessions or compulsions cause marked distress, are time-consuming (take more than an hour a day), or significantly interfere with the person's normal routine, occupational functioning, or usual social activities or relationships with others.

A wider spectrum of life events is now seen as capable of eliciting posttraumatic stress disorder. Classic examples, such as combat exposure, produce the greatest number of recognized cases. However, events such as childhood incest or abuse are now seen as potential causes of the disorder. These exposures appear to have occurred more frequently in patients with a variety of personality disorders and are more common in female patients with substance dependence and antisocial behavior.

BIBLIOGRAPHY

Bodnoff, S.R., Suranyi-Codotte, B, Quirion, R., Meany, M.J.: A comparison of the effects of diazepam versus several typical and atypical antidepressant drugs in an animal model of anxiety. Psychopharmacology (Berlin) 97(2):277-279, 1989.

Braestrup, C., Nielsen, E.B.: Future directions in anxiety research. Psychopharmacol. Ser. 5:180-186, 1988.

DeRobertis, E., Pena, C., Paladini, A.C., Medina, J.H.: New developments on the search for the endogenous ligand(s) of central benzodiazepine receptors. Neurochem. Int. 13(1):1-11, 1988.

File, S.E.: Animal models for predicting clinical efficacy of anxiolytic drugs: Social behavior. Neuropsychobiology 13:55-62, 1985.

File, S.E.: Tolerance to the behavioral actions of benzodiazepines. Neurosci. Biobehav. Rev. 9(1):113-121, 1985.

Geller, I., Siefter, J.: The effects of meprobamate, barbiturates, D-amphetamine, and promazine on experimentally induced conflict in the rat. Psychopharmacologia 1:482-492, 1960.

Guttmacher, L.B., Murphy, D.L., Insel, T.R.: Pharmacologic models of anxiety. Compr. Psychiatry 24(4):312-326, 1983.

Havoundjan, H., et al.: A physiological role of the benzodiazepine/GABA receptor-chloride ionophore complex in stress. Adv. Exp. Med. Biol. 221:459-475, 1987.

Hoehn-Sarie, R.: Neurotransmitters in anxiety. Arch. Gen. Psychiatry (39):735-742, 1982.

Iversen, S.D.: Animal models of anxiety and benzodiazepine actions. Arzneim.-Forsch./Drug Res. 30(I):862-867, 1980.

Iversen, S.D.: 5-HT and anxiety. Neuropharmacology 23(12B): 1553-1560, 1984.

Johnston, A.L., File, S.E.: 5-HT and anxiety: Promises and pitfalls. Pharmacol. Biochem. Behav. 25(5):1467-1470, 1986.

Kandel, E.R.: From metapsychology to molecular biology: explorations into the nature of anxiety. Am. J. Psychiatry 140(10):1277-1293, 1983.

Karobath, M., Supavilai, P., Borea, P.A.: Distinction of benzodiazepine receptor agonists and inverse agonists by binding studies in vitro. Adv. Biochem. Psychopharmacol. 38:37-45, 1983.

Lal, H., Emmett-Oglesby, N.W.: Behavioral analogues of anxiety: Animal models. Neuropharmacology 22(12B): 1423-1441, 1983.

Lydiard, R.B., Roy-Byrne, P.P., Ballenger, J.C.: Recent advances in the psychopharmacological treatment of anxiety disorders. Hosp. Community Psychiatry 39(11):1157-1165, 1988.

Miller, L.G., et al.: Benzodiazepine receptor occupancy in vivo: Correlation with brain concentrations and pharmacodynamic actions. J.P.E.T. 240(2):516-522, 1987.

Mineka, S.: Animal models of anxiety-based disorders: their usefulness and limitations. In Anxiety and the Anxiety Disorders, A.H. Tuma and J. Maser, (eds.). Hillsdale, N.J., Lawrence Erlbaum Associates, 1985.

Minichiello, W.E., Baer, L., Jenike, M.A.: Behavior therapy for the treatment of obsessive-compulsive disorder: theory and practice. Compr. Psychiatry 29(2):123-137, 1988.

Nutt, D.: Benzodiazepine dependence in the clinic: reason for anxiety? Trends Pharmaceut. Sci. 7:457-460, November 1986.

Perse, T.: Obsessive-compulsive disorder. A treatment review. J. Clin. Psychiatry 49(2):48-55, 1988.

Rainey, J.M., Nesse, R.M.: Psychobiology of anxiety and anxiety disorders. Psychiatr. Clin. North Am. 8(1):133-144, 1985.

Saano, V.: Central-type and peripheral-type benzodiazepine receptors. Ann. Clin. Res. (Finland) 20(5):348-355, 1988.

Saano, V.: GABA-benzodiazepine receptor complex and drug actions. Med. Biol. 65(2-3):167-173, 1987.

Shephard, R.A.: Behavioral effects of GABA agonists in relation to anxiety and benzodiazepine action. Life Sci. 40(25):2429-2436, 1987.

Stahmer, S.: Pharmacodynamics of benzodiazepines. S. Afr. Med. J. 26(Suppl.):14-22, 1985.

Stavrakaki, C., Vargo, B.: The relationship of anxiety and depression: a review of the literature. Br. J. Psychiatry 149:7-16, 1986.

Stein, L.: Behavioral neurochemistry of benzodiazepines. Arzneim.-Forsch./Drug Res. 30(1):868-873, 1980.

Stein, L., Belluzzi, J., Wise, C.D.: Benzodiazepines: Behavioral and neurochemical mechanisms. Am. J. Psychiatry 134:665-669, 1977.

Thiebot, M.H.: Are serotonergic neurons involved in the control of anxiety and in the anxiolytic activity of benzodiazepines? Pharmacol. Biochem. Behav. 24(5):1471-1477, 1986.

Treit, D.: Animal models for the study of anti-anxiety agents: A review. Neurosci. Biobehav. Rev. 9(2):203-222, 1985.

Weissman, M.M., Merikangas, K.R.: The epidemiology of anxiety and panic disorders. An update. J. Clin. Psychiatry 47(suppl 6):11-17, 1986.

Williams, M.: Molecular aspects of the action of benzodiazepine and non-benzodiazepine anxiolytics: A hypothetical allosteric model of the benzodiazepine receptor complex. Prog. Neuro-Psychopharmacol. Biol. Psychiat. 8(2):209-247, 1984.

Wolkowitz, O.M., Paul, S.M.: Neural and molecular mechanisms in anxiety. Psychiatr. Clin. North Am. 8(1):145-158, 1985.

Chapter 26

Pathogenesis of Mood Disorders

Larry J. Siever, M.D., Kenneth L. Davis, M.D., and Lauren Kantor Gorman, M.D.

The term *depression* is often applied to a wide range of states, from relatively mild and transient states of feeling "let down" or disappointed to a severe and persistent state of hopelessness and low self-esteem that interferes with effective personal and occupational functioning, sometimes to the point of requiring hospitalization. Although only the latter might properly be termed clinical depression by a psychiatrist, the point at which ordinary human unhappiness ends and depression begins is a boundary not always easy to define. Although clinical depression is often regarded as an extreme intensification of unhappiness or sadness, many depressed patients are unable to express sadness; rather, they experience a severe blunting of interest in or enjoyment of usually pleasurable activities. In contrast, transient disappointments or losses rarely prevent someone who is not depressed from "cheering up," for example, in the company of friends.

Symptoms of Depression

It may be useful to consider clinical depression as a sustained state of lowered mood and activation that is not easily reversible by environmental events. Often, this state is accompanied by guilt, anxiety, feelings of inadequacy, inability to concentrate, ruminations, suicidal ideation, and somatic symptoms. The somatic symptoms may be "vegetative," that is, disturbances in normal bodily regulatory functions, such as sleep and appetite. Difficulty falling asleep, difficulty staying asleep, early morning awakening, or hypersomnia (increased sleeping) may be part of the depressive syndrome. Decreased or increased appetite is common, as is weight loss and slowing of movements. Other somatic symptoms include fatigue, heaviness in the legs and back, and constipation.

Depression and Loss

Depression is often conceptualized in terms of an extreme reaction to loss or disappointment. Grief or mourning is often accompanied by feelings of lowered mood but is not usually accompanied by the extreme loss of self-esteem and guilt observed in depression. In individuals prone to experience depression, seemingly minor losses or disappointments are often precipitants to the depressed state, in contrast to the major losses that invariably precede grief reactions. However, not uncommonly, it may be difficult to identify a clear precipitant to the depression, particularly in people prone to recurrent depressions.

Prevalence of Depression

Depression is a relatively common clinical condition affecting a significant proportion of the population at one time or another. It has been noted throughout history, suggesting that it is not a condition that has emerged with the advent of modern postindustrial society. It is currently estimated that over one fourth of the population will experience a clinically significant depression at one time or another in their life, while 3 to 5 percent of the population may be depressed at any given point in time. The rate of suicide in the depressed population is 30 times that of the general population, indicating that depression is a disorder with a serious morbidity.

Subtypes of Depression

Major depression described above may be distinguished from minor depressions, in which the duration and pervasiveness of the symptoms are less severe. Although depression has been divided into reactive or neurotic depressions versus psychotic depressions, the latter term is best reserved for depressions with psychotic symptoms whether or not initiated by environmental events. In fact, the existence of precipitating events is probably not a good discriminating feature of subtypes of depression, since such events are difficult to establish and may be demonstrable in depressives with a range of severity. The existence of neurotic or characteriological features also is probably not a good discriminator of meaningful subtypes of depression. The term endogenous depression or depression with melancholia may be applied to a subtype of depression in which vegetative symptoms are prominent and biologic factors are presumed to be more important.

Some individuals who experience depression at other times may develop mania, a clinical syndrome characterized by elated mood or irritability, hyperactivity, pressured speech, and flight of ideas, sometimes with grandiose delusions. Individuals with a history of depression and mania are termed bipolar depressives or manic-depressives, and those who have a history of depressive episodes only are termed unipolar depressives. Some unipolar patients may later have manic episodes and thus must be reclassified as bipolars. "Primary" depressions are sometimes distinguished from "secondary" depressions; in the latter the depression appears to be a consequence of another underlying psychiatric disorder.

Seasonal Affective Disorder

Some patients who develop depression do so on a "seasonal" basis; that is, they are more likely to become depressed in a specific season. For most, it is winter. These individuals may respond to therapy with bright lights that extend the hours of bright illumination during the short winter days. The seasonal affective disorders may be grounded in alterations of daily rhythms.

Psychobiologic-Psychosocial Model of Depression

In this chapter, it is assumed, consistent with available evidence, that some individuals are biologically predisposed to develop a depressive disorder. Such a biologial predisposition is based on as yet not fully understood genetic factors or, in some events, perhaps, early congenital biological environmental insults. Such persons' vulnerability may be sensitized or ameliorated by developmental influences throughout their life. These individuals may develop depressive episodes in the face of severe psychosocial stressors or losses (for example, leaving home or loss of spouse) or biological stressors (for example, medical illness or medications with psychoactive effects, such as steroids). The threshold stressors for some individuals to develop a clinical depression may be lower than for the majority of the population.

The emergence of the depressive state may be identified by a characterizable set of behavioral subjective and somatic symptoms that reflect detectable biological alterations in the central nervous system. "State markers" reflect these biological alterations, whereas "trait markers" may be observed in individuals who are in remission from a past depression and reflect biological predisposing characteristics. Psychobiological factors predisposing to depression may be heterogeneous, and so too may psycho-social precipitants, which can be extremely idiosyncratic; that is, there may be no single path to depression in the general population.

GENETIC FACTORS IN DEPRESSION

Numerous studies indicate that there is a genetic basis for at least some forms of depression. The concordance rate for affective illness is greater for monozygotic twins (69 percent) than for dizygotic twins (13 percent). Monozygotic twins reared apart also show a concordance of 67 percent for affective illness, suggesting that genetic rather than environmental factors account for this concordance. The prevalence of affective illness in the first-degree relatives of affectively ill probands is greater (6 to 32 percent) than is the general population prevalence for affective illness (39 percent). These prevalences are lower than would be expected for a fully penetrant single major gene inheritance, suggesting a polygenic inheritance or reduced penetrance of a major gene. Although there are few bipolar relatives of unipolar patients, unipolar illness is not uncommon in the relatives of bipolar patients, suggesting that a subtype of unipolar illness may be related to bipolar illness.

An attempt has been made to determine genetic linkage markers for the affective disorders, that is, markers reflecting genetic loci in contiguity with one of the genes for mood disorder (affective illness). Evidence for linkage markers within the ABO blood group system or HLA tissue antigen system has been reported but, in most cases, has not been consistent. Some but not all studies have suggested that bipolar affective disorder is linked to color blindness or the Xg blood group. Recently, genetic linkage to the short arm of chromosome 11 has been demonstrated in an Amish pedigree, but lack of such linkage in other pedigrees and failure to replicate linkage in an extension of the original pedigree suggest genetic heterogeneity of the affective disorders.

Often, attempts to study the genetic underpinnings of affective illness in a more specific manner have utilized biological markers in twins and families that include probands with affective illness. Relevant results are noted in the sections on psychobiological factors. See under the heading Mood Disorder (Affective Illness) in Chapter 3: Behavior Genetics.

PSYCHOBIOLOGY OF DEPRESSION

Neurotransmitters

Since disturbances in mood and vegetative functions are central to the psychopathology of depression, investigations of psychobiological factors in depression have focused on neurotransmitters and neurohormones that play a role in the modulation of affect and arousal. These include the biogenic amine neurotransmitters: norepinephrine, dopamine, and serotonin; the neurotransmitter acetylcholine; and hormones such as cortisol, growth hormone, and prolactin. Neurotransmitters such as norepinephrine have been shown to be particularly important in mediating the organism's arousal in response to meaningful environmental stimuli and have been hypothesized to play an important role in learning and memory. Abnormalities in this system have been demonstrated in animal models of depression and anxiety. The serotoninergic system seems to play an important role in inhibition of other neurobehavioral systems. The dopaminergic system is implicated in stereotyped behavior and reinforcement behavior. The cholinergic system may also play an important role in punishment-induced behavioral inhibition and, in a more general way, learning and memory. Thus, these neurotransmitter systems are logical systems to investigate in the affective disorders.

Noradrenergic System in Depression

The noradrenergic system has been implicated for two decades in the pathogenesis of depression. The catecholamine hypothesis of the affective disorders posits that depression is associated with a relative deficit of catecholamines in the central synapses of neuronal systems regulating mood, whereas mania is associated with a relative excess of these amines. This hypothesis was based on the observation that psychoactive drugs such as amphetamine or cocaine, which enhance the concentrations of these catecholamines in the synapse, result in euphoria and activation in humans. Conversely, pharmacological agents such as reserpine, which deplete catecholamine stores, may lead to depression in susceptible individuals. L-Dopa, a metabolite precursor to norepinephrine, when administered in high doses to bipolar patients, may precipitate a manic episode, while α-methyl-paratyrosine, which inhibits norepinephrine and dopamine synthesis, has antimanic properties.

In an attempt to test this hypothesis, investigators studied the concentration of norepinephrine or its metabolites, or both, in biological fluids, reasoning that alternating metabolite concentrations reflected corresponding alterations in noradrenergic activity. Early studies focused on the measurement of the 24-hour excretion of urinary 3-methoxy-4-hydroxyphenylglycol (MHPG), the major metabolite of norepinephrine in the central nervous system. Urinary excretion of MHPG was found to be decreased in bipolar patients in the depressed state compared to the manic state. In most studies the MHPG excretion was lower than that observed in normal controls. These results appeared consistent with the catecholamine hypothesis.

Evidence that clinically effective antidepressants had pharmacological effects that might result in increases in intrasynaptic norepinephrine also supported the catecholamine hypothesis. The tricyclic antidepressants block reuptake, which is the major route of activation of the antidepressants, while the monoamine oxidase (MAO) inhibitors metabolize norepinephrine intraneuronally.

More recently, the catecholamine hypothesis has been questioned because these pharmacological effects of the antidepressant medications occur immediately, whereas the onset of clinical antidepressant action requires 2 to 3 weeks of antidepressant administration. Furthermore, studies of norepinephrine and its metabolities have not always found significant differences in the concentration of noradrenergic metabolites in urine, plasma, or cerebrospinal fluid between depressed patients and controls. In fact, some recent studies have found increases in plasma norepinephrine, cerebrospinal fluid MHPG and norepinephrine, and urinary MHPG and other metabolites in unipolar depressed patients.

Thus, modifications in the original catecholamine hypothesis have been proposed. While studies have fairly consistently indicated that noradrenergic activity may be decreased in bipolar depressives, accumulating evidence suggests that many unipolar patients, particularly those with increased anxiety or chronic characterological depressions, or both, have increased noradrenergic activity. The latter group may require higher doses of antidepressants. Thus there seem to be subgroups of depressed patients with regard to noradrenergic activity. Noradrenergic abnormalities in both subgroups

may reflect a poorly regulated or buffered noradrenergic system. Alterations or shifts in the phase of the daily rhythms of noradrenergic activity have been demonstrated, suggesting abnormalities in the timing of the noradrenergic and other biological systems. Since norepinephrine appears to be important in arousal, activity, vegetative functions, and affective responses to the environment, poor regulation of this system may contribute to the altered activity and vegetative symptoms of depression.

As understanding of the complexity of the alterations in the noradrenergic system in depression increases, there has been an increasing emphasis on the role of adrenergic receptors in the affective illness. There are both α-adrenergic receptors and β-adrenergic receptors in the central nervous system that mediate norepinephrine's effects on postsynaptic neuronal systems.

α-Adrenergic receptors are divided into α_1- and α_2-adrenergic receptors, which may be either postsynaptic or presynaptic. α_2-Adrenergic receptors appear to be feedback inhibitory receptors that dampen the output of noradrenergic neurons when norepinephrine is released. β-Adrenergic receptors consist of β_1-adrenergic receptors and β_2-adrenergic receptors, which are found primarily on blood vessels. Central β-adrenergic receptors have not been studied in vivo in acutely depressed patients, although postmortem studies suggest increased β-adrenergic receptor number. Peripheral blood cell β-adrenergic receptors appear to be less numerous and responsive in depressed patients compared to controls.

Blunted biochemical and neuroendocrine responses to the α_2-adrenergic agonist clonidine suggest that central α_2-adrenergic receptors are less responsive in depression, particularly in unipolar patients with high "noradrenergic output." Since these receptors apparently have an important regulatory function, altered responsiveness in this system may contribute to a poorly regulated noradrenergic system. Altered responsiveness in noradrenergic α_2-receptor systems thus may contribute to abnormalities in noradrenergic transmission and release.

Many antidepressants seem to alter noradrenergic neurotransmission, also suggesting that abnormalities in this system may be important in the pathophysiology of the affective disorders. As noted previously, both reuptake blockage and MAO inhibition occur within several days of antidepressant administration, but the therapeutic effects of these medications may take 2 to 3 weeks or more. More recently, it has been determined that a number of adaptational changes in receptors take place after long-term antidepressant administration. The most consistent is the development of β-adrenergic receptor subsensitivity. These receptors seem particularly involved in anxiety and alarm reactivity in primates. It also appears that the inhibitory α_2-adrenergic receptors are subsensitized. α_1-Adrenergic receptors may be involved in the reinforcement of behavior, and α_1-adrenergic receptors become more responsive with antidepressant treatment. α_2-Adrenergic receptor subsensitivity can permit an increase in norepinephrine released per nerve impulse. These adaptational changes may permit the medications to achieve their maximal therapeutic effectiveness. Cumulatively, these changes might increase the responsiveness of the system to specific stimulation and dampen potential alarm reactions.

Noradrenergic abnormalities of a somewhat different character may be observed in patients with anxiety disorders. These patients may also respond to antidepressants. Some studies suggest a genetic relationship between panic disorder and depression.

In summary, it seems likely that abnormalities in the regulation of the noradrenergic system may contribute to the pathophysiology of both anxiety and depression, particularly to the altered arousal, activity, and vegetative functions observed in endogenous depression. Antidepressants may restore more efficient regulation of this system. The underlying eitology and exact character of these abnormalities remains to be determined. See under the heading Norepinephrine in Chapter 8: Neurophysiological and Neurochemical Basis of Behavior. See also Chapter 9: Neurotransmitter Receptor Function.

Serotoninergic System in Depression

The serotonin system has also been postulated to be abnormal in depression, with a decreased serotoninergic activity contributing to a diathesis to depression. Strategies designed to test this hypothesis are similar to those used to test the noradrenergic hypothesis of depression.

For example, a serotonin hypothesis of depression would predict that levels of serotonin or its metabolites would be deficient in postmortem brains, urine, cerebrospinal fluid, or plasma of depressed patients. Studies of postmortem brains of suicides have suggested decreases in serotonin and its metabolites, although these studies have not been entirely consistent. Concentrations of plasma tryptophan, a precursor of serotonin, decrease when patients are depressed and normalize with recovery. 5-Hydroxyindoleacetic acid (5-HIAA), a metabolite of serotonin, is decreased in the cerebrospinal fluid of a subgroup of depressed patients characterized by suicidal behaviors often involving violent methods. Some studies have found that lower 5-HIAA concentrations in cerebrospinal fluid are associated with greater severity of depression.

The psychopharmacological challenge strategy suggests that agents which enhance serotoninergic activity, such as L-tryptophan or fenfluramine, lead to decreased neuroendocrine responses, suggesting net functional decreases in the serotoninergic system in depression. Direct measurement of serotonin receptors on platelets also suggests alterations in depressed patients. The specific role of serotoninergic receptor alterations in the affective disorders has yet to be specifically clarified.

Serotonin is taken up into nerve cells by a specific serotonin reuptake site that is associated with a binding site for the antidepressant imipramine. Thus, the binding of imipramine to neuronal tissue of depressed patients may serve as a marker for the availability of reuptake sites for serotonin. Post mortem brains of suicide victims have been demonstrated to have a reduced density of imipramine binding sites. Platelets also have specific serotonin reuptake sites that are labeled by imipramine, and both imipramine binding and serotonin uptake are also diminished in the platelets of depressed patients compared to controls. These findings have been reported rather consistently, although it has yet to be established how specific they are for depressed patients. They might imply reduced reuptake of serotonin in depressed patients, although it is not yet clear how this might affect intrasynaptic concentrations of serotonin. Although these results might suggest increased serotonin in the synapse due to less inactivation by reuptake, most investigators have interpreted the decreased imipramine binding as reflecting less extensive serotoninergic terminals or a compensatory response to decreased intrasynaptic serotonin. Increased numbers of postsynaptic serotonin receptors in the brains of suicide victims are consistent with the latter possibility. Serotonin receptors are currently a subject of increasing investigation in peripheral cell, postmortem, and challenge studies.

The therapeutic response of depressed patients to pharmacological agents enhancing serotoninergic activity also has been used as a strategy to test the serotonin-deficiency hypothesis. Many of the tricyclic and monoamine oxidase—inhibiting antidepressants increase serotoninergic turnover. Therapeutic responses to these agents have been reported to be enhanced by the administration of serotonin precursors such as L-tryptophan; L-tryptophan has been suggested to have a prophylactic effect in depressed patients in remission. However, the use of such precursors alone to treat depression has led to inconsistent results. Conversely, agents that block serotoninergic activity or a diet free of tryptophan may increase depressive symptoms.

Evidence to date is compelling in suggesting a role for the serotoninergic system in depression. However, similar abnormalities observed in alcoholic and personality disordered patients suggest that serotoninergic abnormalities may not be specific for depression. The association of low serotoninergic activity with self-directed aggression in depressed patients and with aggressive actions toward others in personally disordered patients, in conjunction with animal evidence showing an association between aggressive behavior and reduced serotonin synthesis, raises the possibility that altered serotoninergic activity may be associated with a disinhibition of aggressive behaviors. In some individuals, these aggressive behaviors turned inward may be associated with the pathogenesis of depression and suicidal behavior. See under the heading Serotonin in Chapter 8: Neurophysiological and Neurochemical Basis of Behavior.

Cholinergic System in Depression

Centrally acting cholinergic agents may precipitate a behavioral syndrome resembling depression in some individuals, implicating the cholinergic system in the pathophysiology of depression. These clinical observations are consistent with animal evidence suggesting that cholinomimetics produce depressant effects, including lethargy, decreased locomotion, and decreased self-stimulus.

Physostigmine, a centrally acting anticholinesterase, when given intravenously to a susceptible individual, produces a syndrome characterized by lethargy, anergy, psychomotor retardation, decreased perceived ideation, and social withdrawal. These symptoms can be reversed by atropine, a centrally active muscarinic drug. In manic patients, physostigmine may cause a brief but dramatic reduction in their subjective elation, talkativeness, and hyperactivity. Other cholinomimetic drugs that produce such a depressed mood are the acetylcholine precursors choline and lecithin and the muscarinic receptor agonist arecholine. Patients who are depressed or who have been depressed in the past seem to be particularly vulnerable to these behavioral effects.

Neuroendocrine responses such as cortisol, prolactin, and β-endorphin to cholinomimetic agents may also be enhanced in depressed patients compared to controls. Since acetylcholine plays an excitatory role in cortisol secretion, cholinergic overactivity may play a role in the elevated cortisol concentrations observed in depressed patients.

The latency time from sleep onset to the first period of REM sleep (REM latency) is decreased by cholinomimetic agents such as physostigmine and arecholine. In some, but not all, studies, REM latency is reduced by those cholinergic agents to a significantly greater degree in depressed patients than in controls, even in depressed patients in remission, as well as in some relatives of depressed patients. Furthermore, the magnitude of the cholinomimetic-induced REM latency decrease shows concordance between monozygotic twins, suggesting that increased sensitivity to cholinomimetics may be a genetically determined trait marker for depression. The sleep disturbances of depression, including a reduced REM latency in depressed patients compared to controls (in the absence of cholinomimetic agents), may be related to this cholinergic overactivity. See under the heading Sleep in Chapter 13: Biological Rhythms and the Neuroendocrine System.

It is unclear whether cholinergic overactivity is a function of increased availability of acetylcholine or increased responsiveness of cholinergic receptors. The enhanced sensitivity to arecholine, which is a selective cholinergic agent, suggests the latter. However, the acetylcholine precursor choline has been found to be elevated in the red blood cells of a subgroup of affectively ill patients compared to controls. The transport of choline is inhibited in the red blood cells of patients receiving lithium, resulting in increases in red blood cell choline. Red blood cell choline levels in bipolar patients in long-term lithium treatment are increased compared to controls.

A cholinergic hypothesis of depression might suggest that antidepressants reduce cholinergic activity. Many antidepressants have potent anticholinergic effects, although these do not necessarily correspond to therapeutic efficacy. Preliminary trials of anticholinergic agents suggest beneficial results in some patients. It is also possible that antidepressants reverse associated state-related abnormalities in other neurotransmitter systems that are associated with a trait-related cholinergic supersensitivity, which itself is not reversed by antidepressants.

One hypothesis linking the cholinergic system to other neurotransmitter systems is the cholinergic-adrenergic hypothesis. This hypothesis postulates that affective disorders reflect an imbalance between cholinergic and adrenergic activity. According to this model, depression represents a disease of cholinergic excess, and mania represents one of adrenergic predominance. This model is supported by animal behavioral evidence suggesting that cholinomimetics depress psychomotor and reward-related activity, while adrenergic agents enhance it. Furthermore, reserpine, which depletes monoamines, also causes an increase in cholinergic activity, evidenced by a syndrome of miosis, lacrimation, salivation, diarrhea, akinesia, tremor, and sedation. There are only preliminary indications that decreased responses to challenges enhancing catecholamine system activity may be accompanied by reductions in responsiveness to cholinomimetics. However, the animal evidence and convergence of decreased adrenergic and enhanced cholinergic activity in depressed patients make this an appealing hypothesis. See under the heading Acetylcholine in Chapter 8: Neurophysiological and Neurochemical Basis of Behavior.

Dopaminergic System in Depression

The dopamine system has also been implicated in the affective disorders, particularly mania. Exploration of dopamine's role in the affective disorders grew out of observations that neuroleptics, which block dopamine receptors, also are an effective treatment for mania and may induce depression. Conversely, L-dopa treatment of Parkinson's disease may, in some individuals, precipitate a manic episode. Some studies report that concentrations of the dopamine metabolite homovanillic acid (HVA) in cerebrospinal fluid are reduced in depressed patients and increased in mania, but these findings have not been consistently replicated.

Psychopharmacological agents such as L-dopa and amphetamine, which enhance dopaminergic activity at postsynaptic sites by increasing the availability or release of dopamine, or both, have definite effects on mood. L-Dopa seems to affect arousal or activation more than mood itself but can precipitate hypomania in patients with a prior history of mania. Although L-dopa is not universally effective as an antidepressant, patients with low cerebrospinal fluid HVA or

marked retardation may respond to its administration.

Some depressed patients may have supersensitive dopamine receptors, as suggested by neuroendocrine responses to challenges that enhance dopaminergic activity, such as L-Dopa or apomorphine. These responses seem largely to be attributable to the bipolar patients, while unipolar patients may show blunted responses, similar to subgroup differences observed with noradrenergic challenges. However, many of the agents used have effects on both systems, so it has been difficult to examine independently the responsiveness of these two systems until more selective probes became available.

Although tricyclic antidepressants do not uniformly block dopaminergic reuptake, several antidepressants can significantly inhibit dopamine's reuptake. Furthermore, a variety of tricyclics may include a subsensitivity of presynaptic dopamine receptors, even after single doses.

Thus, it appears that dopamine may play a role in the pathophysiology of the affective disorders. See under the heading Dopamine in Chapter 8: Neurophysiological and Neurochemical Basis of Behavior.

Neurohormones

Cortisol

Cortisol is released in response to stress, particularly stresses over which an organism has no control. Depressed patients show consistently increased concentrations of plasma cortisol, increased urinary excretion of cortisol and its metabolites, and disturbances in the circadian rhythm of concentrations of plasma cortisol. In contrast to normal controls, depressed patients, particularly "melancholic" or endogenously depressed patients, also do not consistently suppress their plasma cortisol levels in response to dexamethasone. Dexamethasone suppresses cortisol secretion by acting on glucocorticoid receptors at the hypothalamopituitary level to "turn off" adrenocroticotropic hormone (ACTH) and, in turn, cortisol. Thus, this feedback mechanism is deficient in depressed patients.

The response to dexamethasone has been studied extensively in depressed patients, and a standardized test has been devised in the hope that such a test will aid in the diagnosis of the melancholic form of depression. Such a test might have diagnostic utility, since melancholia is the form of depression more responsive to somatic treatments such as antidepressant medication or electroconclusive therapy. In this test, dexamethasone is administered at 11:30 P.M. at a dose of 1 mg, and blood samples are drawn at 4 P.M. and 11 P.M. (also at 8 A.M., if possible). A plasma value greater than 5 μg/dl defines the criterion for nonsuppression. This test seemed helpful in distinguishing endogenous from nonendogenous depression and other psychiatric disorders. However, it has become clear that nonsuppression on the dexamethasone test is observed in a variety of other disorders, including obsessive-compulsive disorder, Alzheimer's disease, anorexia nervosa, and alcoholism. Nevertheless, serial dexamethasone tests may be helpful in predicting relapse in known dexamethasone test nonsuppressors, since failure of suppression following antidepressant treatment, even in the face of apparent clinical improvement, may signal an impending relapse.

The origin of the dexamethasone test abnormality in depression has not been clarified, although some evidence suggests excessive secretion of cortisol-releasing factor (CRF) and the responsiveness of adrenals to secrete cortisol. Increased secretion of CRF might be driven at the hypothalamic level by neurotransmitter imbalances. For example, norepinephrine appears to play an inhibitory role in the hypothalamic-pituitary axis, whereas acetylcholine and serotonin are usually excitatory. Thus, a relative deficiency of noradrenergic activity and excess of cholinergic activity might result in overactivity of the hypothalamic-pituitary axis. Although abnormalities in this axis remain among the most robust observed in the affective disorders, the exact mechanisms underlying them remain to be further clarified.

Thyroid

Abnormalities in the secretion of thyroid hormone may sometimes be observed in depressed patients. Usually hyposecretion of thyroid hormone T3 or T4 is associated with depression, but thyrotoxicosis may also be accompanied by depression or, in other instances, mania. Infrequently, elevations of thyroid-stimulating hormone (TSH) in the presence of normal plasma concentrations of T3 and T4 may be observed.

Depressed patients also show a blunted TSH respone to thyroid-releasing hormone (TRH). In this test, 500 mg of synthetic TRH is given by intravenous push over 30 seconds, and blood samples are taken at 15-minute intervals up to 60 minutes. The exogenous TRH acts like endogenous TRH released from the hypothalamus to stimulate the release of TSH at the pituitary. A change from baseline TSH to a peak TSH of less than 5 μU/ml is considered abnormal. Absent or blunted TSH responses to TRH may be observed in slightly less than half of depressed patients. Unipolar patients show consistently blunted TSH responses to TRH, whereas bipolar patients sometimes show increased responses. Manic patients, but not schizophrenics, also show a blunted TSH response to TRH as do depressed alcoholics. It is possible that this test may also prove helpful in identifying patients who are more prone to relapse, since abnormal TRH tests after treatment may be observed more frequently in patients who go on to relapse than those who remain well. Furthermore, evaluation with both the TRH test and dexamethasone test may identify a majority of depressed patients who are abnormal in their response to one or the other test or both.

It is possible that the blunted TSH responses to TRH are a function of abnormal norepinephrine activity. Unipolar depressives and manics may have increased release of hypothalamic norepinephrine, which would excessively stimulate TRH, ultimately downregulating pituitary TRH receptors, which mediate the release of TSH. In contrast, bipolar depressed patients may have decreased availability of norepinephrine in the hypothalamus, decreased TRH, and resultant upregulation of TRH receptors in the pituitary.

Observations that the addition of thyroid hormone to antidepressant medications may enhance their therapeutic effect strengthen the proposal that thyroid abnormalities may sometimes play a role in the pathogenesis of depression.

Growth Hormone

Growth hormone is released episodically in a pulsatile fashion; these pulses may occur more frequently in depressed patients than in normal controls. However, agents that stimulate growth hormone generally induce less of a growth hormone increase in depressed patients than in controls. For example, challenges with insulin-induced hypoglycemia, amphetamine, methamphetamine, L-dopa, and clonidine, all of which appear to initiate growth hormone release via α-adrenergic receptors, may lead to a deficient growth hormone response, with more selective α₂-adrenergic agents showing the most consistent deficiency. Deficient growth hormone responses to 5-hydroxytryptophan (5-HTP) mediated serotoninergically and to apomorphine mediated dopaminergically are less consistent. Some studies suggest a reduced growth hormone–releasing factor (GRF). The same patients may show a normal respone to a dopaminergic challenge but not to a noradrenergic challenge. The results suggest that alterations in growth hormone may not be due solely to a primary disturbance in the growth hormone system but seem to reflect abnormalities in the neurotransmitter systems that modulate growth hormone release.

Prolactin

Prolactin secretion in humans is quite responsive to stress, so that under stressful conditions depressed patients may have elevated plasma prolactin concentrations. If stress is not a major factor, there may be a subgroup of depressed patients with abnormally low prolactin concentrations and those with abnormally high prolactin concentrations. Prolactin responses to TRH and insulin-induced hypoglycemia are generally normal. The prolactin response to morphine is blunted, as are prolactin responses to serotoninergic agents. As with the other hormones, prolactin abnormalities may not reflect intrinsic pituitary abnormalities but more likely represent abnormalities in facilitatory or inhibitory neuromodulators.

Gonadotropins

Alterations in the secretion of the gonadotropins may occur in depressed patients. These alterations may contribute to the abnormalities in the menstrual cycle observed in depressed females. Luteinizing hormone and follicle-stimulating hormone responses to gonadotropin-releasing hormone do not consistently distinguish depressed patients from controls, although abnormal follicle-stimulating hormone responses to gonadotropin-releasing hormone may be observed in some depressed patients.

See under the heading Neuroendocrine Mechanisms in Chapter 13: Biological Rhythms and the Neuroendocrine System.

CONCLUSIONS

Depression is an illness with important genetic determinants that confer a vulnerability to depressive episodes. The state of depression appears to be characterized by multiple abnormalities in the neurotransmitters and neurohormones that play in the modulation of stress, arousal, and mood. Although the specific etiological factors in depression remain to be established, such "vulnerability" factors may interact with internal or external stressors to produce the altered neurobehavioral state that is experienced subjectively and observed clinically as "depression."

BIBLIOGRAPHY

Carroll, B.J., et al.: A specific laboratory test for the diagnosis of melancholia. Arch. Gen. Psychiatry 38:15-22, 1981.

Davis, J.M., Koslow, S.H., Gibbons, R.D.: Cerebrospinal fluid and urinary biogenic amines in depressed patients and healthy controls. Arch. Gen. Psychiatry 45:705-717, 1988.

Janowsky, D.S., Risch, S.C.: Role of acetylcholine mechanisms in the affective disorders, in Psychopharmacology: The Third Generation of Progress, H.Y. Meltzer (ed.), pp. 527-533. New York, Raven Press, 1987.

Jimerson, D.C.: Role of dopamine mechanisms in the affective disorders, in Psychopharmacology: The Third Generation of Progress, H.Y. Meltzer (ed.), pp. 503-511. New York, Raven Press, 1987.

Meltzer, H.Y., Lowy, M.T.: The serotonin hypothesis of depression, in Psychopharmacology: The Third Generation of Progress, H.Y. Meltzer (ed.), pp. 513-526. New York, Raven Press, 1987.

Siever, L.J., Davis, K.L.: Overview: Towards a dysregulation hypothesis of depression. Am. J. Psychiatry 142: 1017-1031, 1985.

Wehr, T.A., Rosenthal, N.E.: Seasonality and affective illness. Am. J. Psychiatry 146:829-839, 1989.

Chapter 27
Psychodynamic Aspects of Mood Disorders

Emil F. Coccaro, M.D.

The two major, and interdependent, approaches to the study, evaluation, and treatment of depressive disorders are the psychobiologic or physiologic and the psychodynamic. The former approach is discussed in Chapter 26: Pathogenesis of Mood Disorders; the latter approach is discussed in this chapter, which focuses on the development of the psychodynamic model and approach to depression. This chapter begins with the earliest psychoanalytic concepts and concludes with a more contemporary, and integrative, overview of the psychodynamic aspects of the disorder.

The syndrome of depressive disorder has remained essentially intact since its first description by Hippocrates in the fourth century B.C. At that time, depression was referred to as *melancholia,* a term that represented Hippocrates' conceptualization of a disorder resulting from an excess of black bile in the brain. Two centuries later, Aretaceus of Cappadocia revised and expanded the concept of melancholia by stating that it was primarily psychological in nature and etiology. Further, he noted the etiologic contribution of interpersonal relationships and stresses on the development and course of a disorder that he recognized as recurrent and associated with the converse state of mania in some individuals (for example, those with manic-depressive, or bipolar, disorder).

This strikingly modern view of depressive disorder, however, did not take hold in the general thinking of the subsequent observers of mental illness. Theoreticians from the second century A.D. on up to those of the eighteenth century returned to Hippocratic concepts and focused on the affect of "humors" and the alignment of the planets on their patients. While the spread of the scientific revolution in the eighteenth and nineteenth centuries led to a less mystical and primitive view of mental illness, investigators continued to focus on physical, as opposed to psychologic, contributions to the etiology of such disorders. It remained, then, until the development of psychoanalytic thought, in the late nineteenth and early twentieth centuries, before serious consideration of psychological factors and/or processes could come to the fore.

EARLY PSYCHOANALYTIC THEORETICIANS: FREUD AND ABRAHAM

The earliest writings regarding the psychoanalytic theory of depression were done by Sigmund Freud and Karl Abraham.

Freud

Freud first wrote on the subject of depression in his classic paper "Mourning and Melancholia." In this brief but highly significant paper, Freud compared and contrasted these two seemingly similar states of behavior. While both conditions share a painful dejection over a loss, decreased interest in the outside world, decreased capacity to love, and an inhibition of purposeful activity, Freud noted that melancholics display a decrease in self-regard and a tendency toward self-reproach, with an irrational expectation of punishment. Further, melancholics appear to be unclear as to the specific nature of their loss. While in mourning the loss is clearly the physical and irretrievable loss of a loved one, in melancholia the loss appears to be internal and unconscious. Accordingly, Freud (1917) stated that "in grief, the world becomes poor and empty; in melancholia, it is the ego itself."

Freud hypothesized that this inner state of emptiness, characterized by self-reproach, results from a split in the melancholic's ego such that the observed clinical picture of self-reproach in fact represents reproaches against an inner mental representation of a lost and/or rejecting love object (for example, a parent) that was incorporated into the ego at an early stage of ego development in childhood. At this stage the ego was split into a critical or judgmental ego ("conscience") and an ego identified with the early lost love object. This then results in an unleashing of critical feelings and ideation from the "critical ego" to the ego identified with the early lost love object. At times the fury of these feelings is so great that the melancholic sets out to destroy this ego identification and commits suicide. Usually, however, the fury is less intense and serves only to devalue the ego identification through self-reproaches to the point that it may be abandoned. At this point the episode passes until a future loss reactivates the process.

In later writings, Freud revised the concept of the critical or judgmental ego into "superego." By this time, Freud had proposed that melancholia results from harsh criticism by the superego. This criticism occurs because aggressive impulses reactivated by a loss would be turned, unless outwardly expressed (as they cannot be), against the self (the ego).

Abraham

As a contemporary of Freud, Abraham published several papers on the subject of depression. Initially, Abraham posited that the state of depression results from a repression of unopposed sexual and aggressive ("libidinal") drives so great that the individual utimately gives up his or her hope of satisfying these impulses. This repression then leads the individual to the awareness that he or she is unable to love or be loved. While this is similar to the dynamic posited for the state of anxiety, Abraham suggested that the libidinal repression experienced in depression is much greater, and more complete, than that experienced in anxiety states. In the latter, libidinal repression is less severe, allowing the individual to maintain some degree of hope that he or she will ultimately attain libidinal gratification.

Abraham compared and contrasted the dynamics of depressives with those of obsessives. In particular, he noted that both groups are profoundly ambivalent in their relatedness to themselves and others. He hypothesized that the strivings toward love and toward loved ones are blocked by feelings of hatred that are, in turn, repressed as unacceptable. These hateful and destructive wishes, kept unconscious, lead to the feeling of guilt in these patients.

While depressives and obsessives may be similar in this regard, Abraham noted that they differ significantly in the way their repressed libidinal impulses find expression. Obsessives find substitutive expression in repetitive rituals, and depressives find theirs through a process of ascribing their unacceptable feelings to others, called "projection." The depressive projection is characterized by the dynamic: "I am incapable of loving; therefore, I must hate." However, since open hatred of others is unacceptable, the depressive represses this feeling and projects this hostility onto others so that it is perceived as being directed back at the self: "I am not lovable; therefore, people must hate me."

In later writings, Abraham attempted to integrate and support Freudian theories of sexuality in his conceptualization of depression. In these, Abraham posited that depression represents a regression to an early psychosexual phase of development referred to as the "oral phase."

In this phase the infant characteristically attempts to "ingest" or "incorporate" its external world through the use of its mouth or other orifice. This phase is characterized by processes referred to as "introjection" and "incorporation." Abraham felt that future depressives have an unconscious "tendency to devour and demolish the [love] object." He believed that this specific dynamic accounts for the anorexia seen in depression (here there is an equation of food with the love object, which the individual fears he or she will destroy if he or she ingests its representation—the food).

Structural Theorist: Rado

In a structural revision of the previously discussed psychoanalytic model, Sandor Rado postulated that depression occurs after a breakdown in the balance of tensions among the ego, superego, and the love object. Rado suggested, as did Abraham earlier, that the depressive is fixated at the oral phase of psychosexual development and thereby has a tremendous need for external emotional sustenance. The configuration of a passive-dependent individual and an all-giving parent who may withdraw, either physically or emotionally, leads to an "anger-guilt-atonement" sequence, with the parent as a love object that becomes set in early development so as to persist and be repeated with subsequent love objects. The child learns that his or her anger at the parent for withdrawing nutritional or emotional support drives the parent away. The child then learns that this support may be reinstated if he or she displays appropriately remorseful behavior. On the structural intrapsychic level, the child, due to the immature nature of his or her cognitive abilities, introjects the esteem-giving parent love object and the withdrawing parent love object as two separate mental representations and incorporates the former into the superego and the latter into the ego.

Later in life, the depressive, who is torn between his or her rage at, and submissive fear of, the love object, intermittently behaves so as to drive the love object away. Once the love object is driven away, the depressive falls back upon the anger-guilt-atonement sequence in an attempt to win back the love object. If this does not succeed, the struggle shifts to the intrapsychic level, where the "bad" ego (self) seeks forgiveness from the internalized "good or esteem-giving" superego. During this period, the depressive withdraws largely from the interpersonal world, giving rise to the symptoms of decreased interest and activity. After a period of atonement, the ego regains the lost esteem of the superego and the episode resolves, until reactivated by the provoked loss of another love object.

Object Relations Theorist: Klein

Further development of a psychodynamic model of depression was made by Melanie Klein through her conceptualization of ego organization, object relations, and the resolution of "depressive" anxiety.

According to Klein, there are two basic developmental stages, or "positions," in the first year of life. The first, a schizoparanoid position, is characterized as a time when the infant can only perceive part objects as opposed to whole objects. At this time, the infant internalizes the mother's breasts as two completely separate objects: a "good" feeding breast and a "bad" nonfeeding breast. When the infant internalizes these objects, it initially does so without differentiating between the "good" and the "bad." However, once the objects are internalized, the infant becomes frightened that the "bad" objects, identified with the nonfeeding or depriving breast, will destroy the "good" objects, identified with the feeding breast. To alleviate this conflict, the infant projects back to the environment these "bad" objects. This leads to the perception that the danger is outside and may come from without.

At about 5 months into the first year of life, the second, or depressive, position takes hold. At this time, the infant, beginning to perceive objects as whole rather than as parts, becomes aware that the same external objects may be a source of pleasure and pain. The conflicts arising from the infant's ambivalent feelings regarding these objects becomes intense as the earlier, and more primitive, defense of external projection is found to be inadequate. Accordingly, once the breasts are identified as belonging to the mother, the infant's hostility can no longer be safely projected to an isolated "bad" object in the environment. As the conflict proceeds, the infant recognizes that the hostility is its own and that the hostility may be powerful enough to destroy the "good" objects, both external (parents) and internal (ego or self). The anxiety this then produces is referred to as *depressive anxiety*.

How the child resolves the anxiety of the depressive position determines the nature of further development. If the child gives in to his or her depressive anxiety, he or she becomes depressed and inhibited, since he or she will fear that his or her (aggressive) action will destroy the "good" objects. If the child denies the value of the "good" objects, he or she may assume the opposite stance characterized by the perception that he or she needs no other object besides himself or herself—the manic defense. Alternatively, the healthy child acknowledges his or her hostile or aggressive impulses and realizes that, while they may temporarily drive away the "good" objects, they will not truly destroy them and that, through appropriate restitutive behaviors, these objects will return, along with a restored sense of self-esteem and well-being.

Self-Esteem Regulation Theorists: Jacobson, Bibring, Sandler

Following Freud's observation that melancholia may be uniquely characterized by a decrease in self-regard, or esteem, a series of later theorists, including Jacobson, Bibring, and Sandler, chose to promote a view of depression as a disorder whose central abnormality resided in a faulty regulation of self-esteem.

Jacobson

The most complex elaboration of this concept was proposed by Jacobson, who theorized that depression occurs when esteem regulation is impaired by an abnormal regulation of investments (cathexes) of psychic energy. In this model, the ego, or self-representation, has specific relationships with the higher psychic structures known as the ego ideal and the superego. Specifically, Jacobson proposed that the ego looks to the ego ideal as the standard against which it must measure itself and to the superego to regulate the distribution of libidinal (ego or esteem building) and aggressive (ego or esteem destroying) energies to the ego. In healthy individuals, the superego theoretically exists as an abstract, depersonalized structure. In depressives, however, the superego is poorly formed and tinged with representations of significant earlier objects; there is interference by these contaminating representations, and the superego is hampered in its ability to properly distribute its libidinal and aggressive energies.

Jacobson theorized that the rage arising from frustration or loss is directed at the ego. The aggressive cathexis into the ego devalues the ego and results in a disparity between the perceived ego and the desired ego ideal, which in turn leads to a fall in self-esteem. As a defense, the depressive attempts to find new sources of libidinal (esteem-building) energy from other objects. If not successful in this regard, the depressive retreats from outside objects and reactivates an internal, but libidinally cathected, image from the past that may merge with the superego. Once this powerfully cathected image has merged, the depressive may then attempt to draw on the newly charged superego's libidinal energy reserves so as to libidinally energize the ego and, as a result, raise its self-esteem.

Bibring and Sandler

The later theorists Bibring and Sandler espoused a simpler and less metapsychological view of depression: like anxiety, depression is a primary experience that cannot be further broken down.

Although Bibring and Sandler agreed that depression is associated with a loss of self-esteem, they differed on the causal mechanism. For Bibring, "depression can be defined as the emotional expression of a state of helplessness and powerlessness of the ego, irrespective of what may have caused the breakdown of the mechanisms which established his self-esteem" (1953, p. 24). Bibring further suggested that the depressive is particularly vulnerable to these blows on his or her self-esteem, unrealistic aspirations that he or she cannot possibly fulfill.

For Sandler, decreased self-esteem is due more simply to a loss of "narcissistic" integrity. Specifically, "when a love object is lost, what is really lost is the state of well-being implicit, both psychologically and biologically, in the relationship with the love object" (1965, p. 91). In this model, as in Freud's, aggression is directed at the self but only because the self was not effective in maintaining the love object.

Heinz Kohut proposed that the organization of the infant psyche is bipolar, with tendencies toward grandiosity and exhibitionism (the beginnings of assertiveness and ambition) at one pole and tendencies toward idealization of the parents (the beginnings of ideals and values) at the other pole. Both groups of tendencies contribute to the strong self-object ties between infant and parent, which are the foundation for the building of a healthy self. He held that the real mover of psychic development is the self, rather than Freudian sexual and aggressive drives. Kohut used the term *selfobject* to describe an object in an infant's surrounding that the infant regards as part of himself or herself. People with narcissistic personality disorder cannot separate adequately from the selfobject and thus cannot perceive or respond to the individuality of others. For Kohut, a lack of empathic response between parent and infant is the cause of later psychologic illness in the growing child rather than isolated drive or superego predispositions.

Family or Cultural Theorists: Cohen and the Washington School

The first and most empiric work to deal with the potential impact of familial or cultural (as opposed to classic psychoanalytic-dynamic) factors on depressive disorders did not appear until 1949. This work, an intensive study of the families of 12 manic depressives by M. B. Cohen and the Washington School of Psychiatry, found that the families of depressives were isolated from, or ostracized by, the general community. In all cases, these families longed for community acceptance and expected their children (the future identified patients among them) to maintain a high level of achievement to "undo" the families' perceived lower community standing. In doing so, the families devalued the children by using them as an instrument for social status elevation.

Within the family unit itself the mother, as opposed to the father, was the stronger parent. Curiously, the father, who was often socially or economically unsuccessful, was implicitly held up by the demanding, critical, and depreciating mother as an example of what fate would befall the children if they did not live up to the mother's high standards. Although this implicit warning was not appreciated by the children until later childhood and adolescence, they experienced a more primal threat of maternal abandonment in the toddler years. The toddler's normal "rebellious," individuating behavior was met by the mother's clear withdrawal of love or approval and threats of abandonment.

Identified patients among the children were found to have developed according to these dynamics in the most extreme form. In fact, the patients were most often found to hold a special place in the family because of better developed talents or a greater willingness to please, both of which were valued for their ability to elevate the social standing of the family.

Ultimately, the patients were found to develop into interpersonal manipulators, viewing relationships as a means of achieving their own (their family's or mother's) ambitions. If the pa-

tients did not achieve, they would be subject to the disapproval of, or the abandonment by, the powerful authority figure (mother), face a great loss of sustenance, and slip into a depression. This group of investigators concluded that the development in such families left the patients with a pervasive sense of inner emptiness that only strong external figures could possibly rectify. When not depressed, the patients attempt to please these external figures to meet their dependent demands for sustenance. If such a relationship is terminated, for whatever reason, the patient plunges into a depressive episode, which may be interpreted as a manifestation of the patient's attempt to win back the lost external figure (see preceding discussion on the structural theorists).

Cognitive or Behavioral Theorists: Beck and Seligman

Two of the most recent theories regarding the psychologic etiology of depression are of a more cognitive or behavioral nature. The first is the cognitive theory as developed by Beck, and the second is the learned helplessness model as developed by Seligman and colleagues.

Beck

Beck's cognitive theory proposes that feelings of depression arise out of a specific cognitive stance that leads depressives to a systematically pessimistic view of themselves, others, the environment, and the future. The etiologic role of this stance is to set off a self-reinforcing chain reaction such that these negative or pessimistic cognitive sets lead to sadness, as well as to the view that the individual is lacking in "some element or attribute that he considers essential for his happiness." Recovery from an episode is thought to occur when the depressive is shown how these negative cognitive sets distort reality and how, by his or her adopting more positive views, these distortions can be lessened.

Seligman

The learned helplessness model of Seligman is behaviorally empirical in nature. The model developed out of animal experiments involving the administration of inescapable shock to dogs. After repeated trials of inescapable shock, these experimental animals "gave up" the possibility of escape from (that is, did nothing to avoid) future shock, even when escape was made possible. On the basis of these and other experiments, Seligman proposed that a "learned helplessness" might explain some aspects of depression in humans. In this model, depression results from the perception that the depressive has no control over the nature of behavioral or emotional reinforcement in his or her environment. As a result, unable to change the unsatisfying circumstances, he or she "gives up."

Overview of Psychodynamic Model

Most psychodynamic models of depressive disorder speak to the etiologic interplay between psychic development and functioning and the mood-regulating infant or child relationship to powerful parental figures. All but perhaps the most recent, most empiric models stress the importance of the nearly inevitable loss of consistent and constant parental love and nourishment as the infant or child matures. The way in which the immature psyche responds to this loss appears to shape the borders and functioning of the intrapsychic structures (id, ego, and superego) in their regulation of self-esteem.

Also critical to several models are the regulation and disposition of aggressive, hostile, and socially unacceptable impulses and drives, existing from infancy or in response to parental loss or future disappointment by a love object. Such impulses and drives are thought to be turned against the self (or its intrapsychic representation) either directly or indirectly— directly through projection (Abraham) or by direct assault (Freud, Jacobson), or indirectly as a consequence of expressing one's rage at the disappointing or rejecting love object (Rado). In some models (Klein), the mere realization that such highly destructive impulses exist within oneself is sufficient to create a vulnerability for depression.

While some models may make little mention of factors related to aggression or hostility, all point to the etiologic significance of an injury, real or perceived, to one's psychic or narcissistic integrity. Such injuries are often precipitated by a significant loss of a love object, goal, or security. In the case of the learned helplessness model, for example, the loss may be considered to be a loss of options (that is, the freedom to make effective choices).

Few of these models adequately address the question of why some individuals develop episodes of major depression and some do not.

Many of the models suggest that the intrapsychic development is upset by early disappointments by parental love objects. However, it is doubtful that this alone is sufficient; even healthy child development cannot proceed without some significant parental disappointments. Other models allude that there may be a "genetic" or "constitutional" defect in the intrapsychic structure of some depressives that creates a psychologic vulnerability to depressive attacks.

Current psychiatric thought generally holds that factors related to impaired intrapsychic development, environmental loss or stress, and real or perceived assaults on self-esteem, as well as biologic defects in the neuronal regulation of mood and vital bodily functioning (for example, appetite, sleep, energy, motor activity), are important in the setting up of vulnerabilities toward, and the precipitation of, the depressive attack in various mood-disordered patients. It is likely that each factor interacts to progressively lower the threshold for the occurrence of depressive episodes. Further, the separate impact of any particular factor is likely to depend upon the severity of the psychic or biologic defect. Depressives with a severe psychological vulnerability (for example, severe dependency on the esteem-giving properties of a love object) may require little in the way of a biologic defect (for example, subsensitivity of the monoaminergic receptors involved in limbic neuronal pathways) to plunge into a depressive episode after rejection by the love object. Similarly, depressives with a severe biologic defect may enter an episode after little, and possibly no apparent, psychologic stress. This seeming dichotomy in regard to etiologic factors is analogous to the "reactive" and "endogenous" classifications of depressive illness as espoused by theorists and clinicians before the development of the DSM-III diagnostic criteria in the late 1970s.

Regardless of specific etiology, however, nearly all depressives display some degree of premorbid psychologic vulnerabilities, as outlined above, that need to be explored and addressed during treatment of the acute attack and during recovery. An assessment of the nature and severity of these vulnerabilities allows the physician to determine the relative priority of psychic versus biologic factors and thus to design the optimal treatment plan for the patient in question. However, cases of severe or recurrent depression often benefit from pharmacotherapy, regardless of the presence of strong psychological vulnerabilities.

BIBLIOGRAPHY

Abraham, K.: Selected Papers on Psychoanalysis. New York, Basic Books, 1960.

Arieti, S.: Psychotherapy of severe depression. Am. J. Psychiatry 134:864-868, 1977.

Beck, A.: Cognitive Therapy and the Emotional Disorders. New York, International Universities Press, 1976.

Bibring, E.: The Mechanism of Depression, in Affecive Disorders, P. Greenacre (ed.), pp 13-48. New York, International Universities Press, 1953.

Cohen, M. B., et al.: An intensive study of twelve cases of manic depressive psychosis. Psychiatry 17:103-138, 1954.

Freud, S.: Mourning and melancholia (1917), in Sigmund Freud: Collected Papers, vol. 4. New York, Basic Books, 1959.

Jacobson, E.: The effect of disappointment on ego and superego formation in normal and depressive development. Psychoanal. Rev. 33:129-147, 1946.

Klein, M.: Mourning and its relation to manic-depressive states. Contributions to Psychoanalysis, 1921-1945, London, Hogarth Press, 1948.

Lewis, A.: Melancholia: A historical review. J. Med Sci. 80:1, 1934.

Rado, S.: The problem of melancholia. Collected Papers, vol. 1, New York, Grune & Stratton, 1956.

Sandler, J., Joffe, W.G.: Notes on childhood depression. Int. J. Psychoanal. 46:88-96, 1965.

Seligman, M., Maier, S.: Failure to escape traumatic shock. J. Exp. Psychol. 74:1-9, 1967.

Veith, I.: Elizabethans on melancholia. J. A. M. A. 212:127, 1970.

Chapter 28

Biology of Schizophrenia

Kenneth L. Davis, M.D., and Blaine Greenwald, M.D.

The development of phenothiazines as a treatment for schizophrenia in the 1950s revolutionized psychiatry. The question of how these drugs work stimulated a search for the biological mechanisms that underlie this illness. Consequently, the last 25 years have brought a wealth of neurochemical, psychopharmacological, behavioral, and neuroendocrine data supporting specific neurotransmitter involvement in the pathogenesis of schizophrenia (Fig. 28-1). The major theory focuses on the neurotransmitter dopamine. Other neurotransmitters and neuromodulators have also been implicated, including GABA, acetylcholine, norepinephrine, endorphins, and so-called endogenous psychotogens. Much of this chapter reviews the evidence for a biochemical basis of schizophrenia.

A structural basis for schizophrenia can be theorized through recent progress in neuroradiology. Morphologic brain abnormalities and associated findings in schizophrenic patients are discussed in the last part of this chapter.

Emil Kraepelin described an illness, the typ-ical symptoms of which were hallucinations, delusions, and thought disorder. In 1908, E. Bleuler named the same illness schizophrenia, meaning split mind. This is not the same as the popular concept of split personality; the split in schizophrenia refers to abnormal relationships between thought, emotion, and behavior, not multiple personalities. Bleuler's four basic symptoms of schizophrenia became standard in America for diagnosis of the illness; over the years, they became elaborated into the current DSM-III-R criteria (Table 28-1).

Five types of schizophrenia are generally recognized:

1. *Catatonic type.* Psychomotor disturbance is present, often in the form of stupor, excitement, or rigid or bizarre posture.

2. *Disorganized type.* Incoherent thought, inappropriate emotion, and disorganized behavior are typical.

3. *Paranoid type.* The person is preoccupied with systematized delusions or frequent auditory hallucinations on one theme.

4. *Undifferentiated type.* Strong symptoms of

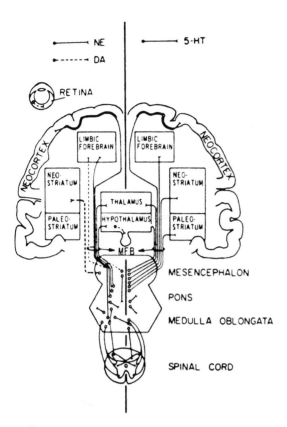

FIGURE 28–1. Diagram showing the distribution of the major neurotransmitter systems of the brain and demonstrating the vulnerability of these systems to disruption by appropriately placed limbic and subcortical lesions. (From Anden, N.-E., et al.: Ascending monoamine neurons to the telencephalon and diencephalon. Acta Physiol. Scand. 67:313-326, 1986. With permission from the publisher.)

psychosis are present and cannot be categorized in any other type.

5. *Residual type.* Strong symptoms are absent, but other symptoms are present.

The onset of schizophrenia usually takes place in adolescence or early adulthood. The course of the illness varies with the individual, and experts differ on the frequency of full remission. People at lower socioeconomic levels suffer more frequently from schizophrenia; there may be a genetic predisposition to it; it seems to occur equally often in both sexes.

DOPAMINE HYPOTHESIS

Stated simply, the dopamine hypothesis proposes that schizophrenia is the result of a functional hyperactivity of dopamine in the brain. The hypothesis is derived from pharmacological evidence: (1) drugs that decrease dopamine neu-

rotransmission (neuroleptics) have antipsychotic efficacy, and (2) agents that stimulate dopamine activity are psychotomimetic.

Anatomy and Related Physiology of Dopaminergic Pathways

Dopamine is localized in several discrete tracts in the brain. These pathways have been defined by histofluorescent and biochemical studies in the brains of laboratory animals and in postmortem human brains. The major dopaminergic neuronal tracts are the nigrostriatal, tuberoinfundibular, mesolimbic, and mesocortical.

Nigrostriatal Tract

The cell bodies of this pathway are located in the substantia nigra, a pigmented nucleus in the midbrain, designated A-9 in the rat. Axons projecting from these nerve cells terminate in the caudate-putamen of the neostriatum, synapsing with neurons containing receptors for dopamine. The primary function of the nigrostriatal dopaminergic tract is the regulation of extrapyramidal motor activity. Degeneration of nigral dopaminergic neurons underlies the pathogenesis of Parkinson's disease, with its characteristic movement disorders—bradykinesia, cogwheel rigidity, and alternating tremor. Pharmacological blockade of neostriatal postsynaptic dopamine receptors results in the parkinsonian-like extrapyramidal side effects of neuroleptic (antipsychotic) medication. Amphetamine-induced dopamine release from nigral cells and direct postsynaptic striatal dopamine receptor stimulation by apomorphine are thought to induce in laboratory animals the syndrome of motor hyperactivity—sniffing behavior with repetitive licking, biting, and gnawing—known as *stereotypy.* This syndrome in rats has been analogized to the repetitive purposeless behavior seen in human amphetamine abusers.

Drugs that block dopamine receptors (neuroleptics) inhibit amphetamine-induced stereotypy. In fact, this ability to block stereotypy has been used as a screening test for antipsychotic activity. However, two neuroleptic agents, thioridazine and clozapine, raise questions about the validity of this test. Their ability to block stereotypy is less potent than their antipsychotic efficacy would predict. One explanation for this discrepancy is that since clozapine and thioridazine rarely precipitate extrapyramidal symptoms, their ability to block stereotypy is actually

---

TABLE 28–1.   Diagnostic Criteria for Schizophrenia

A. Presence of characteristic psychotic symptoms in the active phase: either (1), (2), or (3) for at least one week (unless the symptoms are successfully treated):

   (1) two of the following:

      (a) delusions
      (b) prominent hallucinations (throughout the day for several days or several times a week for several weeks, each hallucinatory experience. not being limited to a few brief moments)
      (c) incoherence or marked loosening of associations
      (d) catatonic behavior
      (e) flat or grossly inappropriate affect

   (2) bizarre delusions (i.e., involving a phenomenon that the person's culture would regard as totally implausible, e.g., thought broadcasting, being controlled by a dead person)

   (3) prominent hallucinations [as defined in (1)(b) above] of a voice with content having no apparent relation to depression or elation, or a voice keeping up a running commentary on the person's behavior or thoughts, or two or more voices conversing with each other

B. During the course of the disturbance, functioning in such areas as work, social relations, and self-care is markedly below the highest level achieved before onset of the disturbance (or, when the onset is in childhood or adolescence, failure to achieve expected level of social development).

C. Schizoaffective Disorder and Mood Disorder with Psychotic Features have been ruled out, i.e., if a Major Depressive or Manic Syndrome has ever been present during an active phase of the disturbance, the total duration of all episodes of a mood syndrome has been brief relative to the total duration of the active and residual phases of the disturbance.

D. Continuous signs of the disturbance for at least six months. The six-month period must include an active phase (of at least one week, or less if symptoms have been successfully treated) during which there were psychotic symptoms characteristic of Schizophrenia (symptoms in A), with or without a prodromal or residual phase, as defined below.

Prodromal phase: A clear deterioration in functioning before the active phase of the disturbance that is not due to a disturbance in mood or to a Psychoactive Substance Use Disorder and that involves at least two of the symptoms listed below.

Residual phase: Following the active phase of the disturbance, persistence of at least two of the symptoms noted below, these not being due to a disturbance in mood or to a Psychoactive Substance Use Disorder.

Prodromal or Residual Symptoms:

(1) marked social isolation or withdrawal
(2) marked impairment in role functioning as wage-earner, student, or home-maker

TABLE 28–1. Diagnostic Criteria for Schizophrenia—continued

(3) markedly peculiar behavior (e.g., collecting garbage, talking to self in public, hoarding food)

(4) marked impairment in personal hygiene and grooming

(5) blunted or inappropriate affect

(6) digressive, vague, overelaborate, or circumstantial speech, or poverty of speech, or poverty of content of speech

(7) odd beliefs or magical thinking, influencing behavior and inconsistent with cultural norms, e.g., superstitiousness, belief in clairvoyance, telepathy, "sixth sense," "others can feel my feelings," overvalued ideas, ideas of reference

(8) unusual perceptual experiences, e.g., recurrent illusions, sensing the presence of a force or person not actually present

(9) marked lack of initiative, interests, or energy

Examples: Six months of prodromal symptoms with one week of symptoms from A; no prodromal symptoms with six months of symptoms from A; no prodromal symptoms with one week of symptoms from A and six months of residual symptoms.

E. It cannot be established that an organic factor initiated and maintained the disturbance.

F. If there is a history of Autistic Disorder, the additional diagnosis of Schizophrenia is made only if prominent delusions or hallucinations are also present.

Classification of course. The course of the disturbance is coded in the fifth digit:

1-Subchronic. The time from the beginning of the disturbance, when the person first began to show signs of the disturbance (including prodromal, active, and residual phases) more or less continuously, is less than two years, but at least six months.

2-Chronic. Same as above, but more than two years.

3-Subchronic with Acute Exacerbation. Reemergence of prominent psychotic symptoms in a person with a subchronic course who has been in the residual phase of the disturbance.

4-Chronic with Acute Exacerbation. Reemergence of prominent psychotic symptoms in a person with a chronic course who has been in the residual phase of the disturbance.

5-In Remission. When a person with a history of Schizophrenia is free of all signs of the disturbance (whether or not on medication), "in Remission" should be coded. Differentiating Schizophrenia in Remission from No Mental Disorder requires consideration of overall level of functioning, length of time since the last episode of disturbance, total duration of the disturbance, and whether prophylactic treatment is being given.

0-Unspecified.

a test that predicts extrapyramidal effects rather than antipsychotic action. Another hypothesis claims that the anticholinergic properties of these drugs antagonize the neuroleptic-induced blockade of stereotypy. The ability of clozapine to block serotonin type 2 receptors may also contribute to its absence of extrapyrimidal effects.

A most important additional problem in relating the ability of a neuroleptic to block animal stereotypy to antipsychotic effect is the fact that, in some test schemas, neuroleptic ability to block stereotypy decreases with time. Tolerance to the antipsychotic effect of a neuroleptic in schizophrenia is not seen.

Tuberoinfundibular Tract

The tuberoinfundibular dopaminergic pathway originates in neuronal cell bodies in the arcuate nucleus of the hypothalamus, designated A-12 in the rat, and terminates in the median eminence. These tuberoinfundibular dopaminergic neurons exert a tonic inhibitory effect on prolactin secretion from the posterior lobe of the pituitary gland. Dopamine may either promote the release of a prolactin inhibitory factor (PIF) into pituitary portal vessels, which consequently suppresses prolactin release, or dopamine itself inhibits prolactin release directly. Therefore, dopaminergic agonists like apomorphine and L-dopa decrease serum prolactin levels, and dopaminergic antagonists (neuroleptics) increase serum prolactin levels. This neuroleptic-induced rise in prolactin explains an often troublesome side effect of these drugs in some female patients—galactorrhea.

Hence serum prolactin levels can be used as an indirect measure of a central dopaminergic system in humans and as a means to monitor the effects of drugs on tuberoinfundibular dopaminergic neurons. Prolactin increase correlates with the antipsychotic activity of most neuroleptics. Again, clozapine presents a problem. Though an effective antipsychotic, clozapine is not a consistent prolactin stimulator in humans. Clozapine does elevate prolactin in rats, which suggests either that the ability to increase serum prolactin levels in rats by drugs with neuroleptic-like chemical structures is not an invariable guide to antipsychotic activity or that the pituitary dopamine receptors that influence prolactin secretion in the rat are significantly different from those relevant to the antipsychotic action of the neuroleptics. Nevertheless, tuberoinfundibular dopaminergic neurons may provide a model for investigating dopaminergic effects of drugs that have a significant influence in schizophrenia.

Since prolactin levels are elevated by dopamine blockers, if schizophrenia is a consequence of dopamine hyperactivity that extends to the tuberoinfundibular dopaminergic neurons, one would predict that, in unmedicated schizophrenic patients, prolactin levels would be reduced as compared to controls. However, when measured in untreated patients, prolactin levels were within normal limits. One explanation for this finding may be that since acute stress increases prolactin, the proposed tuberoinfundibular pathological dopamine hyperactivity during schizophrenic psychosis is suppressing the stress effect and normalizing the serum prolactin. Another explanation is that dopamine increase in schizophrenia is not generalized throughout the brain.

Mesolimbic Tract

The mesolimbic dopaminergic neuronal cell bodies are located in the ventral tegmental area of the midbrain, designated A-10 in the rat, with axons projecting to terminals in the nucleus accumbens, stria terminalis, and tuberculum olfactorium—structures comprising the limbic forebrain. The outflow from this limbic region is to the septum, hypothalamus, frontal lobe, and other cortical areas. The function of the limbic system has not been fully elucidated; however, circumstantial evidence supports limbic mediation of various autonomic, neuroendocrine, memory, learning, affective, and behavioral functions. This system has also been implicated, along with the nigrostriatal system, in mediating apomorphine- and amphetamine-induced stereotypy in rats; it has been suggested as the dopaminergic pathway responsible for amphetamine psychosis. Additionally, injection of dopamine intracerebrally into the tuberculum olfactorium and nucleus accumbens elicits an increase in the locomotor activity of the rat. Neuroleptic agents antagonize dopamine-induced hyperactivity. Thus, reversal of this increased locomotor activity by neuroleptics is a reflection of their mesolimbic and perhaps antipsychotic action.

Tolerance to neuroleptic effects, such as increased dopamine turnover following acute neuroleptic injection, develops later and requires higher dosages in the mesolimbic system than in the nigrostriatal system. These observations indirectly support a greater role of the mesolimbic system as compared to the nigrostriatal system in schizophrenia, since tolerance to the antipsychotic effect of neuroleptic is not seen.

Other animal and human evidence exists to suggest that the mesolimbic dopaminergic system is involved in schizophrenia. Disturbance in affect and behavior and impairment in ability to filter out multiple stimuli may be the consequence of limbic lesions in animals and are commonly seen in schizophrenia. Hallucinations and disturbances in thinking have been reported after electrical stimulation of limbic structures. Additionally, catatonia, paranoia, perceptual distortion, and mood changes have resulted from either stimulation or ablation of the limbic system in humans.

Viral encephalitis, particularly the kind involving the temporal lobe, often presents with behavioral symptomatology; and clinical manifestations of temporal lobe (psychomotor) epilepsy resemble schizophrenia.

Neuropathologists have often concentrated their attention on the mesolimbic structures of schizophrenic patients. A wide variety of nonspecific abnormalities has been found, including dendritic disarray, gliosis, and hypocellularity. Modern immunohistochemical and norphometric analyses have been brought to bear on mesolimbic regions and are likely to help resolve the question of whether there are histological abnormalities in schizophrenia.

Mesocortical Tract

Histochemical studies have demonstrated the existence of dopaminergic terminals in the cerebral cortex. The cell bodies for these terminals have been postulated to lie in the A-9 and A-10 areas of the mesencephalon. Tolerance to the increase in dopamine turnover following repeated doses of neuroleptic does not develop as readily in the mesocortical dopaminergic system as in the other dopaminergic systems. As stated above, tolerance to the antipsychotic effects of neuroleptics is not seen; hence, the mesocortical system may be the dopaminergic tract most relevant to schizophrenia. Furthermore, pathology of this dopaminergic pathway may underlie the disturbances in associations, formal thought processes, and symbolism seen in schizophrenia, since these cognitive processes are cortical functions. Particular attention has been directed to the dorsolateral prefrontal cortex. Psychometric testing suggests that this region may function quite poorly in schizophrenics and that its dysfunction may be correlated with mesocortical dopaminergia.

However, these abnormalities may actually be a function of hypodopaminergic activity in the cortex of schizophrenics, rather than hyperdopaminergia. Indeed, the role of dopamine in the cortex of schizophrenics has suggested that hypo- and hyperdopaminergia could exist in different brain regions of the same patient, a hypothesis supported by data derived from rodents demonstrating a reciprocal relationship between dopaminergic activity in cortical and subcortical regions.

See under the heading Dopamine in Chapter 8: Neurophysiological and Neurochemical Basis of Behavior.

Neuroleptics and Schizophrenia

The dopamine hypothesis of schizophrenia is based in large part on evidence that the mechanism of the antipsychotic effects of neuroleptic drugs is antagonism of dopaminergic neuronal activity. Several lines of evidence regarding neuroleptics support this view.

Dopamine-Receptor Binding

Dopamine-receptor binding has been demonstrated in brain membranes by labeling the receptor both with the agonist, tritiated dopamine, and with the antagonist, tritiated haloperidol. Tritiated dopamine and tritiated haloperidol seem to label specific agonist and antagonist conformations of the receptor, respectively. Therefore, dopamine and other agonists have a greater affinity for dopamine sites than haloperidol sites, while dopamine antagonists have a greater affinity for haloperidol sites. Antagonist binding has been proposed to be of more direct relevance to the clinical effects of antipsychotic drugs. The relative affinities of an extensive series of antipsychotic agents, which includes butyrophenones, phenothiazines, and other dopamine antagonists, in competing for tritiated haloperidol binding to the dopamine receptor, predict these drugs' clinical potencies in psychotic patients. Spiroperidol, a butyrophenone, is the most potent of the drugs studied and is also the most potent inhibitor of tritiated haloperidol binding. Spiroperidol possesses a fivefold higher affinity for tritiated haloperidol binding than fluphenazine (Prolixin), a potent phenothiazine, and a fortyfold greater affinity than chlorpromazine (Thorazine):

- Affinity for tritiated haloperidol binding:
  Chlorpromazine 40 times less than spiroperidol

Chlorpromazine 35 times less than fluphenazine
- Potency as antipsychotic agent:
Chlorpromazine 40 times less than spiroperidol
Chlorpromazine 35 times less than fluphenazine

The close correlation between the clinical potencies of neuroleptics and their affinities in
competing for the binding of tritiated haloperidol to dopamine postsynaptic receptors argues
that these drugs exert their actions by blocking
postsynaptic dopamine receptors.

Dopamine Turnover

When postsynaptic dopamine receptors are
blocked by neuroleptic drugs, a feedback mechanism has been postulated that activates the presynaptic dopaminergic neurons to release more
dopamine in an attempt to overcome the blockade. This hypothesized increase in dopamine
synthesis and turnover secondary to neuroleptic
is reflected in an increase in brain homovanillic
acid (HVA) levels that may show in the cerebrospinal fluid. Other methods for measuring dopamine turnover, which also increases following
acute neuroleptic administration, include the accumulation of dopamine after inhibition of the
degradative enzyme monoamine oxidase; depletion of dopamine after inhibition of the synthetic
enzyme tyrosine hydroxylase; appearance of radioactive dopamine after intravenous infusion of
radioactive tyrosine; and disappearance of radioactive dopamine after previously labeling
brain storage sites by intraventricular injection.

Most neuroleptics with antipsychotic efficacy
have a substantial effect on HVA. Chemically
related substances without antipsychotic action
have negligible effects on HVA. Thus, the increase in dopamine turnover, as reflected by
HVA increase secondary to neuroleptic, is probably relevant to neuroleptic antipsychotic properties.

Three neuroleptics—thioridazine, clozapine,
and thiethylperazine—do not have the predicted effect of increasing HVA levels in the
brain. Thioridazine, an antipsychotic agent generally regarded as equipotent with chlorpromazine, has a much lesser effect on HVA than
chlorpromazine. Clozapine, an effective antipsychotic, also has less effect on HVA than would
be expected. In contrast, thiethylperazine, an
antiemetic phenothiazine generally not used to
treat psychosis, although it may prove to have

antipsychotic activity, has a very substantial effect on HVA levels at clinical dosages.

Another problem in associating increased dopamine turnover with antipsychotic activity
arises from studies demonstrating that the increases seen in cerebrospinal fluid HVA levels
after acute neuroleptic administration are reduced following chronic neuroleptic exposure.
In other words, tolerance develops to this effect. Yet, as noted, there is a lack of tolerance
to the antipsychotic effects of neuroleptics. A
possible explanation for this discrepancy is that
the increase in cerebrospinal fluid HVA levels
following neuroleptic administration may reflect
enhanced *striatal* dopaminergic neuron turnover. This is substantiated clinically by reported tolerance to neuroleptic-induced, striatal-
mediated extrapyramidal reactions. Hence, the
mesolimbic or mesocortical dopaminergic system, or both, which develop tolerance to
neuroleptic-mediated increases in dopamine
turnover more slowly than the nigrostriatal system, may be more likely loci of dopamine-me-
diated psychotic symptoms.

Neuroleptics and Dopaminergic
Neuron Firing Rate

Further evidence demonstrating a relationship between neuroleptic action and dopamine
transmission is provided by recording the electrical activity of dopaminergic neurons after neuroleptic administration. Neuroleptics cause an
increase in the firing rate of nigral dopaminergic
neurons. This finding corroborates the afore-
mentioned feedback stimulation of dopaminergic neurons as evidenced by increased turnover following neuroleptic dopamine receptor
blockade. In contrast, the dopamine agonist
amphetamine suppresses dopaminergic neuron
activity. Amphetamine may increase dopamine
receptor stimulation, thereby activating a feedback mechanism that suppresses dopamine synthesis and turnover. Antipsychotic agents reverse amphetamine-induced suppression of
presynaptic dopaminergic neuron activity.

A real problem in extrapolating from the acute
effects of neuroleptics to their mechanism of action in diminishing psychotic symptoms is that
these drugs require chronic administration to be
effective. Rarely are psychotic symptoms diminished in hours, or even a few days. The more
common time course is weeks. Indeed, with
weeks of treatment, firing rates of dopamine
neurons in nigrostriatal and mesolimbic regions
are substantially diminished, a phenomenon

termed *depolarization block*. Atypical neuroleptics only induced depolarization block in mesolimbic areas, sparing nigrostriatal regions and offering some explanation for the relative absence of extrapyramidal effects with atypical neuroleptics.

Dopamine-Stimulated Adenylate Cyclase

Neurotransmitters are believed to promote their physiological effect by interacting with receptors. The exact nature of the dopamine receptor is unclear; however, in one type of dopamine receptor, the action of dopamine seems to be mediated postsynaptically through stimulation of a dopamine-sensitive membrane-bound enzyme, adenylate cyclase. In other words, the dopamine receptor possibly is linked to dopamine-sensitive adenylate cyclase. This enzyme's activity is increased by dopamine and decreased by neuroleptic drugs. Furthermore, in general, the capacity of a neuroleptic drug to inhibit this enzyme correlates with its antipsychotic potency. For example, a low-dose, high-potency phenothiazine like fluphenazine (Prolixin) is a tenfold to twentyfold more potent inhibitor of dopamine-sensitive adenylate cyclase than digh-dose, low-potency chlorpromazine (Thorazine). Additionally, compounds that are structurally related to neuroleptics but that lack clinical efficacy as antipsychotics either fail to or only weakly inhibit the enzyme.

However, inconsistencies exist. Butyrophenones (haloperidol), indole derivatives (molindone), and benzamide neuroleptics (metoclopromide and sulpiride) are all less potent inhibitors of dopamine-sensitive adenylate cyclase than might be predicted on the basis of their clinical potency as antipsychotics. One explanation for these exceptions is the existence of multiple dopamine receptors. Those coupled with adenylate cyclase are designated D-1, and those not coupled with cyclase activation by dopamine are termed D-2. That clinically effective antipsychotics like those mentioned have little activity as antagonists of the cyclase system implicates D-2 receptor mechanisms in schizophrenia. However, molecular studies indicate that there are at least two types of D-2 receptors. The relative contribution of each to neuroleptic activity is still to be determined.

Antagonists specific for D-1 receptors have been synthesized and widely studied. A complex picture is now emerging of cooperativity between D-1 and D-2 receptor sites, with impor-

tant implications for any conceptualization of dopamine and behavior. With the inevitable isolation of the dopamine receptor as molecular biological techniques are applied to the dopamine system, a more precise understanding of the interactions of all the various subtypes of the dopamine receptor is sure to be forthcoming. However, the role of the D-1 receptor in schizophrenia remains unresolved, a role made particularly important by its relative prominence, compared to D-2 receptors, in the cortex.

Several tricyclic antidepressants, which lack antipsychotic activity, are as potent inhibitors of dopamine-sensitive adenylate cyclase as some clinically effective neuroleptics. Additionally, receptor *supersensitivity* to dopamine is not accompanied by an increase in dopamine-sensitive adenylate cyclase activity. This may indicate that behavioral supersensitivity following the discontinuation of long-term antipsychotic drug treatment is mediated by a nonaldehyde cyclase mechanism. Finally, no difference has been shown in dopamine-sensitive adenylate cyclase activity in the striatum between chronic schizophrenic and control autopsy brain tissue, although the number of D-1 receptors may be diminished. Thus, the significance of D-1 receptors in schizophrenia is not clear.

Summary

Antipsychotic drugs are believed to exert their clinical effect through the blockade of dopamine receptors. This effect can be monitored by the following test systems:

1. Increase in dopamine turnover
2. Inhibition of dopamine-stimulated adenylate cyclase activity
3. Stimulation of prolactin release
4. Blockade of amphetamine- and apomorphine-induced stereotypy
5. Reversal of dopamine-induced locomotor activity
6. Increase in dopaminergic neuron firing rate and reversal of amphetamine-induced depression in firing rate, acutely, with depolarization block, chronically
7. Competition for dopamine binding sites

These effects generally correlate with the antipsychotic effect of the neuroleptic medication. However, the inconsistencies noted highlight the limited understanding of these processes and raise doubts about a single biochemical mechanism underlying schizophrenia.

Other Pharmacological Evidence for Dopamine Hypothesis of Schizophrenia

The dopamine hypothesis of schizophrenia is lent further support by an examination of the clinical effect of both direct and indirect dopamine agonists. L-Dopa, the precursor of dopamine, has been reported to induce psychosis in some Parkinson's disease patients, as well as worsen psychotic symptomatology in schizophrenic patients. A psychosis resembling acute paranoid schizophrenia has been reported in human amphetamine addicts; and in clinical studies, amphetamine has produced a paranoid psychosis in normal volunteers. Additionally, in some active schizophrenic patients, amphetamine intensifies preexisting psychotic symptoms, as does methylphenidate, an isomer of amphetamine, and high-dose apomorphine, a direct dopamine receptor agonist.

A dopaminergic mechanism is believed to underlie psychostimulant initiation and exacerbation of psychosis. Recently, this amphetamine-induced aggravation of psychosis has been shown to be state dependent. Schizophrenic patients whose symptoms worsened following amphetamine challenge were more psychotic at baseline than those patients who did not change. Additionally, patients treated with neuroleptics who worsened with amphetamine also had shown higher baseline psychotic ratings than those who remained stable. Thus, chronic pretreatment with a dopamine receptor blocking agent did not consistently prevent an amphetamine-induced increase in psychosis. These data suggest that responsiveness to amphetamine reflects changes in clinical state but that mechanisms underlying amphetamine activation of psychosis are not dependent solely upon dopamine receptor actions.

The ability of a pharmacological challenge to predict the duration of a period of remission is further evidence for the involvement of dopamine in state-dependent processes. The degree of acute exacerbation in symptoms of schizophrenia produced by either L-dopa or amphetamine administration to remitted and drug-free schizophrenics predicts how long these patients will remain in remission. Those schizophrenics with the most drug-induced worsening of their condition, albeit quite brief, tended to relapse far more quickly than patients who handled these indirect dopaminergic challenges without any symptom enhancement.

Alpha-methyl-para-tyrosine (AMPT) is an in-hibitor of the enzyme tyrosine hydroxylase and diminishes central dopaminergic activity. This drug has been evaluated in schizophrenia. AMPT alone did not produce a consistent antipsychotic effect; however, it potentiated the antipsychotic effect of neuroleptics and permitted a reduction in neuroleptic dosage. Thus, AMPT effects are consistent with the hypothesis of dopamine hyperactivity in schizophrenia. AMPT is too toxic, however, for routine clinical use.

Nonpharmacological Evidence of Dopamine Hyperactivity

The hypothesis that schizophrenia may be associated with an overactivity of postsynaptic dopamine receptors has been tested by measuring the specific binding of radiolabeled dopamine antagonists (tritiated apomorphine) and antagonists (tritiated haloperidol and tritiated spiperone) to synaptic membranes. In postmortem brains of schizophrenic patients, there is an increase in tritiated neuroleptic binding as compared to nonpathological human control brains. To determine whether this enhancement in tritiated neuroleptic binding is due to an increase in the density of binding sites (that is, the number, or concentration, of binding sites; B_{max}) or in the affinity of these sites for the radiolabeled neuroleptic (K_d or dissociation constant), these parameters have been measured. Normal and decreased receptor affinities have been reported in schizophrenia, whereas the density or number of dopamine receptors is significantly increased.

A central question when reviewing these data is whether these dopaminergic changes reflect a disease process or the effect of chronic neuroleptic exposure. The fact that some schizophrenic brains assayed were from patients who had received a negligible amount or no neuroleptic medication, yet also exhibited an increase in tritiated neuroleptic binding (increase in B_{max}), supports a primary effect. Furthermore, enhanced nigrostriatal dopaminergic activity is compatible with the tics, mannerisms, and posturing commonly seen in schizophrenics. Nevertheless, chronic neuroleptic effects cannot be ruled out. For example, the reported decreased *affinity* of the schizophrenic brain's dopamine receptors for radiolabeled neuroleptic *has* been ascribed to residual neuroleptic drug contamination of the assay.

Other efforts have been made to document nonpharmacological markers of increased dopamine activity in schizophrenia. Several biological parameters have been evaluated in schizophrenic patients free of neuroleptic treatment. These include plasma prolactin levels, brain dopamine and HVA concentrations, cerebrospinal fluid HVA levels, activity of synthetic and degradative catecholaminergic enzymes, and platelet monoamine oxidase activity. In the nucleus accumbens and anterior perforated substance of the limbic forebrain, dopamine concentrations have been reported to be increased in postmortem analysis of brains from schizophrenic patients. An area of particular interest appears to be the amygdala on the left side of the brain. On the other hand, HVA and dihydroxyphenylacetic acid (DOPAC) concentrations in the nucleus accumbens, caudate, and putamen were the same in the schizophrenic patients as in the controls. It must be noted that residual neuroleptic effects may confound these results.

Other postmortem catecholaminergic enzymes have been studied in schizophrenic brains. Activities of catechol-O-methyl transferase (COMT), an enzyme that metabolizes dopamine extraneuronally, and monoamine oxidase (MAO), an enzyme that metabolizes dopamine intraneuronally and extraneuronally, did not differ in patients and controls in 14 different brain areas. The activity of tyrosine hydroxylase, the rate-limiting enzyme for catecholamine synthesis, was similar in patients and controls in the caudate, putamen, and nucleus accumbens. DOPA-decarboxylase, which converts DOPA to dopamine, was also unchanged between schizophrenic and normal brains.

Cerebrospinal Fluid HVA Levels

The most extensive attempt to identify an antemortem biologic marker of dopamine hyperactivity has been the evaluation of cerebrospinal fluid HVA, the major dopamine metabolite. If schizophrenic symptoms are associated with an increase in brain dopamine turnover in the nigrostriatal pathway, HVA levels should be elevated in unmedicated patients. However, several studies have been unable to demonstrate differences in HVA levels between such patients and normal controls. It has been noted, though, that this absence of increased levels of cerebrospinal fluid HVA in schizophrenics does not mean that there is not an increased dopamine turnover in dopaminergic neurons. It does suggest that those neurons with increased dopamine turnover do not contribute in a major way to *cerebrospinal fluid* HVA. The critical dopami-

nergic neurons in schizophrenia may be mesolimbic or mesocortical, or both, and their contribution to cerebrospinal fluid HVA in schizophrenia remains a complex question. For example, if, as it has been proposed, schizophrenic patients could simultaneously suffer mesolimbic hyperdopaminergia with mesocortical hypodopaminergia, the net effect on cerebrospinal fluid HVA could be quite unpredictable.

Plasma HVA

The measurement of plasma HVA is an alternative to cerebrospinal fluid HVA measurement as a means to assess the status of brain dopaminergic activity. It has been estimated that, under carefully controlled conditions, 50 percent of plasma HVA can originate in the brain. This circumstance has encouraged the detailed evaluation of plasma HVA in schizophrenic patients, and much information has been gathered consistent with a role for dopamine in schizophrenia. For example, symptom severity and plasma HVA concentrations move in parallel. The most symptomatic patients have the highest plasma HVA, and levels decrease with neuroleptic treatment and a patient's improvement.

Serum Prolactin Levels

Serum prolactin levels are elevated by neuroleptics, reflecting dopaminergic blockade in the tuberoinfundibular dopaminergic system. However, as noted earlier, in unmedicated schizophrenic patients, prolactin levels are unchanged. Nevertheless, prolactin levels may have relevance in schizophrenia. Serum prolactin concentrations have been shown to correlate *inversely* with ratings of psychopathology in drug-free chronic schizophrenic patients with normal ventricular size on CT scan. This finding suggests that the severity of psychosis is related to dopaminergic activity insofar as this is reflected by serum prolactin concentrations.

Platelet MAO Activity

Platelet MAO has been hypothesized to reflect characteristics of brain MAO. Investigations have demonstrated a reduction in platelet MAO activity in some chronic but not acute schizophrenics. However, this was confounded by further studies that indicated a prolonged effect of neuroleptics to lower platelet MAO activity.

NOREPINEPHRINE

Noradrenergic mechanisms have also been implicated in schizophrenia. Psychotogenic drugs like amphetamine facilitate the release of both dopamine and norepinephrine from nerve terminals. Of the three major brain amines in the human (dopamine, norepinephrine, and serotonin), norepinephrine has the greatest *limbic* representation. This area, as noted, has been linked to schizophrenic symptoms. Furthermore, in the limbic forebrain of the rat, a norepinephrine-sensitive adenosine-3,5-monophosphate generating system has been identified that, like dopamine-sensitive adenylate cyclase, can be blocked in a dose-dependent manner by neuroleptics with antipsychotic activity. These antipsychotic agents also have the ability to block both peripheral and central catecholamine receptors.

A norepinephrine hypothesis of schizophrenia was bolstered by the report of increased norepinephrine levels in some limbic forebrain regions of four patients with chronic *paranoid* schizophrenia. A later report confirmed an elevated nucleus accumbens norepinephrine level in two drug-free chronic paranoid schizophrenics. The report of elevated norepinephrine concentrations in the cerebrospinal fluid of paranoid compared to undifferentiated schizophrenics and controls, in addition to the predominantly paranoid nature of amphetamine-related psychosis, lends further support to a growing hypothesis that the paranoid subgroup may have a primary norepinephrine abnormality and may be biologically distinct from nonparanoid schizophrenics.

Although only a small number of paranoid schizophrenics were reported upon, the intriguing suggestion that a biochemical parameter might distinguish a subtype (paranoid) of schizophrenia stimulated a more extensive investigation. Levels of norepinephrine and the major norepinephrine metabolite 3-methoxy-4-hydroxyphenylglycol (MHPG) were examined in the nucleus accumbens and hypothalamus of chronic schizophrenics and age-matched controls. Nucleus accumbens norepinephrine levels in chronic paranoid patients were more than double the levels in nonparanoid schizophrenics or controls. Hypothalamic norepinephrine levels were higher in both paranoid and nonparanoid schizophrenics than in controls, whereas free MHPG in the nucleus accumbens was not different in the schizophrenic groups and the controls. In the hypothalamus, however, free MHPG showed a trend to be higher in the paranoid when compared with the nonparanoid schizophrenics. Thus, these initial studies implicating the norepinephrine system in paranoid schizophrenia represent a possible biochemical corroboration of a clinically evident observation: the schizophrenias may be a heterogeneous group of disorders.

It is possible that noradrenergic dysregulation may extend beyond the paranoid subgroup. Provocative data suggest an elevation in noradrenergic transmission at the beginning of a schizophrenic episode. The further evolution of this possibility is eagerly awaited.

See under the heading Norepinephrine in Chapter 8: Neurophysiological and Neurochemical Basis of Behavior.

ENDORPHINS

The identification in the brain of specific opiate receptors and their endogenous ligands—opiate-like peptides called endorphins—has stimulated research into the role of this neuromodulatory system in psychotic illness, particularly schizophrenia. Peptide fragments have been identified, many of which are related to the pituitary hormone beta-lipotropin (β-LPH). The greatest attention has focused on beta-endorphin (β-LPH 61-91); however, the term *endorphin* refers to the entire group of opiate-like peptides.

The hypothesis that dysfunction of the endogenous opioid system is associated with schizophrenic symptomatology has been tested via (1) pharmacological challenges and treatment studies with the opiate antagonist naloxone, or with the opioid peptides themselves; (2) the direct assessment in the cerebrospinal fluid of endorphin activity through radioreceptor assay techniques, which evaluate functional opioid activity, and radioimmunoassay, which determines the level of immunoreactivity of specific opioid peptides; and (3) treatment studies.

Opioid peptides administered into the cerebrospinal fluid or into the periaqueductal gray matter of the rat brain resulted in profound sedation and catatonic behavior with "waxy flexibility," a state in which the animal could be molded to any position and maintain an awkward posture for long periods. This catatonic state induced by beta-endorphin could not be simulated with other endorphin peptides (met-enkephalin, alpha-endorphin, and gamma-endorphin), even at higher dosages.

Parenteral naloxone reversed this effect. These preclinical studies stimulated investigations of this peptide system in schizophrenic patients.

Results of naloxone administration to schizophrenic patients have been equivocal. However, short-term improvements, particularly in auditory hallucinations, have been found. The pharmacological activities in animal studies of gamma-endorphin (β-LPH 61-77) and its fragments have demonstrated similarities to conventional neuroleptic medication, prompting speculation that these nonopiate (that is, nonanalgesic) endorphin peptide sequences are endogenous antipsychotics. Des-tyrosine-gamma-endorphin (DTGE; β-LPH 62-77) and des-enkephalin-gamma-endorphin (DEGE; β-LPH 66-77) have been administered to schizophrenic patients. Although no consistent overall therapeutic effect on schizophrenic symptoms has been observed, beneficial effects have been reported in schizophrenic subgroups. The ability of opioid peptides to modulate dopamine transmission offers some rationale for the possibility that manipulation of endogenous opioid activity could affect the symptoms of schizophrenia.

The direct assessment of endorphins in the cerebrospinal fluid is another strategy in evaluating their role in psychiatric illness. Measures of beta-endorphin immunoreactivity in the cerebrospinal fluid and of general opioid activity by radioreceptor assay have yielded mixed results. Since the endorphin system has been postulated to relate to ability or inability to experience pleasure, it is seductive to argue that a possible decrement in cerebrospinal fluid endorphin activity in chronic schizophrenic patients may be related to their affective blunting and social impoverishment.

GABA

Another biochemical hypothesis has focused on the inhibitory neurotransmitter gamma-aminobutyric acid (GABA). A feedback loop involving GABA inhibitory effects on dopaminergic neurons has been proposed in the nigrostriatal, mesolimbic, and mesocortical dopaminergic pathways. According to this view, a reduction in the activity of GABAergic neurons would decrease the inhibition, resulting in unregulated dopamine hyperactivity and therefore schizophrenic symptoms.

Limited pharmacological manipulations of GABA activity provide some circumstantial evidence for a GABA role in schizophrenia. In the rat, infusion of a GABA antagonist into the nu-

cleus accumbens induced fearful, psychosislike behavior. In the cat, injection of the GABA antagonist bicuculline into certain dopamine-rich brain regions produced catatonic-like symptoms. This reaction was potentiated by amphetamine, inhibited by haloperidol, and prevented by pretreatment with the neurotoxin 6-hydroxy dopamine, which destroys dopamine terminals. The putative GABA_B receptor agonist baclophen reportedly produced a marked enhancement of neuroleptic antipsychotic action in treatment-resistant schizophrenics. However, this effect could not be replicated. Cycloserine, which inhibits glutamic acid decarboxylase (GAD), the enzyme responsible for the conversion of L-glutamate to GABA, has been reported to exacerbate symptoms in schizophrenia, as has muscimol, a potent GABA_A receptor agonist. Valproic acid, which inhibits a GABA degradative enzyme, lacked effect on schizophrenic symptoms, although a decrease in tardive dyskinesia was reported.

GABA levels have been found to be normal in schizophrenic brains by some researchers but to be decreased by others. Brain GAD levels, GABA receptor binding in the cortex, and platelet GABA transaminase have been reported normal in schizophrenia. Findings have been equivocal for cerebrospinal fluid GABA levels in small groups of schizophrenics. However, a more definitive study showed that younger schizophrenic women (under age 30) had significantly lower cerebrospinal fluid GABA levels than age-matched normal control women. Furthermore, GABA levels were shown to increase with time and with long-term neuroleptic treatment. GABA's role in schizophrenia remains theoretical.

See under the heading GABA in Chapter 8: Neurophysiological and Neurochemical Basis of Behavior.

OTHER BIOCHEMICAL THEORIES

Transmethylation Hypothesis of Schizophrenia

Inspired by the observation that certain hallucinogenic agents such as mescaline are structurally related to O-methylated derivatives of the catecholamines, this theory postulates that schizophrenia arises from the abnormal accumulation of a psychotogenic N- or O-methylated biogenic amine derivative. According to this view, the incorrect methylation of biogenic amines (catecholamines and indoleamines) produces these "endogenous psychotogens" that structurally resemble hallucinogenic agents such as mescaline, psilocybin, and LSD. However, studies of methylated biogenic amines have not demonstrated either their exclusive occurrence or existence in high concentration in schizophrenics. On the other hand, one of the most replicable findings about schizophrenia is that the administration of compounds that donate methyl groups (for example, methionine) exacerbates schizophrenia.

Phenylethylamine (PEA)

PEA is endogenously formed by decarboxylation of the amino acid phenylalanine. The suggestion that this substance plays a role in schizophrenia is based on the similarities of PEA and amphetamine. They are structurally similar and, like amphetamine, PEA induces stereotypy in laboratory animals. This effect is ameliorated by neuroleptics in doses proportional to their clinical potency as antipsychotics. Other data implicating PEA in schizophrenia are inconclusive, including the association of phenylketonuric patients—who generate increased amounts of PEA—with schizophrenics and studies of PEA levels in the urine of schizophrenics.

Histamine

The hypothesis of altered histamine metabolism in schizophrenia is based primarily on the reported hyporesponsivity to intradermal histamine in schizophrenic patients. This remains an unexplained phenomenon. Despite the lack of difference in blood histamine concentration between schizophrenics and controls, ongoing studies examine histamine function in schizophrenia in the hope of relating peripheral insensitivity to central histamine dysfunction. See under the heading Histamine in Chapter 8: Neurophysiological and Neurochemical Basis of Behavior.

STRUCTURAL BASIS FOR SCHIZOPHRENIA

After the systematic observation of thousands of schizophrenia patients, Emil Kraepelin, at the turn of the century, conceptualized a pathologic entity, *dementia praecox*. This syndrome was characterized by a complex symptomatology that included a progressive mental deterioration in the presence of an intact sensorium. For Kraepelin, this progressive tendency toward a state of dementia, starting precociously in life, was the fundamental characteristic of the disease that is called schizophrenia today. This feature of mental decline stirred later investigators to search for specific morphologic brain abnormalities in schizophrenic patients.

With this in mind, a series of pneumoencephalographic examinations were undertaken in schizophrenics. Studies in the first half of this century demonstrated both cerebral atrophy and ventricular dilatation in a large percentage of chronic schizophrenics. Subsequent, better designed studies were not definitive in establishing structural differences between schizophrenic and various control populations. Yet in some studies within the schizophrenic group, correlations were reported between ventricular size and state of mental deterioration or social defect.

Gross neuropathological examinations based on visual inspection of schizophrenic and control brains have been undertaken since as early as the 1920s. In 1954, a review of these studies concluded that no consistent neuropathological abnormality characteristic of schizophrenia could be established at autopsy.

Histological studies of schizophrenic brains are limited; however, quantitative disturbances have been reported in the "cytoarchitectonics" of the cerebral cortex, as well as the presence of encephalitic-like lesions, such as glial knots and perivascular infiltration in the brainstem.

CT Scan Findings

As a result of the nonspecific, inconclusive nature of these earlier studies and the advent of neuroleptic treatment of schizophrenia, the research focus shifted in the last two decades to neurochemical mechanisms in schizophrenia. The development of computed tomography (CT) scanning as a noninvasive reliable means of examining brain morphology during life has reawakened interest in structural abnormalities in the brains of schizophrenic patients.

In CT scan studies of schizophrenic patients and controls, the different populations of schizophrenic patients included older patients, chronically hospitalized patients, and younger patients living in the community. Mean ventricular size as measured by the methodologically more precise ventricle-brain ratio was significantly larger in the schizophrenic group compared with controls. Despite this difference, ventricular enlargement in schizophrenic patients is modest; on routine radiological reading, most scans would be interpreted as normal. Also, ventricular enlargement is not characteristic of all schizophrenics. Percentages range from 6 to 53 percent. Evaluation of neuroleptic and electroconvulsive therapy effects suggests that ventricular enlargement is independent of these somatic treatments. Figure 28–2 shows CT scans of enlarged ventricles in schizophrenic patients.

Most controlled studies of brain CT scans in schizophrenia indicate that schizophrenic patients have subtle structural brain abnormalities. This provocative finding has stimulated attempts at further characterization of this subset of patients. Ventricular enlargement has been asso-

ciated with chronic unremitting illness, lower cerebrospinal fluid HVA, poor performance on intellectual and neuropsychological testing, different HLA antigen distribution, poor response to neuroleptic treatment, and poor premorbid social adjustment, suggesting perhaps an early developmental neuropathological process.

Other notable CT scan findings in schizophrenia are the demonstration of decreased density in the anterior left hemisphere of schizophrenics as compared to controls; atrophy of the cerebellar vermis, a region that has been linked to emotional expression; and, in a study of monozygotic discordant twins, structural abnormalities that are readily visible on the scan of the schizophrenic twin, suggesting that nongenetic factors must play a role in the full expression of the schizophrenia phenotype.

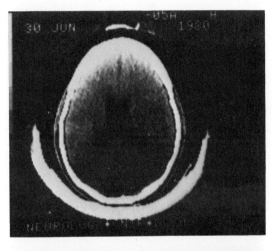 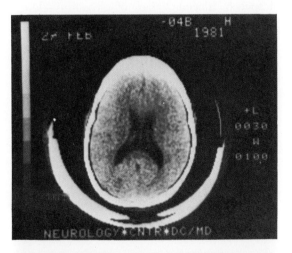
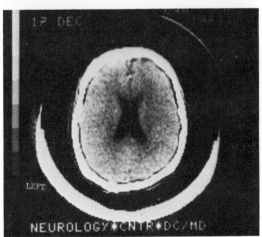 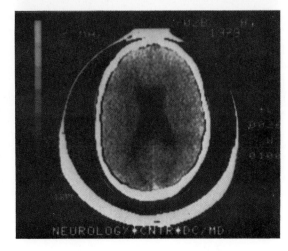

FIGURE 28–2.   Ventricular enlargement in CT scans of four 16- to 18-year-old patients with schizophrenia. (From Grebb, J.A., Weinberger, D.R., Wyatt, R.J.: Schizophrenia, in Diseases of the Nervous System: Clinical Neurobiology, A.K. Asbury, G.M. McKhann, and W.I. McDonald (eds.), Philadelphia, W.B. Saunders, 1986.)

Positive- and Negative-Symptom Schizophrenia

Incorporation of CT scan data with the biochemical understanding of schizophrenia led to a conceptualization of schizophrenia as two syndromes with overlapping features. Positive symptoms of schizophrenia include delusions, hallucinations, bizarre behavior, positive formal thought disorder (derailment, incoherence, pressure of speech, tangentiality, illogicality), and catatonic motor behavior. The underlying pathophysiological process of positive-symptom schizophrenia has been hypothesized to be linked to dopamine, since those symptoms are most responsive to neuroleptics.

Negative-symptom, or deficit-state, schizophrenia is most commonly seen in chronic schizophrenia and is characterized by affective blunting, avolition (loss of drive), alogia (poverty of speech, blocking), lack of pleasure-seeking activity (anhedonia), and attentional deficits. The underlying pathophysiology of negative-symptom schizophrenia has been hypothesized to be associated with cell loss and structural changes in the brain, as evidenced by ventricular enlargement and cortical atrophy on CT scan. Cortical regions have been implicated in deficit-state symptoms. These symptoms appear far more refractory to neuroleptic treatment.

The negative-positive conceptualization attempts to synthesize phenomenology, biochemistry, and morphology. As a theoretical construct, it merits attention; however, it is reductionistic. Schizophrenia is not an illness that can be subdivided into two distinct populations, even overlapping ones. Patients most commonly display mixed profiles. Indeed, the wealth of anatomical and neurochemical data emerging suggests a biological heterogeneity that parallels the clinical diversity of the schizophrenic syndrome.

BIBLIOGRAPHY

Bunney, B.S., Sesack, S.R., Silva, N.L.: Midbrain dopaminergic systems: Neurophysiology and electrophysiological pharmacology, in Psychopharmacology: The Third Generation of Progress, H.Y. Meltzer (ed.). New York, Raven Press, 1987.

Crow, T. J., et al.: Dopamine and schizophrenia. Adv. Biochem. Psychopharm. 19:301-309, 1978.

Gur, R. E., Skolnick, B. E., Gur, R. C.: Brain function in schizophrenic disorders. I. Regional blood flow in medicated schizophrenics. Arch. Gen. Psychiatry 40:1250-1254, 1983.

Losonczy, M. F., Davidson, M., Davis, K. L.: The dopamine hypothesis of schizophrenia, in Psychopharmacology: The Third Generation of Progress, H. Y. Meltzer (ed.). New York, Raven Press, 1987.

Moore, K. E.: Hypothalmic dopaminergic neuronal systems, in Psychopharmacology: The Third Generation of Progress, H. Y. Meltzer (ed.). New York, Raven Press, 1987.

Weinberger, D. R., Berman, K. F., Illowsky, B. P.: Physiological dysfunction of dorsolateral prefrontal cortex in schizophrenia. III. A new cohort and evidence for a monoaminergic mechanism. Arch. Gen. Psychiatry 45:609-615, 1988.

Chapter 29
Psychodynamic Theories of Schizophrenia

Arthur T. Meyerson, M.D.

FAMILY MODELS OF SCHIZOPHRENIA

Schizophrenia often occurs in more than one member of a family. It is a disorder characterized by difficulty with thinking as manifested in communication. Early observers believed that they could frequently identify patterns of family relatedness, communication, and structure. Thus, investigators were stimulated to attempt to understand how family life might give rise to or contribute to schizophrenia.

One of the most important of such family investigations was conducted by G. Bateson, who formulated a theory of schizophrenic communication called the *double bind*. He observed that in certain families the child receives two or more messages that conflict or cancel each other. The child, caught between these messages, may withdraw from the family. Thus, withdrawn, egotistical, and other schizophrenic "behaviors" are seen to result from this double bind communication. The double bind was seen as primarily a maternal communication; the father was

observed as a helpless figure. The child, made to feel terrified, helpless, and frustrated, was seen to withdraw into psychosis.

A number of methodological flaws render the results of all early family studies open to serious question. These methodological flaws gave rise to conclusions on the part of investigators that lack both sensitivity and specificity. Thus, none of the family patterns has consistently and reliably predicted even a majority of schizophrenic patients from observations of families. In addition, the utility of family patterns and their potential linkage with the causation of schizophrenia are brought into serious doubt when identical family patterns have been described as associated with other conditions.

Genetic factors in the etiology of schizophrenia are discussed under the heading Schizophrenia in Chapter 3: Behavior Genetics.

Two aspects of research on family factors in schizophrenia that have not been tainted by logical and methodological flaws are those involved with schizophrenic relapse rates and family burden. In the era of deinstitutionalization, many families must bear the burden of the care of their schizophrenic relatives over long periods of time. Family members take on financial and emotional burdens, give up privacy, and are exposed to schizophrenic behaviors that may be difficult and sometimes violent. Unfamiliar roles must be assumed, including those of nurse, rehabilitation specialist, advocate, and, until recently, psychiatric scapegoat.

These multiple difficulties in coping with a schizophrenic relative may provoke criticism of an overinvolvement with the patient, which have been observed by investigators interested in family environmental factors in schizophrenic relapse. Many studies have now confirmed that if criticism, hostility, and overinvolvement are highly active in family communication and activities, the schizophrenic index patients suffer a higher rate of relapse. The combination of criticism, hostility, and overinvolvement has been called *expressed emotion*. Expressed emotion has been operationalized as a measure of the number of critical remarks and the level of overinvolvement spontaneously expressed by relatives in the course of factual interviews. It is a combination of what is said and the manner in which it is said; raters are taught to evaluate speed, pitch, and intensity of speech, as well as the factual statements and gestures of the family members. A critical comment is one that expresses dislike or disapproval of the patient and must have an intense vocal component. Overinvolvement requires factual evidence of overprotectiveness and a tendency to dramatize events or describe incidents in excessive detail. Displays of emotional distress during the interview are also considered indicative of overinvolvement. Reliability and consistency among raters using these measures have been fairly high, but validity is as yet unproven in that family members who show high expressed emotion on interview may or may not express criticism in their direct dealing with schizophrenic relatives.

A number of studies have correlated expressed emotion measures with physiological responses. Evidence exists from followup studies that family counseling and educative techniques can modify expressed emotion. Several studies report that in families where a high expressed emotion may be associated with a relapse rate in their schizophrenic relatives of upward of 50 percent in a given year, this relapse rate can be reduced to around 10 percent with appropriate intervention. This randomized clinical trial of pychoeducation interventions with "aberrant"

families is the first real evidence of the significance of family factors in successful modification of the course of the schizophrenic illness. Although not directly bearing on the question of causation, the findings are, nevertheless, quite promising. It seems logical to conclude that the family environment can have significant stimulating or dampening effect on the course and expression of a schizophrenic illness. The illness itself seems, in M. Seeman's words, "otherwise patterned by powerful factors which are largely intrinsic and biological."

PSYCHOANALYTIC THEORIES OF SCHIZOPHRENIA

As part of the early development of psychoanalytic theory, Sigmund Freud postulated a conceptual model of schizophrenia analogous to that of neurosis. Conflict and defense were viewed as central to both. The "fixations" in schizophrenia were viewed as occurring earlier in the child's psychosexual development. Later, Freud developed the notion of an "ego defect" as the basis for explaining the observable phenomena in schizophrenia. Thus, these two early and influential conceptual models formed the basis for two separate and irreconcilable approaches to the psychoanalysis and psychoanalytic theory of schizophrenia.

The view that schizophrenia is an illness derived from intrapsychic conflict stresses the dynamic similarity between psychosis and neurosis. Those who hold this view generally believe that the psychopathology of schizophrenia can be explained on the basis of psychodynamic conflicts among instinctual drives (often conceived of as primitive or unneutralized aggression), a prohibition of the expression of these drives imposed by the superego, and a set of defenses that represent a resolution (tenuous or firm) of the conflicts. This in no way conceptually differs from the psychodynamic explanation of neurosis. Signal anxiety is seen as the instigator of the defenses and comes about as a result of the conflicts. The specific symptomatology of a psychosis, as compared with that of neurosis, is most often explained in quantitative terms and is seen as the result of the greater "regression to earlier fixations." Other points of differentiation are in terms of the quantitative strength and resiliency of the defenses, the difficulty of the ego in coping with such conflicts, and the overwhelming strength of the residual anxiety, which is not accounted for by the defenses in psychosis. According to this school, most of the symptomatology then can be seen as a result of "regressions" of reality testing, resulting from a defensive withdrawal at the instigation of anxiety as the signal. Some who subscribe to this general point of view have emphasized the importance of specific fantasies that organize the "psychic structures" of the neurotic or psychotic individual.

The "ego defect" school postulates that the schizophrenic has a defective ego, which, theoretically, may represent an innate deficit or be due to insufficient and inadequate early object relations and child rearing. This ego defect is more often viewed as developmental and characterized by a distortion in the ability to develop "psychic representations" of important objects and to perform other ego functions. Under the impact of early psychological trauma, the child's "psyche" is seen to develop a passive "regression" of major psychological functions. In schizophrenia, this regression is seen as something of a total one, even as a "rout." Many analysts who hold to this position believe that the ego defect is a result of a defect in the "narcissistic" phase of development and consequently in the development of a firm sense of personal identity, as well as clarity of object representation.

Thus, the conflict school of psychoanalytic thinking about schizophrenia appears to fail to distinguish, in any essential way, between neurosis and psychosis. A similar failure to distinguish between schizophrenia and borderline states appears to occur in the thinking of some later psychoanalytic theorists. Although there may be some grounds for explaining brief reactive psychosis and some depressive states on a continuum with borderline character disorders, there appears to be little or no such evidence for a continuum between schizophrenia and these conditions.

Although neither the ego defect nor conflict approach to schizophrenia has successfully integrated data derived from genetic, neurochemical, neurophysiological, and other sources of information about schizophrenia, there have been more recent attempts to integrate such data with psychoanalytic theory. These later investigators have attempted to integrate the observations of psychoanalytic thinkers such as Margaret Mahler and her followers, who have emphasized direct observation of early infantile development, and the school of psychoanalysis derived from the thinking of Melanie Klein and her followers, who have emphasized theoretical psychological structures arising in the early infantile developmental stages. These preverbal experiences are presumed to give rise to paranoid and depressive psychological structures and fixations.

Some investigators have attempted to integrate these psychoanalytic and developmental observations, and these theoretical notions, with observations deriving from the neurochemistry, neurophysiology, and phenomenology of schizophrenia. For example, D. L. Burnham and co-workers pictured schizophrenia as a defect in the utilization of the needed person who is also feared. Thus, they postulated a "need-fear dilemma." This need-fear dilemma was seen to derive from the preverbal psychological development of the infant prior to the age of 2.

Other investigators appeared, at times, to conceptualize the observations of perceptual deficits, stimulus-barrier difficulties, overinclusive thought, and neurotransmitter deficits in schizophrenia as precursors to the development of the ego defect. However, at other times, these same authors appeared to view these same schizophrenic dysfunctions as consequences of early infantile developmental distortions brought about through difficulties with object relations—a perspective that has not been substantiated by data.

The etiology of schizophrenia remains a mystery. It has not been satisfactorily explained by either the biological or psychosocial approaches, and in particular not by the psychodynamic frame of reference. The psychodynamic formulations proffered fail to distinguish between childhood schizophrenia and later-onset schizophrenia; yet any reasonable model must account for this distinction in presentation and etiology. These theories have not led to a reliable, demonstrably valid therapeutic approach to the illness. Psychoanalysis may provide heuristically valuable clinical theory and language for the description of some phenomena associated with schizophrenia, for example, concepts such as ego boundaries and reality testing. However, hypotheses of etiology remain vague and ill formed. Psychoanalytic conceptual notions about experience are certainly applicable to the human being who suffers from schizophrenia, as they are to any stressful life experience, and enrich the approach to all suffering persons.

Schizophrenia may be multiple illnesses in terms of clinical manifestation and etiology, but certainly all "schizophrenics" are different from one another. Each individual requires a unique approach and understanding of his or her experience of illness before a treatment can be rationally planned.

BIBLIOGRAPHY

Appleton, W.S.: Mistreatment of patients' families by psychiatrists, Am. J. Psychiatry 131:655-657, 1974.

Arlow, J., Brenner, C.: The Psychopathology of the Psychoses, in Psychoanalytic Concepts and the Structural Theory, New York, International University Press, 1964.

Bowen, M.: A family concept of schizophrenia, in The Etiology of Schizophrenia, D.D. Jackson (ed.). New York, Basic Books, 1960.

Brown, G., Burley, J., Wing, J.: Influence of family life on the course of schizophrenic disorders: A replication. Br. J. Psychiatry 121:241-258, 1972.

Burnham, D.L., Gladstone, A.I., Gibson, R.W.: Schizophrenia and the Need-Fear Dilemma, New York, International University Press, 1964.

Creer, C., Wing, J.: Living with a schizophrenic patient, Br. J. Hosp. Med. 14:73-83, 1975.

Falloon, I.R.H., et al.: Family management and the prevention of exacerbation of schizophrenia, N. Engl. J. Med. 306:1437-1440, 1982.

Grotstein, J.S.: The psychoanalytic concept of schizophrenia: I and II. Int. J. Psycho-Anal. 58:403-452, 1977.

Kuipers, I.: Expressed emotion: A review. Br. J. Soc. Clin. Psychol. 18:237-243, 1973.

Liberman, R.P., Glynn, S., Phipps, C.C.: Rehabilitation of schizophrenic disorders, in Treatment of Psychiatric Disorders, B. Karasu (ed.). Washington, D.C., American Psychiatric Press, 1988.

Liberman, R.P., Mueser, K.T., DeRisi, W.J.: Social Skills Training for Psychiatric Patients. New York, Pergamon Press, 1988.

Lidz, T., Fleck, S., Cornelison, A.: Schizophrenia and the Family, New York, International University Press, 1965.

Seeman, M.: Schizophrenia and family studies. Psychiatry J. Univ. Ottawa 8, no. 2, 198:38-43, 1983.

Singer, M.T., Wynne, L.C.: Thought disorder and family relations of schizophrenics: III. Methodology using projective techniques; IV. Results and implications. 12:187, 1965; 12:201, 1965.

Vaughn, C.E., Leff, J.P.: The influence of family and social factors on the course of psychiatric illness, Br. J. Psychiatry 129:125, 1976.

Wynne, L.C., Singer, M.T.: Thought disorder and family relations of schizophrenics, Arch. Gen. Psychiatry 9:199, 1963.

Chapter 30

Personality Disorders

Howard Klar, M.D., and Larry J. Siever, M.D.

People differ from one another. They vary widely in their temperaments, talents, weaknesses, likes, and dislikes. By the time a person reaches adulthood, these attributes have been translated into relatively stable, habitual ways of coping. These personality *traits*—stable, characteristic modes of behavior—enable a person to establish satisfying personal relationships and to find satisfaction in work. For the most part, people maintain a degree of flexibility in their characteristic styles of relating to others, as well as to their internal need states, which permits a range of responses to the constantly shifting demands made by an ever-changing world. Some individuals have an extremely small repertoire of responses available to them in their efforts to manage in the world. The nature of their behavior and relating seems rigid, stilted, and inflexible. Although these rigid aspects of personality may be quite adaptive in some of life's arenas, the "one-style-fits-all-situations" nature of these response patterns invariably leads a person into difficulty.

A young accountant who calculates the cost per mile of each and every mile he and his wife travel on vacation and who sticks to a minute-by-minute itinerary thinks he is being thrifty and organized—traits that are certainly laudable and that have served him well in his career. Why, he wonders, is his wife fed up with him and ready to board the next bus home? And why do his secretaries keep applying for transfer when all he does is show them the typos and smudges on their work and point out to them that a coffee break is 10 minutes, not 12 or 15? "Shouldn't things be done correctly?" he asks. "Aren't rules rules?"

All individuals utilize coping strategies to contend with life's events. Sometimes these strategies are conscious and volitional; at other times they are unconscious and outside a person's voluntary control. Most individuals can recognize when a particular coping style is helpful and when their characteristic way of responding is failing. Their responses to life situations can be modulated to fit the demands of the situation. The strategy used by the young accountant described above is notable for its rigidity and maladaptiveness.

While the accountant's symptoms are not as dramatic as those of an acutely psychotic schizophrenic, the degree of impairment in his interpersonal functioning is striking nonetheless. He has alienated his wife and coworkers and may be on the verge of losing his job. His inflexible and maladaptive style has led to impairment of functioning at work and in his relationships. *Chronic, inflexible, maladaptive behavior patterns*, which are often worse under stress, and unawareness of the damage that these behaviors do to oneself or to others are the hallmarks of a personality disorder.

CLASSIFICATION

The concept of personality disorders and the degree of incapacitation patients suffer with these disorders are often difficult to grasp. Unlike most illnesses physicians have to contend with, the boundaries between abnormal and normal personalities are often blurry. When does assertiveness become aggression, caution become suspiciousness, independence become isolation, and spontaneity become impulsivity? At the extremes these distinctions are simple, but most individuals do not exhibit the most extreme forms of these traits. This often makes the assessment of abnormality difficult. The lack of clear boundaries between normal and abnormal personality traits has provided a formidable but not insoluble dilemma for those seeking to study and diagnose personality disorders.

Researchers have approached the study of personality disorders from two different vantage points. One approach has been to study individual traits or *dimensions* found to varying degrees in all people. Dimensional axes allow for quantitative assessment of the relative strength of a particular trait in an individual. Thus, an individual can be located on an axis of tenderness at one extreme and toughness at the other, and similarly along axes of anxious vs. calm, organized vs. chaotic, emotionally stable vs. emotionally labile, and numerous other axes. This approach has the advantage of being comprehensive, highly individualized, and sensitive to idiosyncratic presentations. Its major disadvantages stem from the wide divergence of opinion as to which dimensions should be included for study, the bewildering complexity resulting from such descriptions of personality, and the possibility that an individual's behavior, depending upon circumstances, can vacillate between poles of a dimension. A familiar example of the last phenomenon is the "tough" all pro

linebacker who is a "pussycat" with his children.

The second approach to studying personality disorders, the *categorical approach*, is based on the recognition that certain dimensions of behavior tend to cluster together in identifying categories. A teenager who was always in trouble for lying in school and who had frequent fights with his friends might also be expected to have scrapes with the law and have trouble sustaining intimate relationships as an adult. The organization of dimensions of personality functioning into categories or syndromes is clinically and diagnostically useful. This approach is based on the assumption that certain dimensions have greater importance in the evaluation of a patient's problems. It also assumes that the traits which are used to form the category indicate an important underlying relationship among them, which may be biological or psychodynamic, or both, and lend structural coherence to the diagnostic category. Diagnosing categories of personality disorders allows clinicians to describe patients in a convenient shorthand and to anticipate other traits known to be associated with a specific diagnosis; diagnosis by category also facilitates treatment planning based on experience with similarly diagnosed patients.

DSM-III-R

The categorical model has been incorporated into the revised third edition of the *Diagnostic and Statistical Manual of Mental Disorders* (DSM-III-R), published by the American Psychiatric Association. Although the DSM-III-R categories may not be as discrete as physicians would like—the diagnostic categories overlap and are not mutually exclusive or homogeneous—they represent a considerable improvement over previous diagnostic schemes. The criteria specified for each diagnostic category have led to far greater reliability and clarity of diagnosis of personality disorder.

Twelve specific disorders are described on axis II (personality disorders and specific developmental disorders) of the DSM-III-R classification. They are divided into three broad categories (Table 30–1).

There are other ways to organize the various disorders of personality. Some authors have utilized the degree of impairment found in patients with differing personality disorders and have drawn up hierarchies based on mild, moderate, and severe degrees of impairment. Others have chosen to cluster the disorders based on their similarity to the major psychiatric syndromes

Category	Disorder
Odd (eccentric)	Schizoid
	Schizotypal
	Paranoid
Dramatic	Antisocial
	Borderline
	Histrionic (hysterical)
	Narcissistic
Anxious	Avoidant
	Dependent
	Compulsive
	Passive-aggressive
	Self-defeating

TABLE 30–1. Personality Disorders Described in DSM-III R

with posited biological etiologies, for example, schizophrenia and affective disorders.

This discussion of personality disorders is based on the DSM-III-R organization, since this represents the most current, clear, and clinically relevant approach for the beginning student. The aim of this chapter is to describe and provide a theoretical framework for understanding the multifactorial etiology of personality disorders.

ODD: SCHIZOID, SCHIZOTYPAL, PARANOID

Patients in this cluster—schizoid, schizotypal, and paranoid—tend to live on the fringes of society and to be perceived as strange or quirky by people who know them.

Schizoid

Schizoid patients are distant, aloof people hiding in a remote and protective cocoon of fantasy, seemingly indifferent to the praise or criticism of those around them. Also, these patients are virtually unable to appreciate or empathically respond to the feeling state of another person.

Schizotypal

Schizotypal patients share the characteristics of schizoid patients. They are further impaired by recurrent illusions, for example, thinking a shadow moving on a wall might be a person monitoring their behavior; by odd or eccentric thinking, for example, the belief that they can "read" another person's innermost thoughts; by

profound suspiciousness or mistrust; and by odd speech, for example, referring to a watch as a "time vessel."

Paranoid

Patients with paranoid personality disorder tend to stand out more boldly than either the schizoid or schizotypal patient. Although they have the same strong aversion to intimate human relationships that the other patients in this cluster do, they are most clearly recognized by their chronic and pervasive mistrust of others. Sometimes this mistrust leads patients with paranoid personality disorder to retreat into an isolated existence, although other, more labile patients with this disorder constantly find themselves embroiled in arguments, fights, and legal battles with people they believe to be exploiting them. The exquisite sensitivity to detail and precision that characterizes paranoid patients uniquely suits them to certain kinds of jobs, particularly if they are shielded from social interaction.

Cluster Characteristics

This group of personality disorders is characterized by odd, eccentric behaviors, emotional remoteness, and cognitive disorders, *in the absence of full-blown pyschotic symptoms*. These patients are notable for their lack of interest and enthusiasm for human interaction and the shallowness of their relationships.

More often than not, these patients avoid psychiatric treatment. They come to a physician's attention when seeking medical treatment for nonpsychiatric illness or if they develop a concurrent psychiatric disorder, for example, major depression or a brief psychotic episode. On some occasions, however, their mistrust or suspicion overwhelms them with anxiety and either precipitates their seeking treatment or leads to interactions with others, for example, a boss or teacher, who recommends treatment.

Pathogenesis

Data suggest biological and familial links between schizophrenia and schizotypal personality disorder. Schizotypal personality disorder is significantly more present in the biological relatives of schizophrenics than in other groups. Abnormal smooth pursuit eye movements (SPEM) are found in 60 to 80 percent of schizophrenics. Abnormal SPEM are also associated with schizotypal personality disorder; in randomly selected populations, disordered SPEM seems to be more prevalent in people with social isolation and decreased interpersonal rapport. Abnormal SPEM may be associated with individuals who are vulnerable to disruptions in cognitive organization of incoming stimuli. Under circumstances of interpersonal stress, say face-to-face interactions, these individuals may be unable to recruit the appropriate neuronal pathways and inhibit competing ones required to remain "in contact" with another person, leading to the poor rapport characteristic of schizotypal patients. There has also been an association between paranoid personality disorder and schizophrenia, although a less compelling one than that for schizotypal personality disorder. No solid biological data are associated with schizoid personality disorder.

A rich psychodynamic literature tries to explain the development of these personality disorders. For schizoid and schizotypal patients the prevalent theoretical explanation is that of repeated failures and disappointments in the most basic love relationship (usually in the infant-mother dyad) during an early critical period of the child's development. This empty, frustrating, and ultimately failed attachment leads to an adult without the substrate of a loving attachment upon which to build emotionally satisfying love relationships. The individual then maintains a distant and aloof posture toward the world.

It is not difficult to imagine, then, the following developmental scenario. An infant, subject to the sort of cognitive vulnerabilities described above, does not respond to parental entreaties—cooing and cuddling—as parents would expect; such interactions are overwhelming and frightening. The parents grow increasingly frustrated and respond by redoubling their efforts; they then become intrusive or lose interest and become distant. As the child grows and is faced with the developmental interpersonal challenges common to all children, he or she is forced to adopt a posture of distance and isolation or even paranoia to avoid the stress stemming from such parental encounters. Such a model is, of course, purely hypothetical. However, it does provide an example of how nature and nurture may feed on each other to engender personality characteristics.

Experiential theories for the development of paranoid personality disorder are numerous and highly speculative. No consistent pattern in the interpersonal or family dynamics has been observed.

DRAMATIC: ANTISOCIAL, BORDERLINE, HISTRIONIC (HYSTERICAL), NARCISSISTIC

These patients are linked by their tendency to call attention to themselves with flamboyant, sensation-seeking, emotional, and, at times, threatening behaviors. Clinicians have become increasingly interested in the problems of, and problems caused by, patients with these disorders.

Antisocial

The antisocial person or psychopath is certainly the most well-established, clearly defined, and carefully studied of the personality disorders. While the clinical description is well defined and specific, clinicians must be alert to the presence of *antisocial behavior* in many disorders other than antisocial personality per se. Further, it is important for the physician to be attuned to the behavioral characteristics other than criminality that define antisocial personality disorder. Too often, clinicians search solely for the dramatic conflicts with legal authority in these patients and miss the other characteristic personality traits.

The defining features of psychopathy seem to be present early in adolescence and persist, more or less, on a continuum into adulthood. They include:

- A consistent pattern of behavior that is intolerant of the conventional behavioral limitations imposed by a society
- An inability to sustain oneself in a job over a period of years; for example, frequent job changes that seem independent of seasonal variations
- Disregard for the rights of others, either through downright criminal behavior or through lying or interpersonal or sexual exploitiveness
- Frequent physical fights; quite commonly, child or spouse abuse
- Often a veneer of disarming charm and even sophistication that masks disregard and lack of remorse for mistreatment of others

Although items on this unsavory list describe many easily recognized hard-core criminals, they also describe some elected officials and prominent businessmen whose persistent pattern of disregard for the rights of others and self-centeredness may be well hidden prior to public scandal.

Borderline

Borderline personality disorder has a long and confusing psychiatric history. The term was originally applied to a broad, ill-defined group of patients who shared a vulnerability to psychological disorganization with traditional psychoanalytic technique while appearing, on the surface at least, to be good candidates for analysis. After nearly two decades of empirical research, the term borderline personality disorder, while still very controversial, connotes a definable and diagnosable syndrome. The hallmark of borderline patients is their instability in numerous behavioral arenas. In fact, one characterization of borderline patients is "stably unstable." Their moods are quicksilver, shifting from intense anger to overwhelming anxiety to crippling depression, often all in one day. Their relationships vacillate between adoring, idealized unions and denigrated, contemptible failures. Borderline patients are impulsive, action-oriented people. These characteristics find outlets of expression in the promiscuity, substance abuse, eating disorders, and self-inflicted injuries (wrist cutting, gambling) that are defining features of the syndrome. The impulsive anger and self-destructiveness, in concert with the borderline patient's readiness to devalue or feel devalued by important caregivers in his or her life, pose a major clinical dilemma.

Borderline patients often enact their struggles with their physician, as well as with others in their lives, by threatening or attempting suicide or badgering the other person into abandoning them by provocative and often hostile behaviors. It is important but often hard for clinicians in these predicaments to maintain a physicianly attitude while setting fair, clear, and consistently enforced limits on the disruptive behavior, which will, if unchecked, destroy effective treatment. Extreme reactions by the physician (on the one hand, mollycoddling the patient by yielding to his or her unreasonable demands or, on the other hand, abruptly, preemptively rejecting the patient) do little to help the patient or calm the situation. If consultation with the primary care physician is of no help, referral should be made to a psychiatrist who can provide the stable, predictable treatment relationship the patient is seeking. This interaction protects the patient and may help him or her salvage a job or significant relationships that these behavioral patterns jeopardize.

Histrionic (Hysterical)

Histrionic personality disorder corresponds somewhat to older diagnostic classifications of hysteroid or infantile personality, and represents for some authors a more severe and disabling variant of another diagnostic category—hysterical personality. Whether hysterical and histrionic personality disorders are on a continuum or represent discrete disorders is very much an open question.

Histrionic patients share many features with borderline and antisocial patients, notably a penchant for flamboyant, high-pitched emotional interactions. As a group, histrionic patients are distinguished by their exquisite attentiveness to the emotional responses they elicit from others—and the dependency of their mood on these reactions. In social settings, they "work the room" in their effort to elicit admiration and affection, frequently through the use of seductive, ingratiating behavior. The breezy, uninhibited behavior of histrionic patients can quickly turn into angry, confrontive accusations if the patients fail to elicit the approval and attention they seek.

If pouting or expressions of despair can inveigle an extra phone call or longer consultation from the physician, the physician can count on seeing more of this behavior. Despite the intensity of histrionic patients' feelings, they frequently seem to lack depth or authenticity. Clinicians are often exhausted in dealing with these patients, since they must constantly attune themselves to the patients' strong emotional needs. It is not uncommon for patients, should they fail in their efforts to gain approval or expressions of interest, to threaten or even attempt suicide. The clinician should treat these threats or "gestures" as a serious medical problem. Not to do so is to tacitly agree with the patient that such behaviors are an acceptable part of the currency of interpersonal relations; more important, these threats or gestures can lead to a person's death.

Narcissistic

Narcissistic personality disorder is a relatively new diagnostic category and has not been the object of intensive empirical study. Most data regarding these patients are found in the psychoanalytic literature. Narcissistic patients have a grossly inflated sense of their uniqueness, talents, and importance. Frequently, this sense of specialness leads them to feel exempted from the usual rules of social intercourse. They dominate conversations with tales of their achievements, endeavors, and future plans and poorly tolerate the attempts of others to participate. They seem to expect others to be intrigued by their stories and can become quite indignant when they are not well received. They often feel that their special qualities entitle them to exceptional treatment (for example, skipping to the front of the supermarket line because *their* business meeting is more important than anyone else's) and to exploit others for their own purposes.

The exaggerated notion of self-importance and entitlement that characterizes narcissistic patients serves to mask a fragile and easily punctured sense of self-esteem. Many of the narcissist's behaviors—seeking to be in the company of important and noteworthy people, feeling "above" others without reason—can be viewed as attempts to buttress their enfeebled sense of self-worth. The prevalence of this disorder is still unclear, although clinicians have become increasingly aware of, and sensitive to, the presence of narcissistic traits in many patients. For example, a young athlete who has always taken great pride in his physical prowess may require inordinate external supports for his self-esteem following a career-threatening knee injury. While it would be an error to conclude that his self-centered, prideful recounting of athletic victories yields a diagnosis of narcissistic personality disorder, an understanding of the compensatory nature of this behavior would certainly be helpful in his management.

Pathogenesis

Biological studies of antisocial personality disorder and Briquet's syndrome (an older diagnosis strongly related to histrionic personality disorder) have shown decreased cortical arousal and low levels of platelet monoamine oxidase (MAO) in these patients, which are associated with decreased motor inhibition and sensation-seeking behavior. In addition, recent clinical studies have suggested a link between diminished central serotonergic responsiveness and impulsive aggression, a characteristic of many patients in this particular cluster. Serotonin is a purported inhibitory neurotransmitter involved in the regulation of motor behaviors. The possibility that patients who are predisposed to assaultiveness, and who may also crave motor activity, have an underlying psychobiological vulnerability in this particular neurotransmitter system is an intriguing one and will be the subject of much further study. For further discussion of this neurotransmitter, see under the heading Serotonin in Chapter 8: Neurophysiological and Neurochemical Basis of Behavior.

Evidence of these sensation-seeking tendencies usually punctuates the early history of sociopaths (for example, fights in school) and histrionic patients (for example, temper tantrums). It is interesting to contemplate how the traits described above might shade the developmental experiences of these individuals along particular lines. For a behavior as complex as sociopathy to develop, there must be powerful environmental forces at work to modify an individual's biological predisposition. Histories of patients with antisocial personality disorder are filled with accounts of chaotic families, frequent parental separations from the child, overt parental psychopathology, child neglect and abuse, and ultimately a vicious circle of punitive authority and rejection of authority by the child. Are parental rejection and hostility the last hope of parents dealing with a child who is incapable of responding to reasonable controls? Is such parental behavior a necessary link in the chain that leads from a childhood vulnerability to adult psychopathology? Which environmental factors—such as family chaos, low socioeconomic status, or parental cruelty—lead to sociopathy are unclear. The presence of firm, fair discipline and special talents (for example, athletic ability or intellectual talent) may mitigate the biological predisposition and help channel a child toward experiences that enable him or her to exploit a sensation-seeking predisposition rather than become its victim.

Environmental factors in the development of histrionic personality disorder are unclear but may involve early parental reward for dramatic, seductive, or manipulative behavior. These behaviors are usually spawned in an intense relationship with the parent of the opposite sex. As the child moves through adolescence, these behaviors impel him or her toward frequent and stormy love affairs. Like sociopaths, histrionics build a world for themselves consistent with their hunger for sensation and excitement. Some authors have speculated that antisocial and histrionic patients share common biological vulnerabilities and that the increased prevalence of sociopathy in men and hysteria in women reflects gender-based differences in the socialization of an impulsive predisposition.

Evidence from biological and some family studies has linked borderline personality disturbance with the affective disorders. Abnormalities in dexamethasone suppression tests, thyroid suppression tests, and sleep architecture similar to those in patients with affective illness have been found in borderline patients. Another association has been established between borderline personality disorder and minimal brain dysfunction. Along these lines, evidence from EEG studies suggests a relationship between episodic dyscontrol syndromes and borderline personality disorder. For a discussion of sleep architecture, see under the heading Sleep in Chapter 13: Biological Rhythms and the Neuroendocrine System.

Environmental determinants of borderline pathology have received considerable attention from both psychoanalytic and family theorists. Most psychodynamic theories of borderline personality disorder have related borderline psychopathology to disturbances in the child's relationship to his or her primary caretaker during the first 2 years of life. One theory posits that excessive aggression on the part of the child leads to maternal deprivation or vice versa. This excessive aggression in the mother-child relationship disrupts normal developmental progress and culminates in the child's inability to maintain a stable mental image of a caring, gratifying parental figure. Arrested psychological development in this critical phase of a child's life leads to an adult who is unable to tolerate the frustration inherent in all significant human relationships and who frequently responds to it by excessive expressions of verbal or physical aggression.

A second significant psychodynamic explanation of borderline behavior suggests that the mother is unable to effectively deal with the toddler's early steps toward separation and individuation. Responding with either a suffocating overprotectiveness or terrifying uninterest, the mother makes these early, appropriate steps toward independence painful for, and frustrating to, the child. Consequently, normal adult separations (for example, disappointments in love, therapist's vacations) are marked by profound anger and depression. At these times the sensation-seeking behavior of borderlines is most apparent.

The behavioral difficulties of borderline patients reflect a disruption of the psychological structures that normally regulate an individual's moods and impulses. These autonomous controls of one's behavior usually develop out of a child's early experiences with parenting figures who supply him or her with external controls. When these early interactions are disrupted by innate difficulties in the child, personality difficulties in the parents, or, most likely, an interaction between the child's innate response styles and parental reaction to them, the danger of faulty behavioral regulation looms quite large.

No biological data have been associated with narcissistic personality disorder. Notable for their icy-cool, overly self-assured manner, narcissists treat other people as pawns in their great game of life—merely to be used and exploited, then discarded when they no longer serve any purpose. Most authors trace this behavior to early family interactions in which the child was made the repository of excessive or unrealistic parental ambitions and then overly indulged when he or she realized these ambitions and unloved when he or she failed. This lack of reasonable parental responsiveness leads to egotistical, entitled behavior, with little concern for the welfare of others. Rather, narcissists become engaged in a major struggle to win the love and approval of important parenting figures at any cost. In adult life, narcissists repeat this pattern of setting high, if not impossible, standards for those around them and often themselves, heaping praise on those they deem acceptable and discarding those they deem unsuited in a demeaning, often hurtful manner.

ANXIOUS: AVOIDANT, DEPENDENT, COMPULSIVE, PASSIVE-AGGRESSIVE

This cluster of patients is characterized by their predominantly anxious or fearful presentation. In the course of life, each of these personality types seems quite distinct from one another. However, when these patients' characteristic way of managing life's conflicts breaks down, they all experience profound anxiety. It has been suggested that some patients in this cluster of personality disorders have similar endowments to patients in another DSM-III-R classification, anxiety disorders.

Avoidant

Avoidant personalities eschew social interaction because of a fear of rejection, as opposed to schizoid or schizotypal personalities, who have an impaired capacity for social relatedness.

Avoidant patients are extremely sensitive to rejection, easily embarrassed, and excessively concerned about feeling uncomfortable in everyday situations.

Dependent

Patients with a dependent personality disorder overly rely on others for emotional and practical support; they behave in submissive, even self-deprecatory ways to forestall abandonment and its attendant anxiety. Dependent patients allow others to make important life decisions for them and comply with decisions they disagree with to guarantee the continuation of valued relationships.

Compulsive

Individuals with a compulsive personality disorder are perfectionistic and rigid; they are notable for not seeing the forest for the trees. Their quest for perfection can lead to written tasks being incomplete or decisions not being made because every detail is not available. Each decision can become an agonizing ordeal, with endless rumination and worry about error. The rigidity is emotionally manifest in their cold, often frozen demeanor and inordinate difficulty in expressing affection. These personalities can often function quite well in highly structured work settings but frequently run into problems when faced with open time or tasks that require significant flexibility.

Self-Defeating and Passive-Aggressive

Patients with a self-defeating personality disorder utilize self-sacrifice in an effort to maintain their self-esteem or significant relationships. Such patients frequently complain of being taken advantage of, and, in fact, they often are exploited. They frequently comply with such mistreatment while simultaneously protesting it and rejecting alternative approaches. They often denigrate their significant accomplishments and, at times, undermine their own success.

Patients with a passive-aggressive personality disorder utilize passive or indirect means to resist demands that they find unacceptable. These patients dawdle, "forget" to do things, and claim ignorance or lack of skill about tasks they would sooner avoid. They seek to avoid direct confrontation with authorities and steadfastly deny their anger toward or disagreement with them. Such characteristics are quite common and must be chronic and pervasive to lead to a diagnosis of passive-aggressive personality disorder.

Pathogenesis

While the biogenetic aspects of personality disorders in the anxious cluster await clearer description, numerous psychodynamic explanations exist for these disorders. A detailed explanation of these theories is beyond the scope of this discussion; it can be said, however, that each personality style represents an attempt to master conflicts experienced by the child in early family life. These conflicts emerge to push and pull between a child's temperament and the parental response to them. For example, a child predisposed to tantrums and overemotionalism may have parents who rigidly seek to control his or her behavior; as time passes, the child, seeking to win parental approval, integrates these rigid controls into his or her personality and develops a compulsive style. In another example, a child who is frequently belittled and humiliated by his or her parents may develop strong needs for reassurance or approval before venturing into relationships without them and will consequently avoid and mistrust close personal ties. See Chapter 27: Psychodynamic Aspects of Mood Disorders.

BIBLIOGRAPHY

Frances, A.: Categorical and dimensional systems of personality disorder: A comparison. Compr. Psychiatry 23:516-527, 1982.

Frances, A.: The DSM-III personality disorders section: A commentary. Am. J. Psychiatry 137:1050-1054, 1980.

Frosch, J. (ed.): Current Perspectives on Personality Disorders. Washington, D.C., American Psychiatric Press, 1983.

Gunderson, J.G.: Borderline Personality Disorder. Washington, D.C., American Psychiatric Press, 1984.

Klar, H., Siever, L.J. (eds.): Biologic Response Styles: Clinical Implications. Washington, D.C., American Psychiatric Press, 1986.

Millon, T.: Disorders of Personality: DSM-III, Axis II. New York, Wiley, 1981.

Tyrer, P.: What's wrong with DSM-III personality disorders? J. Personality Disorders 2:281-291, 1988.

Widiger, T.A., Frances, A., Spitzer, R.L., Williams, O.B.W.: The DSM-III-R personality disorders: An overview. Am. J. Psychiatry 145:786-795, 1988.

Index